Biochemistry (all bloo	
Alanine aminotransferase	
♂	
♀	<40IU/L
Albumin	34–50g/L
Alkaline phosphatase	35–120IU/L
Alpha-fetoprotein	<10kIU/L
Amylase	<135IU/L
Aspartate aminotransferase	<40IU/L
Bicarbonate	21–25mmol/L
Bilirubin	<19µmol/L
C-reactive protein (CRP)	<5mg/L
Calcium (total)	2.12–2.65mmol/L
Chloride	96–106mmol/L
Cholesterol	3.9–<6mmol/L
high density lipoprotein (HDL)	0.9–1.93mmol/L
low density lipoprotein (LDL)	1.55–4.4mmol/L
very low density lipoprotein (VLDL)	0.128–0.645mmol/L
fasting HDL-cholesterol reference range	
♂	1–1.5
♀	1.2–1.8
Cortisol	
a.m.:	190–650nmol/L
midnight:	<200nmol/L
Creatine kinase	
♂	<190IU/L
♀	<160IU/L
Creatinine	
♂	70–110µmol/L (17–55yrs)
♀	55–95µmol/L (17–55yrs)
Ferritin	
♂	25–400µg/L
♀ pre-menopausal	6–85µg/L
♀ post-menopausal	20–200µg/L

continued on inside back covers

OXFORD MEDICAL PUBLICATIONS

Oxford Handbook of Genitourinary Medicine, HIV, and AIDS

Oxford Handbooks

Oxford Handbook of Clinical Medicine 6/e
Oxford Handbook of Clinical Specialties 6/e
Oxford Handbook of Accident and Emergency Medicine 2/e
Oxford Handbook of Acute Medicine 2/e
Oxford Handbook of Anaesthesia
Oxford Handbook of Applied Dental Sciences
Oxford Handbook of Clinical and Laboratory Investigation
Oxford Handbook of Clinical Dentistry 4/e
Oxford Handbook of Clinical Haematology 2/e
Oxford Handbook of Clinical Immunology
Oxford Handbook of Clinical Surgery 2/e
Oxford Handbook of Critical Care
Oxford Handbook of Dental Patient Care
Oxford Handbook of Dialysis 2/e
Oxford Handbook of Endocrinology and Diabetes
Oxford Handbook of General Practice
Oxford Handbook of Genitourinary Medicine, HIV, and AIDS
Oxford Handbook of Obstetrics and Gynaecology
Oxford Handbook of Oncology
Oxford Handbook of Operative Surgery
Oxford Handbook of Palliative Care
Oxford Handbook of Patients' Welfare
Oxford Handbook of Practical Drug Therapy
Oxford Handbook of Psychiatry
Oxford Handbook of Public Health Practice
Oxford Handbook of Rehabilitation Medicine
Oxford Handbook of Rheumatology
Oxford Handbook of Tropical Medicine 2/e

Oxford Handbook of Genitourinary Medicine, HIV, and AIDS

Edited by

Richard Pattman

Consultant in Genitourinary Medicine, Newcastle General Hospital, Newcastle upon Tyne, UK

Michael Snow

Consultant in Infectious Diseases, Newcastle General Hospital, Newcastle upon Tyne, UK

Pauline Handy

Clinical Nurse Specialist in Genitourinary Medicine, Newcastle General Hospital, Newcastle upon Tyne, UK

K. Nathan Sankar

Consultant in Genitourinary Medicine, Newcastle General Hospital, Newcastle upon Tyne, UK

and

Babiker Elawad

Consultant in Genitourinary Medicine, Newcastle General Hospital, Newcastle upon Tyne, UK

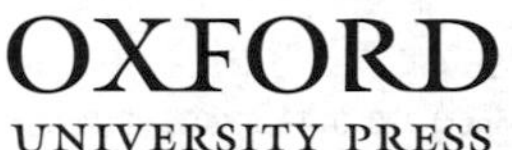

OXFORD
UNIVERSITY PRESS

Great Clarendon Street, Oxford OX2 6DP

Oxford University Press is a department of the Universit
It furthers the University's objective of excellence in rese
and education by publishing worldwide in

Oxford New York

Auckland Cape Town Dar es Salaam Hong Kong Karac
Kuala Lumpur Madrid Melbourne Mexico City Nairobi
New Delhi Shanghai Taipei Toronto

With offices in

Argentina Austria Brazil Chile Czech Republic France Greece
Guatemala Hungary Italy Japan Poland Portugal Singapore
South Korea Switzerland Thailand Turkey Ukraine Vietnam

Oxford is a registered trade mark of Oxford University Press
in the UK and in certain other countries

Published in the United States
by Oxford University Press Inc., New York

First published 2005

A catalogue record for this title is available from the British Library

Library of Congress Cataloging in Publication Data (attached)

Oxford Handbook of Genitourinary Medicine, HIV, and AIDS
edited by Richard Pattman *et al.*

Includes bibliographical references and index.

1. Urology—Handbooks, manuals, etc. 2. Sexually transmitted diseases—Handbooks, manuals, etc. 3. AIDS (Disease)—Handbooks, manuals, etc. 4. Genitourinary organs–Diseases—Handbooks, manuals, etc. [DNLM: 1. Sexually Transmitted Diseases—Handbooks. 2. Urogenital Diseases—Handbooks] WC 39 098 2005. I. Title: Handbook of Genitourinary medicine, HIV, and AIDS. II. Pattman, Richard.

RC872.9.097 2005 616.6–dc22 2005002781

Typeset by Newgen Imaging Systems (P) Ltd., Chennai, India
Printed in Italy
on acid-free paper by Legoprint S.p.A.

ISBN 0–19–852077–8 (Pbk.:alk.paper) 978–0–19–852077–1 (Pbk.)

10 9 8 7 6 5 4 3 2 1

Preface

This handbook provides a wealth of simple and easy to follow information on sexually transmitted infections (STIs), human immunodeficiency virus (HIV), other genitourinary conditions, and the principles to provide a safe, high-quality service. Although designed for the trainee and practitioner in the UK it is envisaged that it will be of global use to all those with an interest in sexual health whatever their level of expertise and wherever they may practice.

The book provides comprehensive practical guidance on genitourinary medicine (GUM), and includes HIV infection in the adult. STIs and related genitourinary problems together with other areas of practical relevance are also covered (e.g. practice within GUM, medico-legal/ethical issues and frequently asked questions).

The continuing rise of STIs has resulted in an extended workforce. This includes the creation of specialist nurses and primary healthcare teams with extended roles. It is intended that the information contained should address their needs as well as the specialist practitioner.

The contents start with service development and administration proceeding to medico-legal and ethical issues, routine patient management and flow charts detailing common clinical situations. This is followed by a series of chapters describing STIs and other problems commonly presenting to GUM in a disease-orientated style. Chapters on HIV infection and the acquired immunodeficiency syndrome (AIDS) follow including an epidemiological overview, basic viral biology, and pathogenesis before proceeding to systematic description of conditions both directly related and opportunistic, their management and concluding with special situations (pregnancy and travel). Commonly used abbreviations are summarized and some useful resources provided.

Feedback on errors and omissions would be much appreciated. Please post your comments via the OUP website: www.oup.com/uk/medicine/handbooks

Contents

Colour plates

Contributors

Babiker Elawad
(editor)

Pauline Handy
(editor)

Jane Hussey
Specialist Registrar in
Genitourinary Medicine
Newcastle General Hospital
Newcastle upon Tyne, UK

Kathryn Kain
Senior Health Adviser
Newcastle General Hospital
Newcastle upon Tyne, UK

Richard Pattman
(editor)

Jane Richards
Staff grade in Genitourinary
Medicine and former
General Practitioner,
Newcastle General Hospital
Newcastle upon Tyne, UK

K. Nathan Sankar
(editor)

Matthias Schmid
Consultant in Infectious Diseases,
Newcastle General Hospital
Newcastle upon Tyne, UK

Michael Snow
(editor)

Symbols and abbreviations

❶, ⚠	Warning
►	Important
►►	Don't dawdle
♂	Male
♀	Female
∴	Therefore
~	Approximately
≈	Approximately equal to
±	Plus/minus
↑	Increased
↓	Decreased
→	Leads to
1°	Primary
2°	Secondary
α	Alpha
β	Beta
γ	Gamma
δ	Delta
σ	Sigma
💣	Bomb (controversial topic)
3TC	lamivudine
ABC	abacavir
ACOG	American College of Obstetricians and Gynecologists
ACTH	adrenocorticotrophic hormone
AGH	anogenital herpes
AHU	arginine, hypoxanthine, and uracil
AIDS	acquired immunodeficiency syndrome
AIHA	autoimmune haemolytic anaemia
AIN	anal intraepithelial neoplasia
AIS	adenocarcinoma *in situ*
ALP	alkaline phosphatase
ALT	alanine aminotransferase
APV	Amprenavir
ARS	acute retroviral syndrome

ASCUS	atypical squamous cells of uncertain significance
AST	aspartate aminotransferase
ATZ	atazanavir
AZT	zidovudine
BAL	broncho-alveolar lavage
BASHH	British Association for Sexual Health and HIV
BCG	Bacillus Calmette-Guerin vaccine
bd	twice daily
BHIVA	British HIV Association
BMA	British Medical Association
BMD	bone mineral density
BSCC	British Society for Cervical Cytology
BV	bacterial vaginosis
BXO	balanitis xerotica obliterans
CAP	chronic abacterial prostatitis
CBP	chronic bacterial prostatitis
CD	cluster differentiation
CDC	Centers for Disease Control
CFT	complement fixation test
CGIN	cervical glandular intraepithelial neoplasia
CHOP	cyclophosphamide, hydroxydaunomycin [doxorubicin], oncovin [vincristine], prednisolone
CIN	cervical intraepithelial neoplasia
CIS	carcinoma *in situ*
CMV	cytomegalovirus
Cmin	minimum concentration
CNS	central nervous system
COC	combined oral contraceptive
CPAP	continuous positive airway pressure
CRP	C reactive protein
CSF	cerebrospinal fluid
CT	computerized tomography
CYP450	cytochrome P450
D4T	stavudine
DDC	zalcitabine
DDI	didanosine
DEXA	dual energy x-ray absorptiometry
DFA	direct fluorescent antibody
DGI	disseminated gonococcal infection
DLV	delavirdine

DMPA	depot medroxyprogesterone acetate
DNA	deoxyribonucleic acid
DOH	Department of Health
DSP	distal symmetric polyneuropathy
EBV	Epstein–Barr virus
ED	erectile dysfunction
EFZ	efavirenz
EGD	endocervical gland dysplasia
EIA	enzyme immunoassay
EM	erythema multiforme
ENF	enfuvirtide
EPS	expressed prostatic secretions
ERCP	endoscopic retrograde cholangiopancreatography
ESLD	end stage liver disease
ESR	erythrocyte sedimentation rate
ESRD	end stage renal disease
EUA	examination under anaesthetic
FBC	full blood count
FGM	female genital mutilation
FI	fusion inhibitor
FPV	fosamprenavir
FTA	fluorescent treponemal antibody
FTC	emtricitabine
FVU	first voided urine
G	gram
G6PD	glucose 6 phosphate dehydrogenase
GBS	Group B streptococci
GCSF	granulocyte colony stimulating factor
GI	gastrointestinal
GMC	General Medical Council
GNDC	Gram-negative diplococci
gp	glycoprotein
GUD	genital ulcer disease
GUM	genitourinary medicine
HA	health adviser
HAART	highly active antiretroviral therapy
HAV	hepatitis A virus
HBV	hepatitis B virus
HCFT	herpes complement fixation test
HCGIN	high-grade cervical glandular intraepithelial neoplasia

HCP	healthcare professional
HCV	hepatitis C virus
hCG	human chorionic gonadotrophin
HDL	high density lipoprotein
HHV	human herpes virus
HIV	human immunodeficiency virus
HIVAN	HIV associated nephropathy
HLA	human leucocyte antigen
HNIG	human normal immunoglobulin
HPA	Health Protection Agency
HPF	high power field
HPV	human papilloma virus
HSV	herpes simplex virus
HT	hydroxy tryptomine
HTLV	human t-cell lymphotropic virus
HVS	high vaginal swab
HZ	herpes zoster
IC50	50% inhibitory concentration
ICC	invasive cervical carcinoma
IDU	injecting drug user
IDV	indinavir
Ig	immunoglobulin
IHD	ischaemic heart disease
IIEF-5	international index of erectile function-5
IM	intramuscular
IMB	intermenstrual bleeding
IN	intraepithelial neoplasia
INR	international normalized ratio
IP	index patient
IRIS	immune recovery inflammatory response
IU	international units
IUD	intrauterine device
IUS	intrauterine system
IV	intravenous
KB	keratoderma blennorrhagica
KC	Koerner code
KS	Kaposi's sarcoma
L	litre
LCGIN	low-grade cervical glandular intraepithelial neoplasia
LDH	lactic dehydrogenase

LDL	low density lipoprotein
LFTs	liver function tests
LGE	linear gingival erythema
LGV	lymphogranuloma venereum
LH	luteinising hormone
LIP	lymphocytic interstitial pneumonitis
LNG	levonorgestrel
LPV	lopinavir
LS	lichen sclerosis
MAC	*Mycobacterium avium* complex
MCV	molluscum contagiosum virus
MHA-TP	microhaemagglutination assay for *Treponema pallidum*
mL	millilitre
MOMP	major outer membrane protein
MOPP	mechlorethamine, oncovin [vincristine], procarbazine, prednisolone
MPC	mucopurulent cervicitis
MRI	magnetic resonance imaging
MRP1	multi-drug resistance associated protein 1
MSSU	midstream specimen of urine
NAAT	nucleic acid amplification test
NAM	multi-NRTI associated mutation
NASBA	nucleic acid sequence based amplification assay
NFV	Nelfinavir
NGU	non-gonococcal urethritis
NHL	non-Hodgkin lymphoma
NHS	National Health Service
NNRTI	non-nucleoside reverse transcriptase inhibitor
NRTI	nucleoside/nucleotide reverse transcriptase inhibitor
NS	necrotizing stomatitis
NSAIDS	non-steroidal anti-inflammatory drugs
NSGI	non-specific genital infection
NSI	non-syncytium producing
NSU	non-specific urethritis
NUP	necrotizing ulcerative periodontitis
NVP	nevirapine
OHL	oral hairy leukoplakia
OI	opportunistic infection
p	protein
PACE	probe assay chemiluminescence enhanced
PCB	post-coital bleeding

PCC	post-coital contraception
PCP	*Pneumocystis jiroveci* (*carinii*) pneumonia
PCR	polymerase chain reaction
PEP	post-exposure prophylaxis
PHI	primary HIV infection
PI	protease inhibitor
PID	pelvic inflammatory disease
PIN	penile intraepithelial neoplasia
PML	progressive multifocal leukoencephalopathy
PMNL	polymorphonuclear leucocyte
PN	partner notification
POC	progesterone-only contraception
POEC	progesterone-only emergency contraception
POP	progesterone-only contraception
PROM	premature rupture of membranes
PUO	pyrexia of unknown origin
RA	rheumatoid arthritis
RCOG	Royal College of Obstetricians and Gynaecologists
ReA	reactive arthritis
RNA	ribonucleic acid
RT	reverse transcriptase
RTV	ritonavir
RVVC	recurrent vulvo-vaginal candidiasis
SARA	sexually acquired reactive arthritis
SCC	squamous cell carcinoma
SCJ	squamo-columnar junction
SDA	strand displacement amplification
SI	syncytium inducing
SIL	squamous intraepithelial lesion
SIV	simian immune deficiency virus
S–JS	Stevens–Johnson syndrome
SQV	saquinavir
SSRT	selective serotonin re-uptake inhibitor
STD	sexually transmitted disease
STI	sexually transmitted infection
TAM	thymidine analogue mutation
TB	tuberculosis
TCA	trichlroacetic acid
TDF	tenofovir
TDM	therapeutic drug monitoring

tid	three times a day
TMA	transcription mediated assay
TP	*Treponema pallidum*
TPHA	TP haemagglutination assay
TPPA	TP particle agglutination
TV	*Trichomonas vaginalis*
TZ	transformation zone
UPSI	unprotected sexual intercourse
UTI	urinary tract infection
VBU	voided bladder urine
VD	venereal disease
VDRL	venereal disease research laboratory
VIN	vulval intraepithelial neoplasia
VL	viral load
VZV	varicella zoster virus
WBC	white blood count
WHO	World Health Organization

Chapter 1

The genitourinary medicine service

Service development

The UK

During the 1914–18 World War there was an alarming increase in legally defined venereal diseases (VD)—syphilis, gonorrhoea, and chancroid. A Royal Commission produced the Venereal Disease Regulations (1916) specifying that local authorities should provide clinics which:

- could be accessed directly (without general practitioner referral)
- enabled voluntary attendance
- assured confidentiality
- provided free treatment.

113 clinics were established in 1917.

During the 1939–45 World War there was a concern that troops were being incapacitated by infection, with a core group of individuals acting as a reservoir. Doctors therefore began to question patients about their sexual partners. An individual named by more than one person could be compelled to have treatment and failure to comply could lead to imprisonment (Defence of the Realm Act 33B 1942). This regulation was subsequently repealed in 1947 but led to the introduction of voluntary partner notification (PN) in the UK, a vital tool in the control of infection.

In the UK there are now over 260 clinics led by consultants specializing in genitourinary medicine (GUM) covering a wide range of sexually transmitted infections (STIs) including human immunodeficiency virus (HIV) and other genitourinary conditions or problems. Their name has evolved from 'VD Clinic', 'Special Clinic', 'Sexually Transmitted Diseases Clinic' to 'Genitourinary Medicine Clinic', 'Sexual Health Clinic' or an eponymous name and some are integrated with contraceptive services.

STIs and genitourinary conditions present in a variety of guises to different specialties (e.g. dermatology, gynaecology, urology, and infectious diseases) therefore cross-referral is common and allows for the establishment of multidisciplinary clinics, e.g. for vulval disorders.

Elsewhere

Europe

Although GUM (previously venereology) is a separate specialty with a dedicated training programme in the UK and Ireland it is combined with dermatology (i.e. dermatovenereology) in the rest of Europe.

In Western Europe provision of services relating to STIs are largely left to individual practitioners, with the exception of the newly independent states, where services are provided by specialists working in the public sector. To date only 33% of European countries have implemented STI-control programmes, but all countries (excluding Greece) have an STI surveillance system. PN activity varies throughout Europe. Services and treatment (including drugs) are generally free with some exceptions, but screening is variable with some tests, such as those for chlamydia, not routinely available in several central European countries. These factors may contribute to the higher incidence of STIs in parts of Eastern Europe and newly independent states than in Western Europe.

USA/Africa/Australasia/Asia

Uniformity, level, and quality of services in other countries are less easy to ascertain, with wide ranging variations in service provision, surveillance, and STI programmes.

Provision

Aims of genitourinary medicine services

The ultimate goal of GUM is to reduce the incidence of STIs within the community. This is achievable by providing accessible and non-judgmental services that provide free and immediate diagnosis and treatment to those who think they may have, or have been at risk of an STI. Epidemiological control of infection remains essential to the sexual welfare of the community. However, clinics must reconcile confidentiality with a need for both 1° care and hospital services to be aware of serious chronic health problems in the individual. Health advising with good community links is important for ensuring that PN issues are dealt with efficiently and sensitively, reducing the continued transmission of STIs.

Comprehensive national surveillance programmes are essential when formulating strategies for national screening and treatment policies. Surveillance data informs clinical practice, allows the planning and allocation of resources and helps identify at-risk populations. This is largely achieved by the collection of reliable data from GUM clinics as information on infection managed elsewhere, including 1° care, is limited.

GUM—core and specialized roles

The core function of GUM is to provide screening, surveillance, diagnosis, treatment, and PN for STIs including HIV. This is combined with sexual health promotion, teaching, training, and research.

In addition some services provide specialized clinics at their main location or outreach venues (e.g. prisons). These are established and resourced to meet local need and may include sessions for:

- chronic or recurrent conditions e.g. HIV, warts, herpes.
- problems involving different specialties e.g. vulval conditions, sexual assault (providing both forensic examination and infection screening), one-stop sexual health (providing contraceptive as well as STI services).
- related problems where service need is identified e.g. psychosexual and sexual dysfunction.
- special groups e.g. young people, homosexual men and women, ethnic minorities, commercial sex workers.

Doctors

GUM is a consultant led service with a dedicated higher medical training programme for specialist registrars. There are some senior house officer posts and many non-consultant career grade doctors either working exclusively in GUM or in association with Contraception and Sexual Health, 1° care etc.

Nurse specialists/practitioners

The role of the nurse within GUM has continued to evolve with specialist (and consultant) nurses now the norm. Nurse led clinics run alongside conventional medically led services with nursing staff working independently taking responsibility for total patient care, including the examination of new patients under protocol and providing medication through patient group directions. No uniform model of care exists with individual centres implementing their own preferred methods.

Health advising and partner notification

The concept of PN in the UK was first introduced in the 1940s with the aim of identifying, diagnosing, and treating the contacts of people with VD. This now extends to all STIs and is an essential part of infection control and has led to the establishment of health advisers (HAs). Their role has evolved to encompass a wide range of healthcare issues as recommended in the Manual for Sexual Health Advisers produced by the Society of Sexual Health Advisers (SSHA). The National Strategy for Sexual Health and HIV recommends that training leading to an HA qualification be in place by 2005.

The Department of Health (2003) Effective Commissioning of Sexual Health and HIV Services recommends that:

- every GUM department should have health advisers
- there should be no single-handed health adviser posts
- there should be at least one whole time equivalent health adviser for every consultant led site in GUM.

Role (varies between clinics) includes:

- providing a holistic approach to patients, with information, education, treatment, and support.
- comprehensive needs assessment of index patients (IPs) and other vulnerable groups (e.g. young people, ethnic minorities, those sexually assaulted) including associated social, emotional, or sexual difficulties.
- effective PN ensuring the attendance and treatment of sexual contacts including settings outside GUM e.g. primary care.
- establishing and maintaining care pathways for patients in primary/acute care diagnosed with STIs.
- pre and post test HIV discussion.
- counselling, information, and support to patients, including those with HIV infection, their partners, friends, and relatives.
- sexual health education provision within GUM and the community liaising with statutory and voluntary services.
- research, audit, and service development.
- support of clinical outreach in non-clinic settings to targeted groups e.g. hepatitis B vaccination for homosexual and bisexual men, STI screening for sex workers.

Partner notification

Infection	PN method		Trace period *s = symptomatic* *as = asymptomatic*
	Patient	Provider	
Cervicitis (mucopurulent), PID, epididymitis	✓	✓	Current sexual partners
Chancroid	✓	✓	10 days from disease onset
Chlamydia	✓	✓	4 weeks (s) 6 months (*as*) or last partner if longer
Donovanosis	✓	✓	40 days from disease onset
Gonorrhoea	✓	✓	2 week (s) males 12 weeks (*as*) males and all females or last partner if longer
Hepatitis A	✓	✓	2 weeks prior to and 1 week after onset of jaundice
Hepatitis B	✓	✓	2 weeks prior to onset of jaundice or based on risk
Hepatitis C	✓	✓	Assessment if asymptomatic and for hepatitis B until surface Ag negative.
Anogenital herpes	✗	✗	Offer advice and STI screening
HIV	✓	✓	Risk assessment informs PN for asymptomatic cases (If 1° infection—3 months)
Lymphogranuloma venereum	✓	✓	30 days from disease onset
Non-gonococcal urethritis	✓	✓	4 weeks (s) 6 months (*as*) or last partner if longer
Pediculosis	✓	✗	12 weeks. Current partner
Scabies	✓	✗	8 weeks. Current partner, house-hold members
Syphilis (early)	✓	✓	12 weeks (1°) Up to 2 years (2°, early latent)
Syphilis (late)	✓	✓	10 years. Vertical transmission possible for a decade post infection therefore includes children born to infected mothers.
Trichomoniasis	✓	✗	Current partner
Anogenital warts/molluscum	✗	✗	Offer to screen current partners

Partner notification

The World Health Organization (WHO) 2003: Notification and management of sexual partners

Contacting the sex partners of clients with an STI, persuading them to present themselves at a site offering STI services, and treating them promptly and effectively are essential elements of any STI programme. These actions, however, should be carried out sensitively and in consideration of social and cultural factors to avoid ethical and practical problems such as rejection and violence, particularly against ♀.

Aim of PN

The ultimate aim is to break the chain and transmission of STIs and rates of infection by:

- stressing the importance of PN to those diagnosed with certain STIs.
- providing them with information on the nature, exposure, and risk of infection. The need to have sexual partners appropriately managed before sexual intercourse resumes must be emphasized.
- identifying, contacting, and screening sexual partners of the IP providing information and offering treatment if appropriate.

Description of terms and methods used in PN

PN should be conducted so that all information remains confidential with the process voluntary and non-coercive. Consultation with the HA should take place in a non-clinical, soundproofed environment free from interruption. Arranging for medication to be provided to patients by an HA emphasizes the importance of PN.

Patient referral: IPs with an STI are encouraged to notify their sexual partner(s) of any infection risk. HAs can help the IP to decide what information should be passed on to partners and how best to do this.

Contact slips: their issue to IPs is a widely used method of notifying sexual partners. Passed onto sexual contacts, they detail:

- IP identification number
- DOH diagnostic (KC60) code or the name of the infection (with the IP's permission) and date of diagnosis
- name and address of the issuing clinic.

When presented at any GUM clinic slips inform staff of the IP's infection, thus initiating appropriate screening and treatment of the sexual contact. Information can be communicated back to the issuing clinic to confirm PN has taken place and indicate infection(s) found, which may be important for the care of the IP. Patient referral may also take place without the issuing of contact slips, e.g. when the contact is only accessible by telephone or lives abroad. KC60 codes are not applicable outside the UK. WHO codes are available but not widely used.

Provider referral: offered to those IPs who do not wish to inform their sexual partner(s) themselves. The IP provides partner details to the HA after reassurance that confidentiality will not be compromised. HAs make direct contact with at-risk sexual partner(s) based on information provided by the IP. Evidence demonstrates that provider referral is more effective than partner referral.

Contract referral: allow the IP and HA to negotiate an acceptable time span in which the IP will attempt to contact sexual partner(s). If unsuccessful, provider referral may follow by agreement.
No referral: Where PN is impractical (involves careful risk/benefit analysis), e.g. when there is insufficient information, a threat of violence to the IP or HA exists.

While partner notification remains a voluntary activity within the UK countries such as Sweden and certain states of the USA have made it a legal requirement.

Availability

Referrals

The majority of patients seen in GUM self-refer or are seen as a result of partner notification. 2° referrals are seen especially from primary care, contraception services, and rape crisis organizations with tertiary referrals from gynaecology, dermatology, infectious diseases, urology, etc. These may be formal, with a letter, or based on verbal advice. By common acceptance there is no correspondence unless the patient has been referred by letter. However, in certain situations it may be in the patient's best interests for there to be an exchange of medical information between professionals providing care, but this should have the patient's agreement.

Access

Easy and timely access to the clinic should be available. When the clinic is closed the use of a pre-recorded telephone message detailing clinic opening hours together with the telephone number for other local GUM services, Accident and Emergency or NHS Direct is of benefit to anyone with an urgent problem. Appointment availability should be linked to staff numbers and experience. Ideally patients should be seen within 48 hours. However testing too soon after an infection risk may produce false negative results, therefore this period should be extended unless prophylactic treatment is required. If this is not possible the careful use of triage may help identify those with urgent problems.

All services should review their location and opening hours to match the need of the local population. Some clinics provide open access without prior booking although most utilize some form of appointment system.

Triage

For clinics operating by an appointment system, a robust triage system should be available for urgent situations. Trained staff should be able to assess and prioritize the patient's condition, including advice on optimum screening time intervals following an infection risk, and then arrange the appropriate attendance.

Disabled

Any assistance required by the disabled should be highlighted at the time of making an appointment, but facilities such as wheelchair access, disabled toilets, minicom systems, etc. should be in place.

Interpreters

Most hospitals are able to provide an accredited interpreting service, but will need time to arrange an interpreter of the appropriate language. If possible avoid family friends or relatives acting as interpreters as information may be withheld by the patient under these circumstances.

The process

Registration

Patients should be allowed privacy during registration by ensuring that they cannot be overheard while providing information or by the use of self-completed registration forms. Help must be available to those with difficulties in completing them. The amount of information required at registration will differ from clinic to clinic, however, collection of the following data may assist the clinic to contact the patient if required and help with service planning, statistics, and surveillance.

Name	Nationality
Address	Country of birth
Date of birth	Ethnicity
Telephone number(s)	Area of residence
General practitioner	Referral source and documentation
Employment status	Name of partner (if attending)

Patients who refuse to give any information about themselves may attend. The right to anonymity is accepted within GUM. The patient should be issued with an individual clinic identification number that will be used on all specimens and request forms. They should be encouraged to provide at least their date of birth which can be used with the identification number as an additional reference when confirming identity, test results, etc.

Appointment cards should be issued at the time of registration showing the patient's identification number and all booked appointments. Details of the clinic opening times and telephone numbers should be clearly printed on the card.

Waiting areas are inevitably areas of stress for those wishing to remain anonymous. Issuing patients with a welcome leaflet on arrival explaining how the clinic operates will hopefully ↓ anxiety. All patients should be seen within 30 minutes of their appointment time (Patients' Charter). Those who are acutely distressed should be moved into a private area. The use of a television or music system in the waiting room may help to distract the anxious patient and also reduce the risk of sensitive information being overheard.

Soundex codes

Soundex codes are commonly used within GUM along with dates of birth to provide clinical information while protecting individual confidentiality (see chart).

The Soundex code

Contains four characters with the first being the first letter of the surname. The remaining three are numbers derived from the name. When the adjacent letters are from the same category, the second is disregarded. An example is Schmid: since the number 2 represents both S and C, the C is omitted. The letters A, E, H, I, O, U, Y, and W only contribute if they start the name. An empty space is represented by a zero. Once the four character limit has been reached, all remaining letters are redundant.

Category	Letter
1	b, p, f, v
2	c, s, k, g, j, q, x, z
3	d, t
4	l
5	m, n
6	r
No Code	a, e, h, i, o, u, y, w

Examples: Sankar S 526 Pattman P 355 Handy H 530 Snow S 500 Elawad E 430.

Confirmation of attendance

Letters confirming attendance for a hospital appointment should be made available for the patient to present to the employer using hospital headed notepaper without reference to GUM. This letter should state the date and time of the visit together with the date and time of any further appointments.

Reimbursement of travel expenses

Patients attending GUM clinics may reclaim their travel expenses upon receipt of bus/train tickets if the distance travelled is >15miles from home. Legislation is unclear about those who travel less than this distance. It is therefore suggested that discretion be used in such cases. This facility is offered to patients irrespective of individual financial circumstances (DOH NHS charges HC11 2002).

Transfer to other GUM clinics

Patients leaving the area may be issued a V15 card which details information on all investigations and treatments carried out while attending the initial clinic. This allows subsequent clinics to assess the need for further management. The V15 will not show the name of the patient but carries only their clinic number on the front cover.

Test results

Various systems are employed throughout the country to provide test results and include:

- returning in person or phoning for all results
- contact by the clinic, usually just for positive results, (letter, phone, text message, e-mail).

Some patients, including those working in the sex industry, may request written proof of the test result. When provided it must be made clear that this may not cover recently acquired infections (e.g. within 'window' periods).

Recall

A computerised system aids the process of recall. Patients are generally reviewed for the following reasons:

- to be given positive test results and treatment
- further management (e.g. ongoing treatment, vaccination, cervical cytology review).

Recall most often takes the form of a letter requesting that the patient contacts the clinic, but may also be by telephone, e-mail, or text-messaging by agreement.

Performance targets

Department of Health Sexual Health Strategy (2001)

Hepatitis B Vaccination

- All homosexual/bisexual men, sex workers, and injecting drug users attending GUM should be offered hepatitis B immunization at their first visit by the end of 2003.
- Uptake of the first dose of vaccine in those not previously immunized to reach 80% by the end of 2004 and 90% by the end of 2006.
- Uptake of three doses of vaccine in those not previously immunized to reach 50% by the end of 2004 and 70% by the end of 2006.

HIV

By the end of 2004 all GUM attendees should be offered an HIV test on their first screening for sexually transmitted infections (and subsequently according to risk) with a view to:

- Increasing the uptake of the test by those offered it to 40% by the end of 2004 and to 60% by the end of 2007.
- Reducing by 50% the number of previously undiagnosed HIV infected people attending GUM clinics who remain unaware of their infection after their visit by the end of 2007.

Specialty Specific Standards for Physicians in GUM

Standard 1

The physician shall ensure that a sexual history is obtained and documented in all persons presenting to a GUM service with a new clinical problem. This shall be done in accordance with the current national guidelines for obtaining such a history. The physician should ensure that a sexual history is re-taken and documented at least every 6 months for persons being followed up for infectious conditions.

Standard 2

Physicians should offer an HIV antibody test to all persons attending a GUM clinic on the occasion of their first screening for STIs, unless the person is already known to be HIV antibody positive. The test shall be offered in accordance with current national guidelines.

Chapter 2

Ethical and medico-legal issues

Introduction

This section deals with some of the ethical and medico-legal aspects specific to HIV infection and GUM. Most medico-legal problems arise from:

- failure to appreciate legal responsibilities
- problems in clinical management
- medication errors
- administrative errors
- failure of communication and inadequate clinical records.

Awareness and adherence to relevant law and General Medical Council (GMC) guidance is essential. If in doubt seek advice from experienced colleagues, professional bodies, or medico-legal defence organizations.

Confidentiality

Common law and the Data Protection Act 1984 protect personal health information. Confidentiality is central to the trust between patient and healthcare professional (HCP). Without its explicit assurance the patient may not volunteer a full history and medical care may be compromised. It is particularly important for those dealing with sexually transmitted infections (STIs) where patients provide highly sensitive information. This is formally recognized by the NHS Trusts and Primary Care Trusts (Sexually Transmitted Diseases) Directions 2000 see p. 38. These apply to any healthcare setting and not just GUM clinics.

To maintain confidentiality the following practices should be adopted:

- anonymize patient data on records/forms/specimens by using identification (ID) numbers, dates of birth, or soundex codes (see pp. 12–13)
- offer the patient a choice on how they would like to be called from the waiting room
- do not discuss patients outside the health team or where the conversation can be overheard by others
- ensure that any consultations are in private e.g. triage patients in a separate room, not at reception
- disclose information to general practitioner only following consent from the patient (unless it falls within the STD Directions 2000).

There are some situations when confidentiality may be broken, however, it may be necessary to justify any decisions in accordance with GMC guidance. Specific regulations apply to 'serious communicable diseases' including HIV, Hepatitis B and C, the latter two (and also hepatitis A) being notifiable. Problems may also be encountered if the patient is unable to take responsibility for his/her management (e.g. prisoners, mental health patients).

Consent

Consent

It is good practice and a legal requirement to obtain consent from a patient before treatment. Failure to do so can result in complaints to the individual's employing authority or relevant professional body, criminal proceedings for assault or indecent assault, and civil proceedings (e.g. if injuries arise following treatment without informed consent). To be valid consent must be given voluntarily by a competent, fully informed patient. A detailed discussion, clearly recorded in the notes is required. To be competent to give consent the patient should be able to comprehend the information that has been given to them and retain it long enough to make a decision. No adult can give consent on behalf of another. However, in the case of incompetent adults a doctor may act in their best interests providing the result will improve medical management, as judged by a responsible body of medical opinion. In the case of those with fluctuating competence, consent should be taken when competent and the discussion clearly documented in the case records. Their decision should then be regularly reviewed during further periods of competence.

Consent is required for investigations, treatment, disclosure of information, research, photography/video recording, and teaching e.g. medical students observing a consultation. In certain situations the use of a signed consent form is required. It must be made clear that refusal to participate in such activities will not compromise clinical care.

The person obtaining consent must be fully aware of the situation, ideally directly involved in it, and be able to answer any queries. To help understanding and therefore the ability to give valid consent, information should be provided clearly, using written or visual aids. If the patient cannot understand English an interpreter, accredited if possible, should be provided and additional time set aside. In certain situations it is helpful to involve another member of the health team such as a health adviser. It may be necessary to provide time, over a number of sessions to allow the patient to reach their informed decision.

To obtain consent for a screening test the patient should be aware of the following:

- description of the test
    - why the test is being taken
    - what it involves
- the likelihood of receiving positive or negative results
- implications of a positive result to the person and partner(s)
- any medical, social, or financial implications
- requirement for follow-up tests/treatment.

Consent: specific issues

Epidemiological studies

Testing for epidemiological purposes (e.g. for HIV, hepatitis C virus) is important for planning disease management, but raises ethical issues. It generally involves screening surplus material (e.g. serum) taken for other tests to allow meaningful epidemiological data to be obtained ensuring that it cannot be linked to the anonymous individual. However, it is acknowledged that the information gained will not directly benefit that person. It is generally agreed that the benefit to public health outweighs the ethical dilemma of testing without consent to avoid biased sampling. Written information should be available to patients explaining the nature of this testing within the clinic as leaflets or posters which must highlight the option to refuse without prejudice.

Testing in error

GMC guidance states that mistakes should be acknowledged, with apology, and appropriate support offered. The patient must be given the choice as to whether they are given the result of the test. If the patient refuses to receive a positive result (with health implications for that individual, partners, and others) then advice should be obtained from professional bodies.

Occupational exposure to infection

In the case of a needle stick injury or other occupational exposure to a HCP it may be important to determine if the patient has a blood borne infection such as HIV. If unconscious the GMC advises that such testing should not be requested until consciousness has been regained and agreement obtained. In the event of a patient being unable for any reason to give consent, testing should only be carried out under exceptional circumstances and should preferably be performed on an existing blood sample. However, experienced colleagues should be consulted and the decision taken may need to be justified before the GMC.

Post-mortem testing for sexually transmitted blood borne infections (HIV, hepatitis B and C, syphilis)

If a member of staff has been exposed to the blood or body fluids of a deceased patient screening is permitted, although the agreement of a close relative or next of kin should be sought. Any person who is brain stem dead and being considered for organ donation requires screening for such infections and this should be explained to the relatives.

Where a postmortem is required the deceased may be screened for these infections if relevant to the cause of death. Information should be disclosed regarding a positive diagnosis to any persons known to be at risk of the infection, e.g. sexual contacts, otherwise it must remain confidential.

HCP/patient relationship

Patients attending GUM can be both physically and emotionally vulnerable due to the intimate details they often have to reveal. Staff must not allow themselves to be influenced by any personal or professional relationship with the patient. It is important for the HCP to explain to the patient precisely what is involved during an examination. Complaints of indecent assault have been made by patients against HCPs irrespective of the gender of either. Therefore all patients should be offered a chaperon for any intimate examination and this should be documented. The use of friends and relatives is not advised as their use could compromise the disclosure of important information. As in any medical setting courtesy and good communication are essential. Should a complaint be made an explanation with a simple apology, if appropriate, may be sufficient to resolve the issue.

Guidelines

National management guidelines are available (see pp. 550–1), however, departmental or regional guidelines may be produced to reflect local variations in clinical practice. Guidelines, whether national or local, must be available to all staff and updated regularly in line with clinical evidence-based expert opinion. Demonstrating that guidelines were followed and therefore a recognized standard of care provided can refute a clinical complaint. As guidelines are updated it is also important to archive old versions which may be required for a retrospective review.

Staff meetings should be used to highlight any guideline changes and discuss any issues regarding them. Where possible services within geographical areas should follow the same or have similar guidelines to allow consistency in patient management. This can be achieved through regional GUM networks which may also help with funding issues over certain management options if regional guidelines advise on them.

Prescribing

Medication errors account for a high level of complaints and claims. This is usually due to errors that can be avoided by simple checking procedures and a clear explanation to the patient. The following are common causes of error: badly transcribed instructions, illegible prescriptions, miscalculation of dosage, prescribing contraindicated drugs, not checking for potential drug interactions, not reviewing repeat prescriptions and failure to act on laboratory results. Good prescribing practice should involve clear verbal and written instructions to the patient, checking for drug interactions and taking a history for any possible contraindications.

In unusual or complex situations or when the treatment advised is unfamiliar check with an experienced colleague or pharmacist before prescribing or dispensing.

General Medical Council guidance on intimate examinations (December 2001)

The GMC regularly receives complaints from patients who feel that doctors have behaved inappropriately during an intimate examination. Intimate examinations, that is examinations of the breasts, genitalia or rectum, can be stressful and embarrassing for patients. When conducting intimate examinations you should:

- Explain to the patient why an examination is necessary and give the patient an opportunity to ask questions.
- Explain what the examination will involve, in a way the patient can understand, so that the patient has a clear idea of what to expect, including any potential pain or discomfort (paragraph 13 of our booklet '*Seeking patients' consent*' gives further guidance on presenting information to patients).
- Obtain the patient's permission before the examination and be prepared to discontinue the examination if the patient asks you to. You should record that permission has been obtained.
- Keep discussion relevant and avoid unnecessary personal comments.
- Offer a chaperon or invite the patient (in advance if possible) to have a relative or friend present. If the patient does not want a chaperon, you should record that the offer was made and declined. If a chaperon is present, you should record that fact and make a note of the chaperon's identity. If for justifiable practical reasons you cannot offer a chaperon, you should explain that to the patient and, if possible, offer to delay the examination to a later date. You should record the discussion and its outcome.
- Give the patient privacy to undress and dress and use drapes to maintain the patient's dignity. Do not assist the patient in removing clothing unless you have clarified with them that your assistance is required.

Patient records

It is a requirement of professional organizations and good medical practice to keep clear, accurate, and legible notes. They are also essential in dealing with complaints and claims. Records should contain information on how a diagnosis was reached and information given to the patient. At all times care must be taken to ensure that there is no unintentional disclosure of third party information. The use of a clinic proforma sheet for general consultations and screening and for more specialized situations such as sexual assault can greatly improve clinical record keeping, by ensuring all essential information is sought and detailed. Notes must be dated and clearly signed by the individual who should also indicate their status.

The Data Protection Act (1984) and the Access to Medical Records Act (1990) allow patients the right to see their medical records. In order to protect third party confidentiality it is wise to record ID numbers rather than names when referring to sexual contacts in a patient's case notes. If patients obtain formal access to their records all third party information must be removed.

Storage of patient's records should be in a secure part of the GUM clinic. Records should be retained for a minimum of 8 years (Public Records Acts 1958 and 1967). In the case of children and young people they should be retained until the individual's 25th birthday (26th if the notes were made when the patient was aged 17). Records of patients attending with syphilis or HIV may be held for the period of time dictated by locally agreed policy and prolonged storage may be required for the case records of those enrolled in research.

Electronic technology

The use of computer records, e-mails, fax, and text messages have the potential for breaching patient confidentiality. The GMC has guidelines for the security of personal information by electronic processing. If necessary, specialist advice should be sought on the security of such information.

To maintain patient confidentiality and confidence in the service, computerized medical record systems must overtly exhibit a high level of security. Many clinics have stand-alone systems but if linked to a network, robust systems must be in place to ensure that sensitive patient information cannot be accessed by any unauthorized personnel which includes HCPs working in other services. Individual computers should be password protected, especially for patient related information, with the level of information accessible appropriate to the staff member involved. As with written records patients have the right of access to all electronically held material with the exclusion of third party information.

Computers and fax machines should be kept in a secure setting, computer passwords should be changed regularly, and any information sent by e-mail should be encrypted as it may be intercepted. The use of prearranged codes can help protect confidentiality.

Partner notification issues

Patient with an STI and an unaware regular sexual partner

In the case of a person infected with an STI being reluctant to inform sexual partners consider the following GMC advice:

'You may disclose information about a patient, whether living or dead, in order to protect a person from risk or serious harm. For example, you may disclose information to a known sexual contact of a patient with HIV where you have reason to think that the patient has not informed that person and cannot be persuaded to do so. In such circumstances you should tell the patient before you make the disclosure and you must be prepared to justify a decision to disclose information' (GMC Serious Communicable Diseases 1997 paragraph 22).

Clear documentation and discussion with colleagues in such circumstances is vital.

Patient with an STI and unaware casual sexual partners

This situation is more difficult. The patient must be counselled that they have the duty to inform any sexual partners of their infection. This is especially relevant to someone who continues to carry a chronic infection such as HIV, hepatitis B and C viruses and remains infectious. It is also essential to document such advice in the patient's case records.

Ethically the same principles apply to the other STIs although the consequences compared to HIV infection are generally less serious.

Criminalization of HIV transmission

- Men, knowing that they were HIV positive, have been convicted under English and Welsh law, for 'biological' grievous bodily harm after infecting ♀ sexual partners with HIV who were unaware of their contact's positive HIV status. In judgment it has been stated that anyone infected must disclose this to any sexual partners and must 'take protection' if sexual intercourse is to occur.
- In February 2001 a ♂ was convicted under Scottish law of reckless conduct after infecting his girlfriend with HIV.
- Three ♂ were convicted in 2003 and 2004 under English law for 'grievous bodily harm by recklessly infecting sexual partners with HIV'.
- Finnish courts gave a ♂ infected with HIV a sentence of 14 years for infecting 5 ♀ by having sex with them without informing them of his HIV status.

Successful prosecutions have also taken place in Denmark and Germany. Over 20 states in the USA have amended existing statutes or introduced new laws to make it a criminal offence to have sexual contact with another when the person is aware they are infected with HIV but when that fact is not known to the partner.

Although the UN programme on aids advises that any criminalization of HIV transmission should be restricted to intentional or deliberate infection most prosecutions so far have been more inclusive.

Under 16 years

Although the legal age for heterosexual and homosexual sex in the UK is 16 years (except for N. Ireland where it is 17 years), an estimated 25% of boys and girls are sexually active below this age.

Any competent person, regardless of age can give consent for medical treatment. A patient is competent if they can understand the choices and their consequences, including the nature, purpose, and possible risk of any treatment or non-treatment. Although parental support should be encouraged, if the patient does not wish the parent's involvement this view should not be overridden. When establishing if a patient under the age of 16 years is competent the Fraser Ruling (Gillick competence) should be followed. The Gillick case (Gillick v West Norfolk and Wisbech Health Authority 1985, 3 A11 ER 402 HL) established the current legal position in England and Wales. Although this ruling is directed towards contraceptive services it can be extrapolated to include the management of STIs and details of the following points:

- the patient should be encouraged to inform their parents of the consultation
- the patient understands the potential risks and benefits of the treatment and advice
- the HCP must take into account whether the patient will engage in sexual activity without contraception
- the HCP must assess whether the patients physical or mental health or both are likely to suffer if they do not receive contraceptive advice or supplies
- the HCP must consider whether the patient's best interests would require the provision of contraceptive advice or methods or both without parental consent.

Consent in minors in Scotland

The Age of Legal Capacity (Scotland) Act 1991 gives statutory power to the minor to consent to medical or dental treatment. This act goes beyond the Fraser Ruling stating children <16 years have legal capacity to consent to any surgical, medical, or dental treatment or procedure so long as that child is capable of understanding the nature and consequences of the proposed treatment or procedure. In England and Wales if a child refuses treatment, this can be overruled by a person with parental responsibility for the child or by the court. This is not the case in Scotland where the above act protects the child's right to refuse examination or treatment, presuming the child has the capacity under the legislation.

Immature patients

GMC guidelines state that if a doctor does not consider the patient to be capable of giving consent due to immaturity, the relevant information may be disclosed to an appropriate person or authority if it is thought to be in the best interests of the patient. However, the following conditions should be met:

- the patient does not have sufficient understanding to appreciate the implications of advice or treatment

- the patient cannot be persuaded to involve an appropriate person in the consultation
- the doctor believes it is in the best medical interests of the patient.

Child protection issues

There is a duty of confidentiality to all patients, irrespective of their age. The exception is when disclosure of information is in their best medical interests or the patient, or other vulnerable persons are at risk of harm. The HCP must be prepared to justify his/her decision to his/her professional body. Under such circumstances, if the patient cannot be persuaded to make a voluntary disclosure, the HCP should explain to the patient that confidentiality cannot be preserved.

The age of a 'child' for child protection purposes has been raised from 16 years to 18 years by the Sexual Offences Act 2003, applicable in England and Wales and, in part, in N. Ireland (see p. 38).

Asylum seekers and refugees

To confirm refugee or asylum seeker status one of the following documents is required:

- a letter from the Home Office stating the patient is a refugee
- a letter from the Home Office confirming that the patient has made an application for asylum
- a travel document issued in the UK in accordance with the convention on the status of refugees.

If these documents are not available the Home Office can be contacted on 020 86860688, ideally in the presence of the patient, to confirm.

Definitions

Asylum seeker—an individual who claims to be a refugee and is awaiting a decision.

Refugee—any person who 'owing to a well founded fear of being persecuted for reasons of race, religion, nationality, membership of a particular social group or political opinion, is outside the country of his nationality and is unable, or owing to such fear, is unwilling to avail himself of the protection of that country' (1951 UN Convention relating to the status of refugees).

Failed asylum seeker—when application has been rejected after an initial decision and appeal. They are either deported or leave voluntarily.

Indefinite leave to remain—given to people recognized as refugees, allowing them to remain in the UK without a time limit.

Exceptional leave to remain—a discretionary status usually granted to someone who does not qualify as a refugee, but has genuine humanitarian reasons for staying in the UK.

Confidentiality

Sometimes health information, for administrative purposes, is requested by third parties. Patients need to know this and that information concerning HIV status can be useful when planning appropriate care if relocated. However, no information can be passed on without the patient's prior consent.

Exception from medical charge

Refugees, anyone who has formally applied for asylum and those with exceptional leave to remain are exempt from charges for medical treatment under the NHS. (Statutory Instrument No 306, NHS Regulations 1989). Treatment for STIs should be available free of charge to any patient. The exception is HIV and AIDS where only the initial test and counselling is free of charge to those not entitled to full NHS treatment. (National Health Service Act 1977, schedule 12, Section 77). However, withholding proper medical care from someone with a serious illness could contravene Article 2 (right to life) or 3 (freedom from torture) of the Human Rights Act 1998.

Details of those entitled to full NHS hospital treatment available at www.doh.gov.uk/overseasvisitors.

Mental health patients

Mental health act

The mental health act only refers to treatment for the mental condition itself and not any physical condition. However, sometimes the two may be closely linked—in advanced HIV or late syphilis, for example. Sometimes the courts may be called upon to determine what is and what is not 'treatment of the psychiatric condition'.

Consent

Any competent mental health patient attending for STI screening or treatment must be consenting. Even if the patient is sectioned under the Mental Health Act consent is still required, unless the STI is directly related to the mental condition. The exception is when the patient is not mentally competent to make a decision when testing or treatment may be performed in the patient's 'best interests' under common law. In such circumstances it is advisable to seek a second opinion from an experienced colleague and the reasons clearly documented.

Confidentiality

If the patient should attend with a mental health nurse, offer an alternative chaperon—the patient may be uncomfortable in discussing sexual health issues in the company of staff responsible for his or her mental health. Only relevant information relating to the mental health or treatment of the patient should be passed on, with the patient's consent. The exception would be a condition causing potential harm to others—e.g. a positive HIV result in a violent mental health patient.

Prisoners

HCPs, whether working in clinics within the prison or outside the prison, should not disclose to security guards anything about the prisoner's state of health. The prisoner is entitled to be examined in private. An exception to this rule (thereby allowing prison guards to be present in the same room) should only be made to prevent any disorder or crime, or for the protection of the HCPs rights and freedoms (Article 8 (1) of the European Convention on Human Rights).

HIV positive HCPs

The GMC advises that doctors or other HCPS with a serious communicable disease, such as HIV, are entitled to the same level of confidentiality and support to which every patient is entitled. However, if there is knowledge or good reason to believe that the HCP is practising, or has practised, in a way which places patients at risk, an appropriate person in the HCPs' employing authority, e.g. an occupational health physician, or a relevant regulatory body must be informed. Wherever possible the HCP concerned must be advised before such information is passed on to an employer or regulatory body. The Public Interest Disclosure Act (1998) protects any employee who discloses concerns about a colleague in the public's best interests.

Death

Living wills (or 'advance statements')

Allows competent people to give instructions about what is to be done should they subsequently lose the capacity to decide or to communicate. This issue received much prominence with AIDS before effective antiretroviral treatment was available. The British Medical Association (BMA) Code of Practice gives guidance on how to draft and implement living wills. Once a document exists, medical staff involved with the patient's care should make themselves aware of its contents for legal and ethical reasons. However, in an emergency treatment should not be delayed if the document is not readily available. An alternative to a living will is the nomination of a healthcare proxy by the patient who can make decisions for them. However, no adult has the legal right to accept or refuse treatment on behalf of another adult and in the absence of a written living will it may be difficult to prove that the opinion of the healthcare proxy reflects the views of the patient.

Death certificates

GMC guidance states that if HIV or any other STI has contributed to the death it is unlawful to omit this from the death certificate.

Release of information after death

Any information recorded after 1 November 1991 is subject to the 'Access to Health Records Act (1990)'. This states that a deceased patient's representative has a statutory right of access to health information which is directly relevant to a claim. However, no information can be provided if the patient has requested non-disclosure and this is recorded in their records. Results of investigations that the deceased believed to be confidential may not be disclosed. It is therefore important to counsel patients on such matters, especially with sensitive diagnoses like HIV. Problems may arise when an insurance company refuses payment under a life insurance policy if a doctor refuses to disclose information. Despite this any information that the doctor believed the patient would have wished to remain confidential should not be disclosed. Information recorded before November 1991 cannot be disclosed as the duty of confidentiality extends beyond death. If further advice is required this should be sought from the medical ethics committee via the BMA.

Writing statements and court appearances

Statements may be required for a variety of reasons—from insurance companies, solicitors, or a police statement.

Before writing a statement the following should be established:

- *What questions the enquirer wants answered.* Exclude irrelevant information.

- Whether the information provided is as a *professional witness* (a factual report concerning a patient who the doctor has provided care to) or *expert witness* (to give an opinion concerning a patient who may not have been under the care of that individual).
- *Has the patient given consent?* Always check that the patient understands what the information is for and that they have consented for it being passed onto a third party, even if the person requesting the information states that the patient has given consent. However, consent is not required for a coroner's statement or if demanded by an order of the court.
- *Is the statement required to deal with criticism regarding the medical management of the patient?* Always consult defence organizations prior to sending any completed statement.

Doctors are usually only required in court if there is dispute as to the contents of any provided statements. If called to court because of the medical management of a patient the doctor involved should contact his or her defence organization for advice.

Legislation pertinent to GUM

► Although there are differences in the legal systems and instruments within the countries constituting the UK the general principles affecting the management of patients are similar.

NHS Trusts and Primary Care Trusts (Sexually Transmitted Diseases) Directions 2000

Came into force on 1 April 2000 replacing the NHS Trusts (Venereal Diseases) Regulations and apply only to England.

Confidentiality of information

Every NHS trust and Primary Care trust shall take all necessary steps to secure that any information capable of identifying an individual obtained by any of their members or employees with respect to persons examined or treated for any sexually transmitted disease shall not be disclosed except:

- for the purposes of communicating that information to a medical practitioner, or to a person employed under the direction of a medical practitioner in connection with the treatment of persons suffering from such disease or the spread thereof; and
- for the purpose of such treatment or prevention.

National Health Service Act 1977 (Schedule 12, Section 77)

The act states that no charge is to be made to patients in relation to any medication or investigation required in the treatment of venereal diseases. Treatment for sexually transmitted infections (referred to as venereal disease in the text) should be available free of charge. The exception is HIV and AIDS where only the initial test and counselling is free to those not entitled to full NHS treatment.

Addendum HM (68)84, section 27 accompanying the 1968 NHS (VD) Regulation SI 1624 Article 3

This states that medical and other staff involved in contact tracing are not liable to defamation.

The Aids Control Act 1987

This act relates to the collection and annual reporting of statistics relating to HIV and AIDS. It further addresses the availability of facilities and staff for testing, consultation, treatment, and health education. Note that HIV and AIDS are not notifiable diseases.

The Sexual Offences Act 1967

Permits male homosexual practices by two consenting adults in private. The age of consent in homosexual behaviour was lowered from 21 to 18, and more recently further reduced to 16 in England, Wales, and Scotland, and 17 in Northern Ireland.

Sexual Offences Act 2003 (enacted May 2004)

This act more closely defines 'consent' and the abuse of trust especially with regards to children. The age of a 'child' set in the Protection of

Children Act 1978 has been raised from 16 to 18 years. Although it should not alter normal practice clinic staff need to be aware that 'children' up to the age of 18 years fall within its protection. It re-defines 'sexual' with, e.g. attention to 'grooming', use of the internet, child pornography, prostitution, administration of a substance with intent to commit a sexual offence, and other miscellaneous offences, including voyeurism and bestiality.

It protects the public, especially children, from sexual harm. Sexual offences prevention orders replace sex offenders and restraining orders. In addition new sexual harm and foreign travel orders have been created.

In view of concerns expressed by those providing sexual healthcare and advice to young people a statute has been introduced to ensure that a person does not commit an offence if the action taken is to;

- protect the child from STIs
- protect the physical safety of the child
- prevent the child from becoming pregnant
- promote the child's well-being with advice.

This is conditional that such action does not cause or encourage a child's participation and is not for the purpose of obtaining sexual gratification.

Anyone who acts to protect a child (e.g. teachers, relatives, friends) and not just HCPs are now covered.

The Prohibition of Female Circumcision Act 1985

This makes female genital mutilation an offence except on specific physical or mental health grounds. A local authority may exercise its responsibility to make enquires under section 47 of the Children's Act 1989 if it has reason to believe that a child is likely to be or has been the subject of female genital mutilation.

The Public Health (Infectious Diseases) Regulations 1988 SI 1988/1546 (England and Wales)

Modification of section 38 of the act as it applies to AIDS states 'justice of the peace may on application of any local authority make an order for the detention in hospital of an inmate of that hospital suffering from AIDS… if the justice is satisfied that on his leaving hospital proper precautions to prevent the spread of that disease would not be taken by him, (a) in his lodging or accommodation or (b) in other places to which he may be expected to go if not detained in hospital.'

The Public Health Regulations (Notification of Infectious Diseases) (Scotland) Regulations 1988 SI 1988/1550:

These regulations make no reference to AIDS.

Public Health (Control of Diseases) Act 1984 or Public Health (Infectious diseases) Regulations 1988

These acts list notifiable diseases. Among the many infections it should be remembered that Hepatitis A, B, and C are all notifiable. Any doctor who makes the diagnosis is required by statute to notify the proper officer of their local authority.

Chapter 3

The standard clinic process

The genitourinary medicine (GUM) patient

It is estimated that 1 in 7 adults over the age of 16 in the UK has attended a GUM clinic at least once. Many who attend may not harbour an active sexually transmitted infection (STI) but wish to exclude one. The 'GUM patient' does not fit a single stereotype. While it may be more common for young people to attend those of a wide age range from <16 to >60 are seen. Their demographic characteristics vary and depend on the risk factors of the local and commuting population and the acceptability and accessibility of GUM services to potential users. Slightly more ♂ than ♀ attend with sexuality and ethnicity varying geographically.

The following groups of people are more likely to attend:

- ♂ aged 25–34
- ♀ aged 16–24
- those who have changed sexual partners recently
- those having multiple sexual partners
- those single, separated, or divorced.

Special situations

The distressed or aggressive patient

While most patients attending may feel anxious and embarrassed some are intensely distressed. The psychological responses to STIs or risk of such include severe anxiety, depression, a strong sense of stigma, shame, guilt feeling, low self-esteem, and anger. Strong negative responses such as these could hamper communication and lead to apparently irrational behaviour. It is necessary to understand and appraise the emotional state of the patient when providing optimum care. If a patient is aggressive the priority should be safety while attempting to de-escalate the situation.

Under-age patient (see p. 88)

Adolescents <16 years attending GUM have a high incidence of STIs and report a low use of reliable contraception. Some may also have suffered sexual abuse.

Survivors of sexual assault or rape (see p. 84)

May attend for sexual health screen and STI risk assessment and due consideration should be given for any post-traumatic stress that may dominate the patient's mood and emotions.

Risk factors

Social and demographic

The following risk factors have been noted in various epidemiological studies. Likely to vary over time and across different geographic regions but useful in planning local service provision and targeting specific sexual health promotion. Clinically they are useful in risk assessment.

- Age <25 years—the highest rates of gonococcal and chlamydial infections occur in age groups 16–19 years in ♀ and 20–24 years in ♂.
- Being single—separated, divorced, or not being in a stable relationship (compared with marital, stable relationship, or widowed status) associated with higher rates of STIs.
- ≥2 partners in preceding 6 months
- Use of non-barrier contraception
- Residence in inner city
- Symptoms in partner
- History of previous STI
- Ethnicity or migration—prevalence of several infections, notably syphilis, gonorrhoea, and HIV infection, is higher in certain ethnic minority groups and immigrants
- Sexual orientation—e.g. syphilis, gonorrhoea, HIV, and hepatitis B virus infections are more prevalent among homosexual ♂.

Sexual

Certain types of physical contact carry higher risks for certain infections e.g. penetrative sex and HIV, orogenital contact, and anogenital herpes.

Types of sexual practice

Knowledge of the wide range of sexual practices and the vocabulary in use is of value in advising those at risk of STIs.

Sexuality and relationship

- Heterosexuality (opposite sex): (heterophilia, 'straight')
- Bigynist (sex between 1 ♂ and 2 ♀), bivirist (sex between 1 ♀ and 2 ♂).
- Homosexuality (same sex)—general: (homophilia, 'gay', iterandria, uranism)
- Cruising describes searching for homosexual ♂ partners in public places e.g. common land, saunas, bath-houses, toilets (cottaging).
- ♀ homosexuality: (lesbianism, cymbalism, gynecozygous)
- Bisexuality (both sexes): ambisexual, amphisexual, androgynophilia, sexoschizia
- Cybersex: use of the internet to deliver sexual pleasure.

'Safe sex' (no penetration by penis into vagina, anus, or mouth)

Arousal from kissing (basoexia); manual genital stimulation (mutual masturbation and heavy petting); body rubbing (frottage and 'dry rooting'); rubbing buttocks (pygotripsis); feet (podophilia); kneading flesh (sarmassophilia); tickling (titillagnia); lap dancing (squatting above a sitting person and non-genital rubbing).

Penile positioning: into the axilla (axillism), between breasts (coitus a mammilla and mazophallate), between legs (coitus interfermoris), between knees (genuphallation).

Genital stimulation using the mouth

- Insufflation—(blowing air into body cavity—usually vagina)
- Penile oral sex—fellatio, 'blow-job', corvus, irrumation, penosugia
- ♀ genital oral sex—cunnilingus, gamahucheur, clitorilingus (clitoral tongue stimulation).

Anorectal stimulation

- General terms for anal sex—anocratism, arsometry, buggery, coitus analis, pederasty, proctophallism, sodomy, sotadism.
- Oral stimulation—analinctus and hedralingus (anal licking), anophilemia (anal kissing), analingus and rimming (anal penetration with tongue).
- Specific penile anal sex—androsodomy (with ♂), anomeatia (with ♀).
- Manual—fisting, brachioprotic eroticism (fist/arm into ano-rectal canal).

Arousal with body fluids

- Urine: golden enema/douche/shower (urine deposited into anus/vagina/over body), urolagnia, urophilia, water sports.
- Faeces (scat): coprolagnia and coprophilia (arousal), coprophagy (consumption).
- Miscellaneous: hygrophilia (body fluids), blood sports (blood), mucophage (ingestion of mucous secretions), salirophilia (ingestion of sweat or saliva), felching (ingestion of semen from vagina or anus), emetophilia and Roman shower (vomit and vomiting over partner).

Sado-masochism

- Sadism—arousal by inflicting pain.
- Masochism (pain translated to erotic feelings).
- Algophilia and doleros (arousal from pain).

Examples: caning/flagellation (using cane/whip), bondage/strangulation (physica restraint/constriction), electrophilia (arousal from electricity), meatotomy (urethral dilation).

Sex with animals

Bestiality, zoophilia. Specific examples include cynophilia (dogs), entomophilia (insects), ophidiophilia (snakes), felching (inserting animals into vagina or anus).

Use of sex-toys and piercings

- Arousal enhancers: penis substitutes (dildos, vibrators, olisbos, anal, butt plugs), and genital piercings (rings, bars, beads, wires, etc).
- Erection sustainers: rings and bands (e.g. cock ring).

Use of drugs during sex

- Amyl nitrite for euphoria and sphincter relaxation.
- Crack cocaine ↑ desire.
- Alcohol and some tranquillising drugs (sometimes used illicitly e.g. 'drug rape') remove inhibitions.

The sexual history

Taking a sexual history and discussing sexual health issues are vital elements of the consultation eliciting essential information on the STI risk. It must be non-judgemental and empathic thereby promoting effective patient participation. When taking a sexual history:

- Put the patient at ease with proper initial introduction and positioning.
- Reassure regarding confidentiality.
- Explain why sexual history is needed.
- Check if patient agrees to be asked personal questions.
- Ideally interview the patient alone but respect the patient's desire to have a third person present which may help to ↓ anxiety.
- Avoid distractions during the consultation.
- Display a non-judgemental attitude.
- Do not make assumptions about patient's sexuality or sexual behaviour.
- Listen actively and maintain adequate eye-contact observing non-verbal communication.
- Use language the patient understands avoiding jargon, with appropriate intonation, pauses, and cues to gain information.
- Reflect what patient says to clarify and confirm.

Proformas ensure a systematic approach to history-taking. Asking when last sexual intercourse took place is a useful way to start the sexual history (details of sexual partners, contraception, and sexual risks). Presence of a third person, especially sexual partner, may inhibit this. Types of sexual practices reported can help in planning which specimens to obtain. Obtain any information patient has on the nature of sexual partner's infection(s). Where mother to child transmission is relevant enquire about clinical presentations in the children.

Conducting the consultation through an interpreter or when cross-cultural issues are relevant may be difficult. It is preferable to use an unrelated interpreter but sometimes this may not be possible.

1. Introduce yourself and your position to the patient. He/she may be anxious or feeling guilty and therefore it is important to put him/her at ease as soon as possible.

2. Determine the presenting problem or concern. There may be information available to you (e.g. contact information) which should be accessed before and not in the presence of the patient.

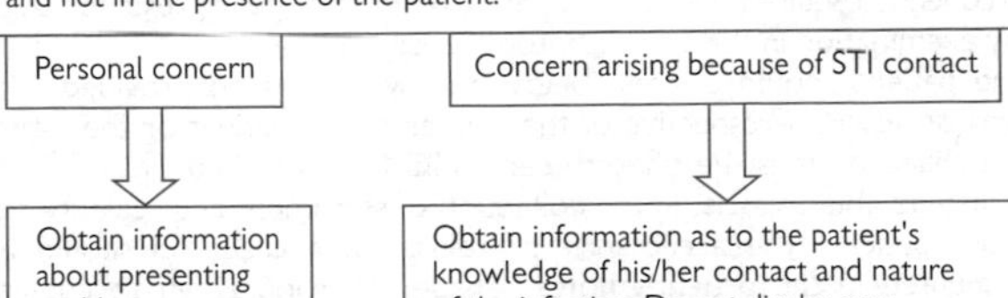

Personal concern	Concern arising because of STI contact
Obtain information about presenting problem or concern (its nature, duration, other relevant symptoms, etc).	Obtain information as to the patient's knowledge of his/her contact and nature of the infection. Do not divulge any sensitive 3rd party information. It may be necessary to explain in some detail the rationale for partner notification and potential benefit to your patient. Enquire about any relevant symptoms etc.

Obtain relevant background information

- Past STIS and other relevant present and past medical history
- For ♀, contraceptive, gynaecological and obstetric history
- Current/recent drug history and drug allergies
- Drug misuse

Sexual history

- Last sexual contact—date, relationship (regular/casual), sex (male/female), country (if relevant). More detailed information may be obtained such as the type of contact and use of protection (condoms) though the latter merely ↓ risk and should not alter immediate clinical practice except for HIV post exposure prophylaxis.
- Other contacts in last 3 months (incubation/ latent period for most symptomatic STIS) and last 12 months (helpful in risk assessment).

Finally

- Thank patient for providing this information (often embarrassing to them).
- Discuss and explain further recommended investigation and management plans based on the information available.

Routine examination: general principles

Prior to the examination the patient should be given an explanation and his/her agreement obtained. Certain procedures require written consent e.g. local anaesthesia, minor surgery, and clinical photography.

The examination room should be warm and comfortable with a screened area allowing privacy while the patient undresses. An examination couch is required with good lighting (with stirrups/leg rests for ♀, to allow examination in the semi-lithotomy position).

The patient should undress below the waist and be provided with drapes or gowns. Irrespective of the gender of the patient or the examiner a chaperon must be offered (see GMC Guidance 2001, p. 25), who may also be able to assist in the collection of specimens and reassure the nervous patient. The acceptance or refusal of a chaperon should be documented in the patient's notes. Chaperons should sign to confirm their attendance during the examination. Although the GMC suggests a patient's friend or relative could act as a sole chaperon this is not advised in GUM as it may compromise confidentiality and the provision of relevant information to the healthcare professional (HCP).

The examination trolley should be set up prior to the examination. Specula should be pre-warmed in water which also acts as a vaginal lubricant. Lubricating gels should be avoided whenever possible as they may inhibit the growth of *Neisseria gonorrhoeae*. The use of lubricants cannot be avoided for proctoscopy but care should be taken to ensure that swabs are not contaminated. During examination the patient should be kept informed of progress but unnecessary or facetious comments must be avoided. Convenient facilities should be available to obtain urine specimens.

Serology

A venous blood sample should be taken from patients at risk of an STI for syphilis and testing for HIV infection promoted and recommended. Because of the sensitivity arising from HIV testing and the implications of a positive result additional discussion is usually required to ensure fully informed consent (see p. 366). Testing for hepatitis B/C virus may also be required.

Examination

General

Skin rashes/lesions, generalized lymphadenopathy, hair loss, jaundice, mucosal lesions (orogenital), conjunctivitis/uveitis, and arthritis may arise from STIs and genital problems may be features of dermatological or systemic diseases.

Women (Fig. 3.1)

- Inspect the entire pubic and anogenital area ensuring that the labia are parted and the clitoral hood gently retracted.
- Palpate the inguinal area for lymphadenopathy
- Urethral specimens. There is doubt about the value of routine urethral samples for Gram-staining and culture for *Neisseria gonorrhoeae*, however, they have been shown to be useful on occasions. Urethral sampling may be deferred until the end of the examination as it may cause discomfort. The addition of a urethral swab to an endocervical specimen ↑ the detection of chlamydial infection.
- Introduce a speculum lubricated with warm water.
- Inspect the vagina and cervix for atypical discharge, mucosal lesions, and signs of inflammation.
- Take vaginal material from the posterior vaginal pool/vaginal walls using a loop or swab and prepare a suspension in normal saline on a slide protected with a cover-slip. An additional swab should be prepared as a Gram-stained smear.
- If cervical cytology is required it is best taken at this stage (see p. 311).
- Before microbiological sampling clean the cervix using a cotton ball held in a sponge-holder to remove vaginal material
- Take an endocervical swab to prepare a Gram-stained smear and to plate onto selective medium for *N. gonorrhoeae* (or send in transport medium, e.g. Amies, Stuart).
- Take an endocervical swab for *Chlamydia trachomatis*, rotating it within the walls of the cervical canal. Although cervical specimens are not essential with nucleic acid amplification tests (NAATs), see p. 130 it is important to inspect the cervix (especially for mucopurulent cervicitis) and to take swabs for *N. gonorrhoeae*, hence it is reasonable to also screen this site for *C. trachomatis*.
- If there are any signs or symptoms to suggest lower abdominal or pelvic pathology offer a bimanual pelvic and abdominal examination.
- Urine specimens should be obtained if pregnancy testing is required or a urinary tract infection (mid-stream sample) suspected. They can also be used for chlamydia testing (1st 20mL) by NAAT, and certain enzyme immunoassays (EIAs).

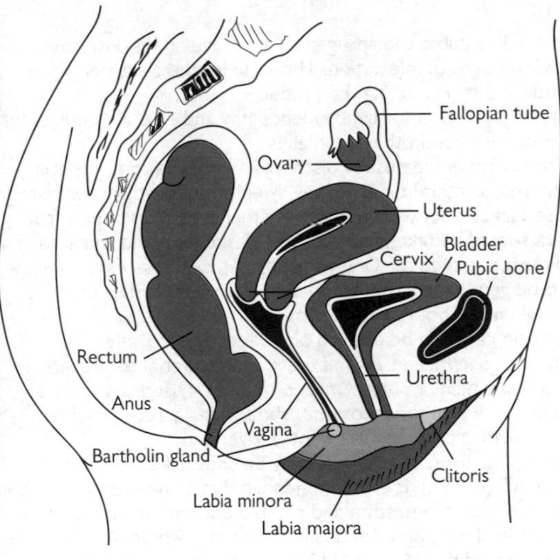

Fig. 3.1 Female genital anatomy

Men (Fig. 3.2)

- Inspect the entire pubic and ano-genital area for skin lesions, masses, discharges, and signs of infestation. This includes the glans penis and sub-preputial sac by retracting the prepuce.
- Palpate the inguinal area for lymphadenopathy and scrotal contents for masses, tenderness, and other anomalies.
- Examine the urethral meatus for discharge and skin lesions, especially warts. If there is urethral exudate, any symptom of urethritis or history of penile sexual contact with gonorrhoea then a gentle scraping from the urethra should be taken using a small plastic loop and smeared onto a microscope slide for Gram-staining. It may be necessary for the urethra to be gently massaged to obtain a specimen. Ideally samples should be taken 3–4 hours after last micturition.
- The same loop can then be used to plate directly onto selective medium for *N. gonorrhoeae*, even if there is no material to prepare a slide. If transport medium (e.g. Amies or Stuart) is used, a separate swab is required which the laboratory should ideally receive within 48 hours for plating provided it is kept refrigerated.
- Urethral sampling for *C. trachomatis* may be undertaken at this time using an NAAT (or EIA). It is recommended that a fine urethral swab is inserted 1–4cm into the urethra and rotated once against the urethral wall although in clinical practice this is often not possible. Alternatively urine can be tested by NAAT or EIA licensed for urine specimens.
- Finally the patient should provide a first voided 20ml urine specimen (ideally having retained their urine for 3–4 hours before testing). As well as providing a test sample for *C. trachomatis* it can also be examined for threads, a possible indicator of urethritis. A second, mid-stream sample can be obtained especially if urinary tract infection needs to be excluded. Samples can also be tested by dipstick for blood, protein, glucose, nitrites, and leucocytes as required.

Extra-genital infection

Rectum: In those at risk, especially homosexual/bisexual ♂ proctoscopy and screening for *N. gonorrhoeae* and *C. trachomatis* (if NAAT available) should be offered remembering that infection may occur without penile penetration. The anal canal and distal 5cm of the rectum should be examined with a proctoscope to check for pus (which can be sampled and prepared as a Gram-stained smear) and other lesions (e.g. warts). This also minimizes faecal contamination when taking swabs. Lubricants should be used with care around the anal sphincter to avoid rectal contamination as they may impair the isolation of *N. gonorrhoeae*.

Rectal testing for *N. gonorrhoeae* should also be offered to ♀ at risk (e.g. with symptoms, urogenital gonorrhoea, contacts of gonorrhoea, and following sexual assault). Chlamydia screening may also be considered.

Pharynx: Swabs for *N. gonorrhoeae* should be offered to those at risk especially if symptomatic, gonorrhea found at other site(s), contacts of gonorrhoea, homosexual/bisexual ♂, and those sexually assaulted.

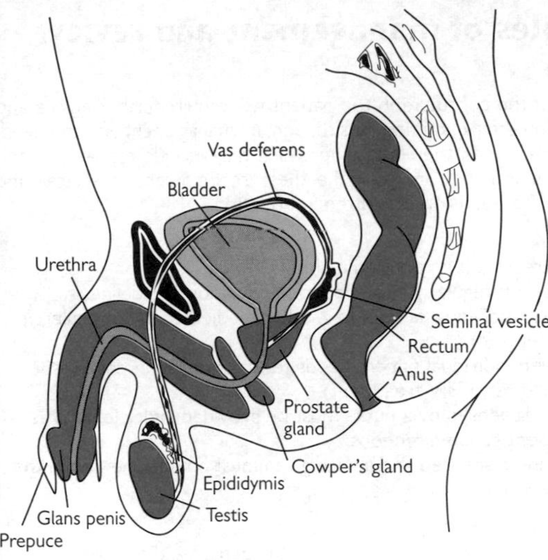

Fig. 3.2 Male genital anatomy

Principles of management and review

General

At the end of the consultation the patient will require further advice and information on their condition or situation, its management and the need, when relevant, for further follow-up which may include repeat or additional tests. It is important to make these recommendations clear and explicit with the provision of written information.

Treatment

- If specific treatment is required it should:
  - be based on regularly reviewed local or national guidelines
  - recognize individual factors (e.g. other medical conditions, allergies, pregnancy, etc)
  - meet with individual patient needs to maximize adherence (especially long-term HIV treatment).
- Treatment dispensed by a nurse must be provided under local Trust ratified patient group directions.
- Any medicine dispensed and advice given must be documented in the patient's records.

Management points

- Confirm that any test results relate to the patient and complete information is available (e.g. antibiotic sensitivity).
- Explain the nature of the condition and its implications.
- Discuss rationale for treatment including a risk/benefit analysis, specific information on the treatment recommended and obtain patient's agreement.
- Ensure full STI screening is offered (explaining possibility of co-existing infections).
- Provide additional advice that may include:
  - avoidance of sexual intercourse even with condoms (until infection cleared and partner treated)
  - possible effects on combined hormonal contraception
  - additional self-help information
  - general sexual health promotion
- Consider sexual partner(s) and partner notification issues when indicated (with health adviser)
- Agree arrangements for obtaining results and/or further review (which may include tests of cure).

Pharmacy arrangements

Ideally medication should be dispensed, free of charge, to the patient while they are in the clinic.

Free treatment

Treatment of STIs excluding HIV/AIDS (but including initial diagnosis of and counselling support for HIV) is free without any prescription charge to all attendees at GUM clinics irrespective of their nationality. HIV/AIDS management after the initial diagnosis and counselling is subject to the standard regulations concerning entitlement to NHS hospital treatment (see p. 32).

Chapter 4

Investigations and microscopy

Laboratory testing

Introduction

Certain infections may be detected or diagnosed within clinics or surgeries but others require microbiological services, also essential for confirmatory and antimicrobial sensitivity testing. If on-site microscopy is unavailable the use of air-dried swabs sent for laboratory staining and microscopy should be considered. This is applicable for vaginal discharge e.g. bacterial vaginosis, candidiasis, and also ♂ urethral discharge for polymorphonuclear leucocytes (PMNLs) indicating urethritis and Gram-negative intracellular diplococci—highly suggestive but not diagnostic of gonorrhoea.

The optimum minimum time to take swabs for screening from asymptomatic patients following a specific incident has not been established. It will depend on the type of test used, the site screened and the presence/absence of infected secretions, however, 7–14 days after a sexual risk is suggested (and is compliant with sexual assault guidelines).

The timing of serological tests should take into consideration the 'window periods' of the respective infections. Final exclusion tests must be advised at the end of this time. Baseline assays soon after the incident may be useful, especially if subsequent repeat tests are positive.

Chlamydia trachomatis

Nucleic acid amplification test (NAAT)

♂ urethra, endocervix, first voided 20mL of urine (especially ♂), vagina, vulva. Although not essential, urethral samples from ♀ enhance the detection rate when combined with endocervical specimens. In addition rectal samples (although unlicensed) have been shown to be useful in homosexual ♂. Important to take if homosexual ♂ present with anorectal symptoms because of recent outbreaks of lymphogranuloma venereum (recently reported in W. Europe). If confirmed genotype for L1, L2, or L3.

Not licensed for oropharyngeal specimens.

Enzyme immunoassay (EIA)

Still widely used but are at least 30% less sensitive than NAAT. Not suitable for urine and vulvo-vaginal testing in ♀ and certain kits not recommended for urine testing in ♂.

Culture

Not widely available now but still considered important in medico-legal situations (e.g. assault and rarely if antibiotic resistance is suspected).

Transport and storage

Specimens for culture should be kept refrigerated at all times. Storage of NAAT and EIA specimens for >24 hours at room temperature may result in sample degradation although absolute data is lacking. If delays are anticipated storage at 4°C is recommended. Manufacturers' instructions should be followed.

Neisseria gonorrhoeae

Culture

Routinely from ♂ urethra and endocervix. Although not essential urethral samples from ♀ enhance the detection rate when combined with endocervical specimens.

Rectal and pharyngeal specimens should also be considered if at risk remembering that rectal gonorrhoea may occur without peno-anal penetration. If a carbon dioxide incubator is available specimens can be plated directly onto selective growth medium (e.g. modified New York City culture medium) although they will require to be transported to the laboratory in a carbon dioxide enriched environment (e.g. in candle jars).

Otherwise specimens must be sent in transport medium (e.g. Amies, Stuart). Their use only reduces sensitivity by ~10% (compared with direct inoculation) providing the specimens are refrigerated and received by the laboratory within 48 hours.

Nucleic acid amplification test

Limited availability but more sensitive compared to culture. From urogenital sites only, positive results need culture for confirmation and antibiotic sensitivity testing.

Bacterial vaginosis (BV)

Swab from posterior fornix. Prepare air-dried smear from the swab or send in transport medium (Amies, Stuart) requesting a Gram-stain for bacterial flora and clue cells. A result suggestive of BV does not necessarily indicate the need for treatment, which must be assessed clinically.

Herpes simplex virus (HSV)

Swabs of vesicular fluid or from ulcers

Culture

Must be sent in transport medium. Standard viral transport systems should be kept refrigerated but some commercial systems (e.g. Virocult®) can be maintained at ambient temperature as HSV will survive for up to 12 days up to 23°C. Local laboratory or manufacturers' instructions should be consulted.

Real time polymerase chain reaction

Highly sensitive (detects 11–88% more cases than culture), specific, allows typing and is rapid. Manufacturers' instructions should be consulted for transport.

Others

- Immunofluorescent antigen detection: provided by some laboratories using material (sample in viral transport medium).
- Type specific serology: of little diagnostic value.

Trichomonas vaginalis

Swab from posterior fornix or urethra/sup-preputial sac (if indicated) in growth medium (e.g. Feinberg-Whittington incubated at ~37°C) or Amies'/Stuart's transport medium, refrigerated, and received within 24–48 hours. Although some laboratories provide a culture service most diagnose on slides prepared from the swabs.

Candida spp.

Swab from vaginal wall or vulva, glans penis, prepuce, anus, etc. if indicated in transport medium (Amies/Stuart) without any special precautions. *Candida* spp. are common skin and genital commensals therefore the need to treat must be based on clinical findings.

Serology

Clotted blood is required with no special arrangements required for transport. Baseline assays are useful, especially if subsequent repeat tests should be positive.

- Syphilis and HIV: seroconversion usually occurs within 2–6 weeks but may take up to 3 months when repeat or initial testing should be recommended.
- Hepatitis B surface antigen and hepatitis C antibody: can usually be detected within 3 months of infection though occasionally may be longer. In high-risk situations a further test at 6 months is advisable.

More detailed information on testing in specific situations and less common infections can be found in the relevant chapters.

Will the tests hurt?

♂: You will feel some discomfort but it should not be painful. The swabs only take a few seconds to take. You may notice slight discomfort on urinating the first time after the swabs have been taken.

♀: We use a speculum inserted into the vagina to take the swabs, similar to when having a smear taken. We also take swabs from the urethra (urinary passage).

Are you going to use the umbrella?

No. This is an old instrument used for ♂ >40 years ago. Modern day swabs are taken with very fine swabs.

Will I get the result today?

No. You will not get all of your results today.

If you are a ♀, microscopy at the time of your appointment may show thrush, bacterial vaginosis or trichomoniasis. We can also sometimes detect gonorrhoea but this needs to be confirmed by swabs taken at the same time and sent to the laboratory. Swabs are also taken for chlamydia at the same time. The results for chlamydia and gonorrhoea are available within a week.

In ♂ we can diagnose NSU or gonorrhoea on the day if microscopy is performed (usually if there is a urethral discharge). Gonorrhoea needs to be confirmed by swabs taken at the same time and sent to the laboratory. We also send swabs to the laboratory for chlamydia and the results of all swabs are available within a week.

Blood tests results take up to 7 days however if there is a particular concern we can obtain a preliminary result within 24 hours.

Do they need repeating?

We rarely need to do tests of cure nowadays. You will be told if you need a test of cure. Swabs do not need repeating unless the first tests were taken too soon after a risk (within 1 week), there is a high infection risk, symptoms persist or there is a risk of re-infection/new infection.

I'm on my period can you still do the tests?

Yes we can still take swabs whilst you are menstruating. However some ♀ prefer to wait until their period has finished.

I need to pee, can I pee first?

♂: It is advisable not to pass urine for 3–4 hours prior to testing.

The microscope

Usually two microscopes are required. One for direct light and phase contrast illumination and the other for dark ground microscopy.

Objective lenses

- 10x, 40x (low power): provide overall magnification of 100x and 400x. Suitable for screening for clue cells, trichomoniasis and candidiasis and fungal infection although may require high power to confirm. Also used to identify scabies mites and threadworm ova.
- 100x (high power): provides overall magnification of 1000x. Must be used with immersion oil.

Used to examine specimens for PMNLs, gonococci, and other bacteria including treponemes. Separate objectives required for direct light/phase contrast and dark ground illumination.

Condensers (Fig. 4.1)

- Direct light
- Phase contrast (must match with the same Ph code on the objective)
- Dark ground (used with immersion oil between lens and under surface of the slide).

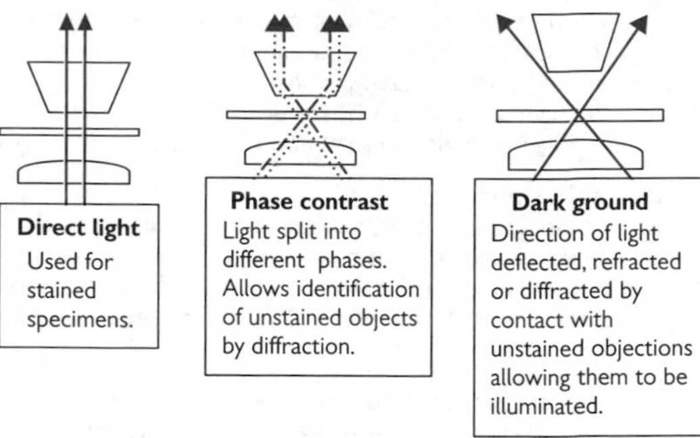

Fig. 4.1 Condensers

►Microscopy—general points

- Ensure lenses are wiped clean of immersion oil and dust with a lens tissue after use.
- To avoid lens damage ensure that high power objective lens is not aligned when slides are moved to and from the microscope.
- When using dark ground microscopy place a drop of oil on the condenser and raise until it just touches the slide.
- When using phase contrast ensure that the Ph codes on the condenser and objective match.
- Start with low power to identify good, wide field, and approximate focus before moving to high power.

Slide preparation

Gram-stain

- Fix the smear by heating the slide or submersing it in 95% methanol for 2 minutes.
- Apply crystal violet, methyl violet, or gentian violet (a combination of the 1st two) for 15 seconds.
- Apply an aqueous solution of iodine for 15 seconds.
- Decolourize slide with acetone for 3 seconds.
- Rinse slide with water.
- Apply red counterstain (e.g. carbol fuchsin, basic fuchsin, or neutral red) for 15 seconds.
- Rinse slide in water.
- Carefully dry the slide.

Preparation of ulcer fluid for dark ground microscopy for *Treponema pallidum* (see p. 100)

- Clean the ulcer with a swab soaked in sterile saline.
- Squeeze lesion gently to release serum.
- Collect serum with the edge of a cover-slip and mount in normal saline.
- Gently press the cover-slip onto the slide.

Clinic-based tests

Examination by microscopy

Gram-stained smear

- ♂ urethra/urine threads: PMNLs, Gram –ve intracellular diplococci.
- Glans penis/subpreputial sac: yeast spores +/– hyphae, mixed Gram +ve and –ve cocco-bacilli +/– curved rods (generally anaerobes).
- ♀ urethra and cervix: PMNLs, Gram –ve intracellular diplococci.
- Vagina: lactobacilli (Plate 1), PMNLs, mixed Gram +ve and –ve cocco-bacilli +/– curved rods (generally anaerobes), Gram +ve cocci, yeast spores +/– hyphae.
- Rectum: PMNLs, Gram –ve intracellular diplococci.
- Ulcers: Gram –ve coccobacillus in shoals (*Haemophilus ducreyi*)—unusual finding.

Saline suspension

- Phase contrast
  - Vagina or subpreputial sac/glans penis: clue cells/motile curved rods, *T. vaginalis*, yeast spores +/– hyphae
  - ♂ urethra: *T. vaginalis*.
- Dark ground
  - Ulcers: *Treponema pallidum*
  - Vagina or subpreputial sac/glans penis: clue cells/motile curved rods, *T. vaginalis*, yeast spores +/– hyphae
  - ♂ urethra: *T. vaginalis*.

Skin samples

- Burrow material for scabies mite
- Skin scales in 10% potassium hydroxide for mycelia (tinea/ringworm)
- Perianal transparent adhesive tape strip—threadworm ova

Vaginal discharge

- 'Whiff test'—addition of 10% potassium hydroxide releases pungent amines
- pH— >4.5

Both indicators of bacterial vaginosis.

►Unnecessary if Hay/Ison diagnostic criteria used (see p. 188).

Urine

Inspection

Urine haze in ♂ (not cleared by addition of 5% acetic acid) +/– threads in first passed suggests anterior urethritis. A second specimen (MSSU) may be of value in suggesting posterior urethritis or UTI (if turbid) and is essential for culture and sensitivity. Urine may also be required for pregnancy testing.

Urinalysis

- Sugar, ketones—diabetes (recurrent candidiasis, balanitis).
- Protein, leukocytes, blood, nitrites—UTI.
- Persistent proteinuria/haematuria—refer to nephrology.

Pregnancy test (immunoassay), urine and serum

First documented in Egypt (1350 BC) when ♀ who suspected that they were pregnant urinated on wheat and barley seeds over a 7 day period. Germination of either seed (probably due to ↑ levels of oestrogen) indicated pregnancy (70% accuracy demonstrated in 1963).

Pregnancy testing may be performed on urine or serum samples. Both tests detect β human chorionic gonadotrophin (hCG), a glycoprotein hormone produced by the placental trophoblastic cells shortly after implantation. A positive result indicates secretory activity of trophoblastic tissue normally associated with the presence of a viable fetus.

Urine (qualitative test)

Urine sampling kits give only a positive or negative result. Samples can detect hCG levels above 25–50mIU/mL. Levels of urinary hCG average 100mIU/mL following the first missed menstrual period and ↑ up to 200,000mIU/mL at 10–12 weeks of pregnancy. There is a dramatic fall in levels after this time. Test read after 3 minutes.

Limitations of urine test

- Unable to distinguish between uterine and ectopic pregnancy.
- Occasional false negative results in ectopic pregnancy.
- Inability to distinguish between pituitary luteinising hormone (LH) and hCG. Positive result may be obtained in the presence of ahydatidiform mole, chorioadenoma, or choriocarcinoma.
- Conditions such as trophoblastic disease and certain non-trophoblastic neoplasms can cause higher levels of hCG.
- ~10% of pregnancies undetectable on the first day of missed menses.
- False positive results estimated at up to 10%.
- False negative may result due to dilute urine.

Serum

More accurate and should be considered if urine testing is negative but there is a pregnancy risk. Tests can detect hCG levels above 5–10mIU/mL. Positive results may be obtained within 7–10 days of conception. Qualitative (just positive or negative) and quantitive tests available. The latter allows exact measuring of the amount of serum hCG, useful in assessing the stage of pregnancy. Serum hCG doubles every 36–48 hours in the early stages. A subnormal response may indicate miscarriage or ectopic pregnancy. Extremely high levels of hCG may suggest multiple pregnancy.

Routine female microscopy

Vaginal Gram-stained smear

1. Are there bacteria present and what are they like?

<table>
<tr><td colspan="2">Grade 0
Epithelial Cells only
• Post-menopause
• Pre-menarche
• Antibiotics
• Intra-vaginal gels</td><td colspan="2">Grade I
Lactobacilli only
• Normal flora</td><td colspan="2">Grade II
Reduced lactobacilli and mixed bacteria
• intermediate transitional phase</td></tr>
<tr><td colspan="3">Grade III
Mixed bacteria/no lactobacilli and 'clue cells'
• Indicates bacterial vaginosis</td><td colspan="3">Grade IV
Gram +ve cocci only (often in chains)
• Usually irrelevant</td></tr>
<tr><td colspan="6">Treatment for bacterial vaginosis required for Grade III (and occasionally Grade II) with symptoms/signs.</td></tr>
</table>

2. Are there any yeast spores and/or hyphae?

<table>
<tr><td colspan="2">Usually associated with vaginal PMNLs if symptomatic.</td></tr>
<tr><td>Hyphae +/– spores</td><td>Usually Candida albicans</td></tr>
<tr><td>Spores alone</td><td>Probably Candida glabrata</td></tr>
</table>

3. Are there vaginal PMNLs?

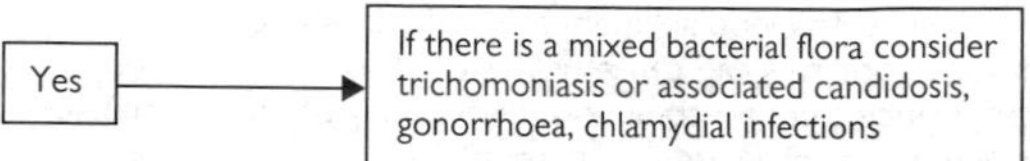

Urethral and cervical Gram-stained smears

Are PMNLs present?

- Urethra: ↑ risk of gonorrhoea therefore check urethral and cervical smears especially carefully for gonococci.
- Cervix: variable depending on menstrual cycle, sexual activity, and contraception (often ↑ with hormonal methods). >30 per high power field correlates best with gonococcal or chlamydial infections.

Are Gram-negative diplococci (GNDC) present?

Examine urethral and cervical smears for intracellular GNDC. Urethral smear of doubtful value if cervix examined. Finding extracellular GNDC ↑ sensitivity by 20% but ↓ specificity by 4%.

Vaginal preparation in saline protected by a cover slip

- Switch light source to phase contrast (or dark ground).
- Screen slide (low power) for motile protozoa, spores +/– hyphae.
- If necessary switch to high power. Place a drop of immersion oil on to cover slip before examining. Can also be used to identify clue cells and motile vibrios (*Mobiluncus* spp.) often found in bacterial vaginosis.

Routine male microscopy

Urethral Gram-stained smear

Are PMNLs present?

Non-gonococcal urethritis diagnosed by finding:

- ≥5 PMNLs per high-power field (averaged over 5 fields with the greatest concentration of PMNLs).
- no GNDC.

Are GNDC present (with intracellular organisms)?

If seen allows for working diagnosis of gonorrhoea. Generally associated with numerous PMNLs.

Gram-stained smear from urine

Useful if urine threads in first-voided urine (FVU) specimen and no urethral material to sample directly. Slide can be prepared from threads or centrifuged FVU. Ideally urine should not be passed for at least 3–4 hours before assessment.

Are PMNLs present?

Non-gonococcal urethritis diagnosed by finding:

- ≥10 PMNLs per high-power field (averaged over 5 fields with the greatest concentration of PMNLs).
- no GNDC.

Are GNDC present (with intracellular organisms)?

Allows for working diagnosis of gonorrhoea.

Saline suspension of sub-preputial, glans penis, or urethral material

Subprepuce and glans

If balanitis/balanoposthitis check for:

- yeast spores +/– hyphae
- clue cells (anaerobic balanitis)
- *T. vaginalis*

} A Gram-stained smear can also be used.

Urethra

T. vaginalis (may occasionally be seen with urethritis).

Microscopy—accuracy

Infection and site	Sensitivity (%)	Specificity (%)
Gonorrhoea		
Urethral Gram-stain from symptomatic ♂	90–95	95–99*
Urethral Gram-stain from asymptomatic ♂	50–75	
Rectal Gram stain from homosexual ♂	35–80[†]	95–100*
Urethral Gram-stain from ♀	20	Unknown
Cervical Gram-stain	23–65	88–100*
Bacterial vaginosis (Hay/Ison criteria)		
Vaginal Gram-stained specimen	97.5	96
Trichomoniasis (saline suspension)		
Suspension of vaginal discharge	40–80	If motile protozoa seen-100
Suspension of male urethral/subpreputial material	30	
Candidiasis		
Vaginal Gram-stain if symptomatic	65	No data Probably near 100
Vaginal saline suspension	40–60	
Primary syphilis		
Dark ground examination of ulcer material in saline	79–86	77–100

* This excludes *Neisseria meningitidis* which rarely may be found (indistinguishable morphologically from *N. gonorrhoeae*).
[†] Higher level if rectal pus.

Commensals and confounders

Genital specimens include various microorganisms which may not be pathogenic. These include hydrogen peroxide-producing *Lactobacillus* spp. which indicate normality and other organisms, usually commensal but pathogenic under certain conditions. Results of routine genital specimens therefore should be interpreted in the clinical context and inappropriate antibiotic treatment should be avoided.

Leptothrix

Elongated chain of lactobacilli that may be mistaken for *Candida* spp. on microscopy. Usually not clinically significant but may be associated with vaginitis.

Group B β-haemolytic streptococci—*Streptococcus agalactiae*

Vaginal carriage rates in ♀ attending GUM clinics 12–36%, usually not clinically significant except in late pregnancy (see p. 320).

Actinomyces israelii

Found in 3% of ♀ genital specimens—4% if using intrauterine device (IUD). Detectable on cervical cytology or vaginal wet mount and Gram-stained smears. If asymptomatic no intervention is required. However, removal (and culture) of IUD and treatment with penicillin or erythromycin may be indicated if otherwise unexplained symptoms e.g. intermenstrual bleeding, dyspaerunia, and pelvic pain.

Actinomycosis (a suppurative upper genital tract infection) is a rare complication, especially associated with long-term use of plastic IUDs (see p. 144).

Neisseria meningitidis

↑ rates of nasopharyngeal carriage in homosexual ♂ and those practising oro-genital sex, reporting multiple sexual partners or diagnosed with anogenital gonococcal infection (>20% in these groups compared with a general rate of 5–15%). High rates also found in university students (up to 34%). Anogenital carriage in up to 2% of homosexual ♂, 0.2% heterosexual ♂, and 0.1% ♀. May rarely cause urethritis in ♂.

Other micro-organisms

- *Gardnerella vaginalis, Prevotella melaninogenica, Peptostreptococci*, and other anaerobic organisms may be detected in genital specimens because of low-level colonization without bacterial vaginosis.
- *Ureaplasma urealyticum, Bacterioides urealyticum*, and *Mycoplasma hominis* may also be found without any clinical manifestations.
- *Corynebacterium species, Escherichia coli*, and coagulase-negative staphylococci in genital specimens are usually of no clinical significance but rarely may be implicated in vaginitis.
- Spirochaetes—*Brachyspira aalborgi* and *Brachyspira pilosicoli* colonize colo-rectal epithelium in up to 30% of people in some developing countries and a similar proportion of homosexual ♂ or those with HIV infection in the developed countries. In addition *Treponema denticola, Treponema vincentii*, and other similar treponemes associated with periodontal infections and *Treponema refringens, Treponema phagedenis*, and *Treponema minutum*, found as commensals in the genitalia, need to be distinguished from *T. pallidum* in rectal, oral, or genital specimens.

Chapter 5

Specific genitourinary situations

Men with symptoms suggesting urethritis

Factors suggesting sexually acquired cause

Presentation: ↑ likelihood if new sexual risk/suspicion about a partner with urethritis arising within 4 weeks (usually).

- Age: most commonly found in ♂ from late teens to 50 years.
- Symptoms: usually prominent dysuria and/or urethral discharge (may just be found on examination). ↑urinary frequency and systemic symptoms unusual.

Management

Urethral smear: ≥5 polymorphonuclear leucocytes (PMNL) per high-power field (HPF) and/or urinary thread from first voided urine (FVU): ≥10 PMNL per HPF. Consider sending air-dried smear to lab, if on-site microscopy unavailable.

Urethral swab for *Neisseria gonorrhoeae*; swab or FVU for *Chlamydia trachomatis*, ideally using a nucleic acid amplification test (NAAT). Consider:

- mid-stream sample of urine MSSU (to exclude UTI), if relevant.
- exposure to other STIs—consider screening, e.g. syphilis and HIV serology.

Treat on microscopy findings or clinical assessment, if microscopy unavailable (while awaiting lab results).

Partner notification/contact tracing must be arranged. Contacts of gonorrhoea, NGU/chlamydia should be treated epidemiologically. No sex until treatment completed and partner(s) treated.

Factors suggesting non-sexually transmitted cause. Consider underlying urinary tract infection

- Sexual history: long-standing stable sexual relationship/not sexually active
- Age: >50 years (prostatism with UTI more common)
- Symptoms: ↑ frequency, loin pain, pyrexia, malaise.

Management

Consider/exclude STI:

- urethral smear for Gram-stain, swab for *N. gonorrhoeae*; swab, or FVU for *C. trachomatis*.
- offer syphilis and HIV serology.

FVU and MSSU typically both opaque failing to clear on acidification (e.g. 5% acetic acid). Dip-stick usually shows leucocytes, nitrites, protein, and blood. Send MSSU for microscopy, culture, and sensitivity.

If suspected—manage as UTI.

Balanitis and balanoposthitis

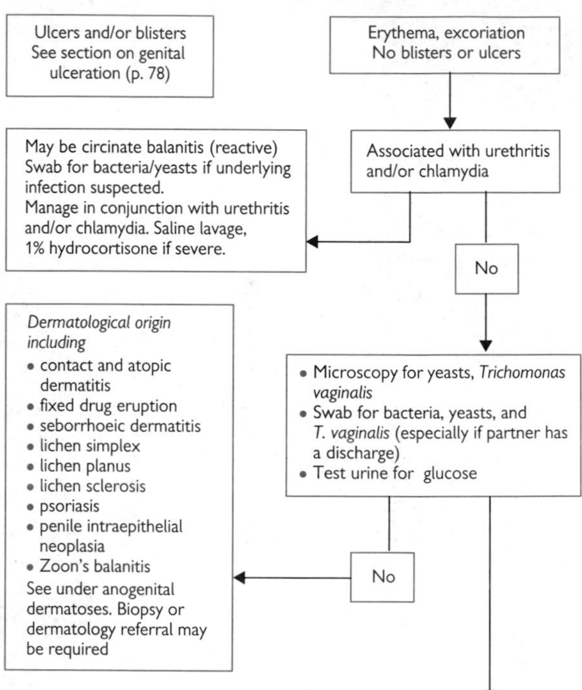

- Candida: azoles, offer check to ♀ partner
- Trichomoniasis: oral metronidazole, treat ♀ partner
- Anaerobes: saline lavage, oral metronidazole if severe
- Aerobes: often found as commensals so only treat if symptomatic
  - *Staphylococcus aureus*—antibiotics dependant on sensitivity.
  - Group A and B streptococci—as above.
  - *Gardnerella vaginalis*—usually found with anaerobes; manage accordingly.

Vulval irritation and pain

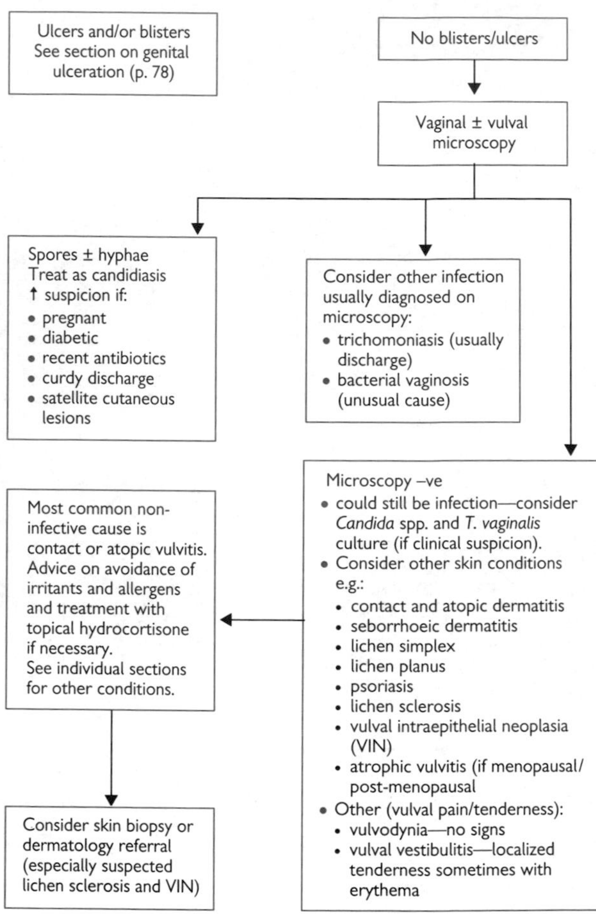

Altered vaginal discharge

The normal physiological discharge will alter with the time of the menstrual cycle, pregnancy and sometimes hormonal contraception. The finding of lactobacilli without other anomalies provides reassurance, pending swab results.

Remember that it is common for infections to co-exist.

Primary vaginal conditions

- Watery white/grey discharge
- Fishy smell often worse after sex or at menstruation

→

Bacterial vaginosis

- Free flowing white/grey discharge, often frothy. Fishy smell, demonstrated if discharge mixed with alkali (10% potassium hydroxide)
- pH of vaginal fluid >4.5
- Microscopy: loss of lactobacilli, replacement with small gram-variable cocco-bacilli (mostly *G. vaginalis*) forming clue cells
- Culture: unhelpful as organisms are commensals

- White curdy discharge
- Pruritus vulvae, vulval rash
- Pregnancy, diabetes, recent antibiotics

→

Candidiasis

- Vulval erythema, satellite lesions, white curdy discharge typical but may be very variable
- Microscopy: spores and/or hyphae
- Culture: dry high vaginal swab (caution—*Candida* spp. commensal in ~20%)

- Sexual risk
- Malodorous green/yellow discharge (mucoid with time)
- Vulval burning/discomfort
- External dysuria

→

Trichomoniasis

- Discharge—as described, vulvovaginitis, 'strawberry cervicitis' in 2–5%
- Microscopy: motile flagellated protozoa on saline suspension using phase contrast or dark ground
- Culture: from vaginal swab sent in Feinberg–Whittington or transport medium

Other causes commonly seen in GUM

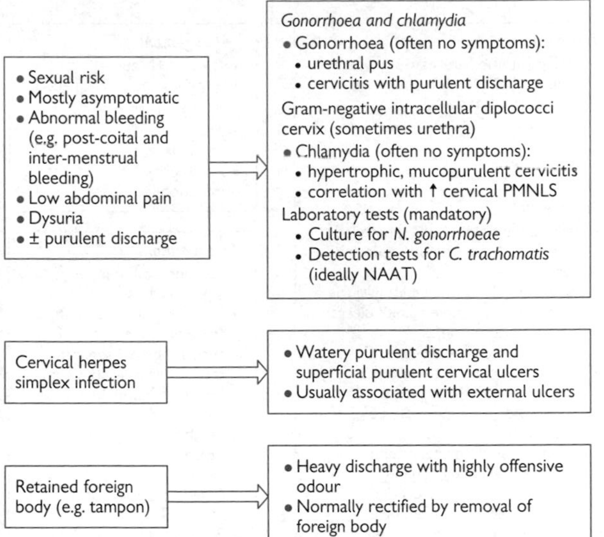

Anogenital ulceration

Traumatic
- Timing—immediately after incident
- Appearance (often irregular—as dermatitis artefacta)

⇒

Management
Exclude STI cause
Bacterial swab (if 2° infection)
General STI screen
Advise
- Saline lavage
- Antibiotics for secondary infection if necessary

Possible STI
- Herpes: multiple, painful, preceded by vesicles. Most common infective cause
- Syphilis: 1° chancre—typically single and painless (multiple painful ulcers now more common):
  2°—'snail track', usually with skin rash
- Tropical: (suspect if travel history or exposure). Typical presentations:
  - chancroid—multiple, soft, painful ulcers
  - lymphogranuloma venereum (LGV)—usually bilateral inguinal lymphadenopathy (preceded by transient, small, painless ulcer)
  - granuloma inguinale—pruritic papule followed by granulomatous ulcer

⇒

Investigations
- Herpes—swab for herpes simplex virus
- Dark-ground examination for treponemes. Consider repeating on 3 separate days if clinically suspicious. Ensure full syphilis serology requested
- Swab for *Haemophilus ducreyi*
- Swab ulcer/bubo pus for *C. trachomatis*; blood for LGVCFT
- Biopsy for Donovan bodies

Other
- Neoplastic: progressive over weeks or months (age usually over 50 years)
- 'Dermatological': e.g. aphthous ulcers/Behçet's disease—usually chronic, relapsing associated with oral ulcers and if Behçet's other systemic symptoms

⇒

Management
Urgent urology referral if carcinoma suspected.
Dermatological referral may be required for other conditions

The most common infective cause in GUM is genital herpes

First episode

- Diagnosis
  - Swab—in viral transport medium
  - Diagnostic confirmation important although treatment should commence on clinical grounds
  - Full STI screen advised. Internal examination in ♀ may be deferred until acute symptoms resolved
- Management
  - If clinically suspected, start oral antiviral treatment
  - Analgesia may be required (e.g. 30–60mg codeine phosphate 4–6 times a day)
  - Recommend saline lavage
  - Suggest micturition in warm bath water if severe dysuria. Supra-pubic catheterization may be required if urinary retention

Recurrence

- Supportive treatment (e.g. saline bathing) unless unusually severe when oral antiviral treatment is justified
- STI screen only if new risk

Frequent recurrence (>6 per year)

- Anticipatory episodic treatment
- Suppressive treatment

Genital lumps and bumps

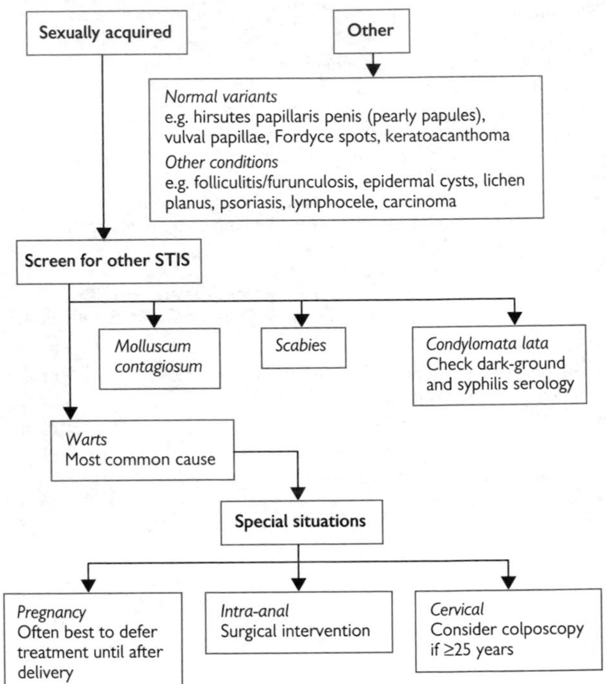

Epidemiological treatment for contacts of STIs

Infection of index case	Treatment need	Contact treatment
♀ candidiasis ♂ candidiasis	✗ ✓	 Antimycotic treatment often required
Chancroid	✓	Ciprofloxacin 500mg twice daily for 3 days Ceftriaxone 250mg single dose, IM
Chlamydia	✓	Doxycycline (100mg twice daily for 7 days, azithromycin 1g stat., erythromycin 500mg twice daily for 14 days
Donovanosis	✓	Azithromycin: to current contacts and those from 30 days prior to onset of symptoms
Epididymitis	✓	Doxycycline, erythromycin (as chlamydia)
Gonorrhoea	✓	Single doses of cefixime 400mg; ciprofloxacin 500mg; amoxicillin 3g + probenecid 1g; ceftriaxone 250mg IM.
Hepatitis A	✓	Hepatitis A vaccine HNIG*—close contacts <2 weeks
Hepatitis B	✓	Specific hepatitis B immunoglobulin (<7 days). Super-accelerated active immunisation
HIV	✗/✓	If <72 hours, consider highly active antiretroviral therapy (HAART)
Lymphogranuloma venereum	✓	Doxycycline: to current contacts and those from 30 days prior to onset of symptoms
Non-gonococcal urethritis	✓	Doxycycline, erythromycin (as chlamydia)
Mucopurulent cervicitis and PID	✓	Doxycycline, erythromycin (as chlamydia). Consider anti-gonorrhoea treatment
Pediculosis	✓	Permethrin or malathion to sex contacts
Scabies	✓	Permethrin or malathion to sex and household contacts
Syphilis—early Syphilis—late	✗/✓ ✗	Consider benzathine penicillin 2.4MU IM stat or oral doxycycline 100mg twice daily for 14 days
Trichomoniasis	✓	Metronidazole 2g single dose or 400mg twice daily for 7 days

* Human normal immunoglobulin

No partner treatment required

Infection	Need	Contact treatment
Bacterial vaginosis	×	Not required
Hepatitis C	×	
Anogenital herpes	×	
Anogenital warts/molluscum contagiosum	×	

NB. These tables only provide information about epidemiological treatment. They do not cover the requirement to offer contacts at risk STI screening, information and advice.

Sexual assault—general principles

Definitions

Include both ♂ and ♀ survivors and apply irrespective of the relationship between those involved, e.g. a ♂ can be convicted of raping his wife.

Rape: non-consensual penetration of the vagina, anus, or mouth by a penis. 'Vagina' is defined as including the vulva.

Assault by penetration: non-consensual penetration of the vagina or anus by the assailants body part (e.g. finger), or anything else (e.g. a bottle), where the penetration is 'sexual'.

Sexual assault: intentional touching of another person intimately without consent.

Causing a person to engage in sexual activity without consent: this offence covers non-consensual activity not within the definition of rape or sexual assault. Applies when a person intentionally causes another to engage in sexual activity without consent. Examples: person 'A' forces person 'B' to masturbate, 'A' forces 'B' to manually stimulate a 3rd person, 'A' compels 'B' to penetrate her/him.

Statistics

Studies have shown that up to 25% of ♀ have experienced rape or attempted rape and 3% of adult ♂ have been sexually assaulted. 91% of ♀ told no one with <7% reporting the assault to the police. 97% of callers to rape crisis lines knew their assailant. Only 6% of those reporting rape see their assailant convicted.

Myths/misconception

♂ who are anally raped may have an erection and ejaculate as a normal physiological response. It does not mean they are homosexual, have enjoyed or consented to it. The absence of physical trauma does not exclude rape. Many victims are too afraid to fight off an attack for fear of further assault or loss of life. A victim can appear calm and even smile following a rape but this does not mean the rape accusation is false, it is a normal coping mechanism. Rape is not committed due to an overwhelming sex-drive with a sexual motivation. It is usually an act of violence and power with the vast majority premeditated.

Good practice

It is important to ensure that there are links with the police and support agencies (e.g. Rape Crisis Centres). The patient should be offered a choice of ♂ or ♀ experienced staff if possible. A suitable appointment with minimum waiting time and private waiting area should ideally be provided if distressed.

Forensic testing

No attempt to perform a forensic examination should be made unless forensically trained and in a suitable environment with the correct equipment to perform it. Forensic examination can be useful up to 7 days following an assault. Local police services should give advice on where this is performed. The person should be advised to retain all clothing ivolved unwashed and not bathe prior to the forensic examination.

Sexual assault—history check-list

▶ Always inform the patient that they only need to give as much information as they feel comfortable with—asking a patient to give full details of an assault can be distressing and can lead to psychological consequences.

- ***Date of assault:*** essential for determining when STI screening should occur and the use of emergency contraception.
- ***Location of assault:*** needed to assess the background prevalence of certain STIs, especially if the attacker is a stranger.
- ***Attacker(s) details:*** assessing the risk of the acquisition of STIs:
  - number
  - known or stranger
  - if known—any risk factors for blood-borne viruses.
- ***Was assault reported to police?/Does the patient want to report?/Has a forensic examination been performed?*** Important as forensic examination should be performed prior to STI screening.
- ***Were alcohol/drugs taken prior to attack?*** To establish the possibility of 'drug rape'.
- ***Is the general practitioner aware of the assault and/or has the patient contacted a rape support agency?*** To assess any treatment given and psychological support arranged.
- ***Details regarding type of attack:*** to determine the exact nature of the attack for legal purposes and the risks/sites of possible STIs or injury.
  - Physical injury
  - Vaginal penetration
  - Anal penetration
  - Oral penetration
  - Was a condom used?

▶ Those assaulted may be too upset to recall this information or may have blanked out the detail as a means of coping. It is therefore wise to offer screening from all sites and this may provide additional assurance to the patient.

Sexual assault—management

► If the patient wishes to report the assault to the police examination and screening for STIs should be deferred until forensic tests have been taken as evidence may be lost.

The management of victims of sexual assault can appear complex and should include screening for STIs, emergency contraception, and psychological support. Occasionally medical evidence may be required in court and well-written clear notes are vital for this. The use of a proforma for rape cases can help ensure no vital areas of management are missed and all the necessary information is recorded.

History taking

This should be taken with a degree of flexibility depending on the emotional state of the patient and be performed in a calm and sensitive manner. In addition to the standard history detailed information should be taken regarding the assault.

Examination

In recent assault cases the presence or absence of visible trauma should be clearly documented with the use of diagrams. Should any injury require medical treatment this should be provided prior to any further examination. Attempted rape can produce more injuries than actual rape. The absence of any injuries does not exclude rape. In cases of recent forced oral penetration examine for haemorrhages on the palate. Offer proctoscopy if recent forced anal penetration for signs of trauma.

Investigations

It is rare for the presence of an STI to legally reinforce a case of rape. As people who have been assaulted may have pre-existing STIs it is advisable to do a full screen at presentation. However, it is recommended that swabs are repeated 1–2 weeks after the assault as early sampling may miss recently acquired infection. Ensure patients fully understand what tests are recommended and their implications. All specimens should be clearly marked to indicate that the result might have legal consequences. Where possible the 'chain of evidence' should be implemented (i.e. every handover of the specimen is signed, dated, and timed). As well as the standard STI screen and microscopy, additional specimens should be considered (see Box). If the patient does not want serological testing at presentation a serum specimen can be stored. This may help to clarify the timing of any subsequent seroconversion.

Management

Offer treatment for any infection found. A health adviser can reinforce information given, provide links for psychological support, and clarify the follow up arrangements. Ensure the patient leaves the clinic with contact numbers of agencies able to provide further emotional support.

Sexual assault—investigations check-list

(NB. swabs should only be taken after forensic samples have been taken, if relevant)

- ***Microscopy***: urethral, cervical, and rectal smears (if relevant) for *N. gonorrhoeae*, vaginal preparations for yeasts, bacterial vaginosis, and *T. vaginalis*.
- ***NAAT testing for C. trachomatis***: urethra and cervix. May also detect rectal infection. However, culture is still required for medico-legal purposes.
- ***Culture for N. gonorrhoeae:*** urethra, cervix, throat, and rectum (advised in 5 even in the absence of forced anal penetration).
- ***Culture for T. vaginalis:*** vagina
- ***Serology***
  - Syphilis
  - HIV
  - Hepatitis B virus
  - Hepatitis C virus (if patient has risk factor or if assailant known to have risk factor)
  - Storage (if patient does not wish baseline testing)

Management check-list

- ***Treat any infection found***
- ***Emergency contraception:*** if indicated (see p. 330)
- ***Prophylactic antibiotics:*** consider for chlamydia and gonorrhoea if the patient cannot tolerate an examination or requires an intrauterine device for emergency contraception.
- ***Hepatitis B immunisation:*** may have a protective effect if given within 3 weeks following an assault.
- ***HIV prophylaxis:*** individual risk assessment needed, including type and location of assault and assailant risk factors.
- ***Support:*** may be provided by a health adviser, specialist nurse, or other agencies.
- ***Consent to write to general practitioner:*** helpful to provide total care.
- ***Review:*** for follow-up of any infection detected, repeat investigations (to cover 'window periods'), hepatitis immunisation, psychological support.

Children

All healthcare professionals working within GUM should remain alert to the possibility of child abuse. The Children's Act 1989 defines a child as a person <18 years of age. The legal age of consent is 16 in England, Scotland, and Wales and 17 in N. Ireland. Penetrative intercourse with a child <13 years is defined as rape.

Sexual abuse involves forcing a young person to take part in sexual activities whether or not the young person is aware of what is happening. If suspected, screening for STIs should be considered. If infection is found in a child aged <3 years vertical transmission from the mother is possible so she should be offered STI screening. This may be extended to the siblings and others in the household.

All GUM clinics should have:

- Guidelines for the management of children.
- A nominated consultant physician to take the lead for children as part of a multidisciplinary team.
- Access to formal child protection training.
- Details of local child protection policies and procedures.
- Chain of evidence procedures (see p. 86).
- Regular audit of adherence to child protection guidelines.

Sexually transmitted infections

► The significance of an STI in children requires careful interpretation. It may be used as corroborative evidence to indicate sexual abuse.

Sampling techniques

The least invasive methods should be used together with the minimum number of swabs. Sterile cotton tipped swabs are recommended, with smaller ENT swabs being useful for urethral or trans-hymenal vaginal sampling. Urethral sampling causes discomfort and should be kept to a minimum. Vulval or vaginal washings are acceptable. Samples should be taken for *N. gonorrhoeae*, *C. trachomatis*, *T. vaginalis*, and in the presence of ulcers, herpes simplex virus (also *H. ducreyi* and dark ground for syphilis if clinically indicated).

Recommended urogenital sites for prepubertal ♀ (usually <11 years)

Vulva and vagina lined with immature epithelium, receptive to infection by *N. gonorrhoeae* and *C. trachomatis*, therefore swab vulva (especially posterior fourchette) and posterior vaginal wall.

Recommendations for post-pubertal ♀ (usually ≥11 years)

- as for ♀ adults if speculum examination can be tolerated.
- if speculum examination impossible — blind vaginal sampling (ideally using NAAT) plus urethral swabs +/– urine NAAT.

Management

Wherever possible treatment for children should be prescribed within the terms of the product licence. However, some conditions may require drugs not specifically licensed for paediatric use. If in doubt, discuss with local pharmacist.

Specific infections

Chlamydia

Found in the rectum, vagina, conjunctiva, or nasopharynx of infants. Estimated risk of perinatal transmission 50–70%. Chlamydia has been found in 1.2–17% of sexually abused children.

Gonorrhoea

Estimated risk of perinatal transmission resulting in gonococcal ophthalmia of 30%. Gonococcal infection has been found in 2.4–11.2% of sexually abused children.

Anogenital warts

Warts which develop within the 1st year of life are likely to be perinatally acquired. In children aged between 1 and 12 years being investigated for possible sexual abuse approximately ~2% have been found to have genital warts. Inconsistent results have been obtained from studies into perinatal transmission, and data on the presence of human papilloma virus DNA in children beyond the neonatal period is variable.

Trichomoniasis

Found in ~5% of infants born to infected mothers. In children being investigated for sexual abuse 1–4% have been found to be infected.

Anogenital herpes

No data on risks of acquiring anogenital herpes following sexual abuse.

Syphilis

Pre-pubertal children presenting with 1° or 2° stages of syphilis occurring beyond the neonatal period should be considered to be victims of sexual abuse. Congenital syphilis is now uncommon in the UK.

HIV

No data on risks of acquiring HIV following sexual abuse.

Bacterial vaginosis (BV)

The significance of finding BV in children is unclear as BV is not classified as a STI. *G. vaginalis* has been cultured from various sites in the newborn and from the vagina in 1–32%. Variable rates of BV, from 7 to 34%, have been demonstrated in sexually abused girls.

Chapter 6

Syphilis

Introduction

The origins of syphilis are unclear but it became an epidemic in Europe in the late fifteenth century (although skeletal evidence suggests earlier endemic infection). The name originates from a poem about the infected shepherd, Syphilis written by Fracastoro in 1530.

Aetiology—*Treponema pallidum*

Delicate spiralled spirochaete, 6–20μm in length by 0.1–0.18μm in diameter. Consists of a cylindrical nucleus and cytoplasm contained within a cell wall and outer envelope with flagella in the periplasmic space. Microaerophilic and can only be grown on tissue culture. Limited viability outside its host (obligate human parasite) so usually transmitted sexually to and from mucosal skin through tiny abrasions.

Epidemiology and transmission

Currently high rates in Eastern Europe. In UK disproportionately high rates of infection in homosexual ♂, especially as outbreaks, through anonymous sex in saunas and 'cruising sites', by orogenital sex and in association with HIV infection.

- Sexual (only from early syphilis) ~30–50% of contacts are infected.
- Accidental infection by inoculation (e.g. healthcare professionals).
- Blood-borne—needle sharing, blood transfusion (very rare as blood is screened and organisms die after 96–120 hours at 4°C).
- Transplacental (from 9th week of pregnancy). More common in early syphilis (80–90% risk), rare after 4 years.

Natural history

Acquired

Early (infectious) syphilis—first 2 years of infection.

- 1°: 9–90 days after infection (average 3 weeks) resolving within 3–8 weeks (occasionally with small pale scar).
- 2°: 6–12 weeks after infection, associated with a persisting 1° lesion in ~33%. Lesions may relapse (in 25% if untreated) and regress over a period of 2 years. Permanent depigmentation of the skin of the neck (leukoderma colli) rarely occurs.
- Early latent

Late syphilis—after 2 years of infection.

- Late latent—(end result of two-third of those who are not treated).
- Gummatous ('benign')—can appear in 2 years, more usual 10–15 years.
  - Musculo-skeletal (10%), visceral and mucosal (15%)
- Cardiovascular (10%)—after ~30–40 years
- Neurological (10%)
  - Meningovascular—after ~15–18 years, general paresis—after ~20–25 years, tabes dorsalis—after ~30 years

► Data from the pre-antibiotic era.

Congenital

- Early, first 2 years of life.
- Late, lesions usually from 2–3 years of age.

Frequently asked questions

Can I catch syphilis from oral sex?

Yes, unprotected oral sex is a risk factor.

Is it true that you can go 'mad' with syphilis?

Neurosyphilis may lead to general paralysis with dulling of the intellect, judgement and insight, with memory loss, antisocial behaviour, grandiose delusions, depression, and dementia. It takes 20–25 years to develop but is prevented by earlier treatment. Fortunately, it is extremely rare nowadays.

When I've been treated am I immune?

No, it is possible to catch syphilis again after re-infection. Having been infected once with syphilis does not give any lasting immunity to that person.

Do I have to have an injection for treatment, can I have tablets instead?

The 1st line recommended treatment is with long-acting penicillin injections. For those who are allergic to penicillin, oral doxycycline is recommended. The dosage and duration of treatment depends on the stage of infection.

My blood tests are still positive after treatment. Does this mean I still have syphilis?

No. Many of the blood tests used for detecting syphilis measure anti-treponemal antibodies, which are usually produced for life even after successful treatment. They do not provide protection against future infection. It is important to measure their nadir after treatment as re-infection will produce a rise in their levels.

Does my partner need treating?

If you have been diagnosed with:

- 1° syphilis—your current partner needs to be seen to be tested for syphilis, and any other partners seen within the previous 3 months.
- 2° syphilis—all sexual contacts within the previous 2 years need to be seen with serological review for 3 months from the last sexual risk.

Partners will only be treated if they test positive for syphilis. If surveillance is not possible epidemiological treatment may be considered.

If you have been diagnosed with late latent syphilis you are not sexually infectious, however we need to work out when infection was most likely acquired and partners from within 2 years of this time should be notified for testing.

Clinical features—early syphilis

Primary syphilis—lesion(s) at site(s) of infection

Classical presentation: initial painless papule at inoculation site, expands and ulcerates producing a round or oval painless chancre, 1–2cm in diameter with an indurated margin and clear moist base exuding serum without blood on pressure (Plate 2). Typically solitary, although multiple lesions may occur. Moderate, usually bilateral, painless enlargement of regional inguinal lymph nodes if chancre within the area of drainage.

Contemporary presentation. it has become more common for multiple, painful ulcers to be found with little induration mimicking genital herpes, especially in ♂ homosexual outbreaks (Plate 3). Orogenital sex is a major vehicle for transmission, with oral ulceration seen more frequently.

Sites

- Genitals: may appear anywhere but more likely on mucosal surfaces, i.e. sub-preputial sac, glans penis, labia, fourchette, and cervix (the latter without inguinal adenopathy and usually asymptomatic). Rarely an intraurethral chancre presenting as urethritis may occur in ♂. Rare reports of balanitis (of Follman).
- Extra-genital: oral (lips, mouth, tongue, tonsils, and pharynx—the last two may be painful); anal margin—often resembling a fissure with local tenderness; rectum (unusual); and rarely other sites (including finger, hand, arm, supraclavicular, nipple, eyelid).

Secondary syphilis—from haematogenous dissemination

- Constitutional: malaise, fever, headache, anorexia, myalgia.
- Skin lesions (syphilides), often polymorphic (~80%), pruritus in ~40%:
  - Macular: pink, 1cm diameter, mostly on trunk, often overlooked.
  - Papular (dull-red with shiny surface) and papulosquamous (with surface scaling). Extensive, typically affecting flexor surfaces and involving palms (Plate 4) and soles (firm non-prominent papules, scaling common). May form condylomata lata, hypertrophied wart-like lesions on moist areas, especially around vulva and anus (Plate 5). Brittle nails.
  - Other: pustular (especially with debility), hyper- or hypopigmented (leukoderma) lesions.
- Lymphadenopathy: 75% inguinal, 60% generalized also splenomegaly.
- Mucous membrane lesions in 30%: 'mucous patch'—ulcer with white/grey border (may coalesce with others forming 'snail track ulcers'). Found in the oral cavity and larynx (sore throat, hoarseness), nasal mucosa (discharge), genitalia, anus, and rectum (diffuse, distal proctitis).
- Alopecia: specific—'moth-eaten'; non-specific—telogen effluvium (diffuse).
- Musculo-skeletal: periostitis—bone pain (25% prior to antibiotic era), especially tibia; bursitis; arthralgia (6%).
- Hepatitis: usually subclinical, raised enzymes, mainly alkaline phosphatase, in 20%.

- Renal: rarely glomerulonephritis; nephrotic syndrome (both mild and self-limiting).
- Neurological: meningism in 1–2%; transitory cerebrospinal fluid (CSF) white cell and protein ↑ in 5–40%; very rarely meningitis/meningovasculitis; perceptive nerve deafness; peripheral neuritis.
- Eyes: iritis (<1%); anterior uveitis (more common in HIV infection); choroidoretinitis, including optic atrophy (usually asymptomatic).

Early latent

No signs or symptoms, positive serology, within 2 years of acquisition.

Differential diagnosis of 2° syphilis

Macular rash

- Pityriasis rosea—initial herald patch.
- Tinea (Pityriasis) versicolor—hypo- or hyper-pigmented scaly macular rash, mostly over trunk. Culture scales for *Malassezia furfur*.
- Measles—oral Koplik spots.
- Rubella—posterior cervical lymph node enlargement.
- Infectious mononucleosis—may be associated with biological false positive cardiolipin test result.
- Drug reaction—associated with drug intake and pruritus.

Papular lesions

- Psoriasis—extensor surfaces, knees and elbows, scalp, nail pitting.
- Lichen planus—oral lesions, Wickham's striae.

Clinical features—late syphilis

Late latent

No signs or symptoms, positive serology, >2 years after acquisition. Proportionately, more common now as active late syphilis has declined with the widespread use of antibiotics for other purposes.

Gummatous (late benign) syphilis

- Gumma formation (syphilitic granulation tissue) due to reactivation of residual treponemes in sensitized host. Gummata are nodules or nodulo-ulcers, indurated and indolent, single or few in number. They commonly heal with central scarring while peripherally still active. Ulcers are described as 'punched out' with a basal 'wash leather' appearance due to slough. They are not contagious.
- Sites
  - Skin: especially below knee, buttocks, thighs, shoulders, scalp, face.
  - Bones: gummatous periostitis (bony proliferation) e.g. sabre tibia; gummatous osteitis (bone destruction).
  - Mouth and throat: palatal perforation; gumma of tongue or superficial glossitis (associated with leukoplakia and malignancy); epiglottis destruction and laryngeal infiltration (hoarseness).
  - Other organs: gummata of liver, testis, oesophagus, stomach, intestine, cerebrum, spinal cord, aortic wall, myocardium. Also reported in bronchi and lungs, kidney, bladder adrenal glands, and breast.

Cardiovascular syphilis

- Conduction defects: if gummatous involvement (e.g. Stokes–Adams syndrome).
- Aortic aneurysm: proximal ascending aorta, fusiform or saccular, without dissection. Presents as chest pain or signs of compression of adjacent structures (e.g. hoarseness, dysphagia).
- Aortic regurgitation (30% of those with cardiovascular syphilis): insidious so well compensated. Typical early diastolic murmur on forced expiration with patient inclined forward.

Neurosyphilis

- Asymptomatic: abnormal CSF findings. 23–87% of cases progressed to clinical neurosyphilis in the pre-antibiotic era.
- Meningovascular: now the most common neurosyphilitic presentation. Consider if cerebrovascular accident in a young adult. Often sudden onset preceded by headache and mental deterioration. Hemiplegia/paresis, aphasia, seizures typical features but ocular palsy and trigeminal neuralgia may occur. Pupillary abnormalities are frequent with a full Argyll Robertson pupil (constriction on accommodation, not to light) in 10%.
- General paralysis: insidious, dulling of intellect, judgement and insight. Memory loss, antisocial behaviour, grandiose delusions (now rare), hand and facial tremor, depression, spastic paresis, and dementia. Full Argyll Robertson pupil in 25%.

- Tabes dorsalis: selective degeneration of the spinal dorsal columns. Lightning pains, paraesthesia, visceral crises (smooth muscle spasm), ataxia with stamping gait and +ve Romberg sign. Diminished or absent reflexes, deep pain, vibration, and position sense. Trophic changes lead to neuropathic joints (Charcot) and painless perforating plantar ulcers. Optic atrophy and bilateral ptosis are common.

Pregnancy and congenital infection

Syphilis in pregnancy

Although fetal infection has been reported from 9th week of gestation it is most likely to arise after the 18th week. Spontaneous abortion typically occurs in 2nd and early 3rd trimester. Outcome in untreated infection varies with stage:

- 1° or 2° syphilis: up to 50% prematurity/perinatal death and 50% congenital infection.
- Early latent syphilis: up to 40% prematurity/perinatal death and 20% congenital infection.
- Late latent syphilis: up to 20% prematurity/perinatal death and 10% congenital infection.

(Normal control: 9% prematurity/perinatal death).

► Despite treatment in early syphilis up to 14% may result in fetal death or congenital infection.

Early congenital syphilis (within first 2 years of life)

Clinical manifestations do not normally appear until 2–12 weeks after birth. Features include:

- Failure to thrive.
- Mucosal lesions—with pharyngeal and nasal involvement (snuffles), progressing to local destruction and perforation.
- Skin lesions:
  - rashes similar to 2° syphilis but prominent around the mouth and body orifices leading to scarring (rhagades).
  - blistering bullous eruption of palms and soles (syphilitic pemphigus).
  - condylomata lata around anus and genitalia.
  - sparse hair and brittle, atrophic nails.
- Hepatosplenomegaly and moderate generalized lymphadenopathy.
- Osteochondritis and later periostitis especially of the long bones (may present as pseudoparalysis).
- Others (meningitis, nephrotic syndrome, choroidoretinitis, anaemia, thrombocytopenia).

Late congenital syphilis (after 2 years of age)

No clinical features in about 60% (diagnosed on serology). Otherwise many features are similar to accelerated late stage acquired syphilis (though the cardiovascular system is usually spared).

Inflammation

- Interstitial keratitis (most common late feature—20–50%).
- Deafness (2° to otolabyrinthitis).
- Clutton's joints (bilateral painless effusion of the knee joints).
- Gummata of nasal septum, palate and throat; skin and bone (as acquired syphilis).
- Neurosyphilis (seizures, mental deficiency, juvenile tabes dorsalis and general paralysis).
- Paroxysmal cold haemoglobinuria.

Malformations

- Craniofacial: frontal bossing; 'bulldog' appearance—hypoplastic maxilla, high arched palate and prominent mandible; 'saddle-nose'; circumoral rhagades.
- Dental:
  - Hutchinson's incisors (usually upper central)—conical, tapered towards the apex and notched. Hutchinson's triad ≈ Hutchinson's incisors, interstitial keratitis and nerve deafness.
  - Moon's (Mulberry) molars—1st lower molars dome shaped with hypoplastic cusps.
- Skeletal: bony sclerosis (generalized) or nodules (localized). Long bones primarily affected especially the tibia with anterior bowing ('sabre tibia').

Frequently asked questions

I am pregnant, is syphilis harmful to my baby?

Syphilis in pregnancy is associated with a high risk of spontaneous abortion, premature delivery, perinatal death, and congenital syphilis. Risks are greater in 1° and 2° syphilis. Despite treatment in early syphilis during pregnancy, up to 14% will have a fetal death or a baby with congenital syphilis.

Can I have passed it on to my children?

There is a high risk of congenital syphilis in offspring of ♀ with early syphilis during pregnancy, and may even occur when the syphilis is treated during pregnancy. Early congenital syphilis occurs within the first 2 years of life, late congenital manifestations occur after 2 years of age.

Diagnosis—regular investigations

Dark ground microscopy (see p. 61 for obtaining specimen)

Material

- 1° syphilis: serum from chancres (79–86% sensitivity)—less reliable for non-genital lesions, especially oral, because of other commensal treponemes.
- Aspiration of a regional lymph node (especially if the chancre is secondarily infected).
- 2° and early congenital syphilis: serum from mucous patches, ulcers, and condylomata lata.

Examination

- Treponemes are very slender with tight spirals moving forward and backward, rotating about longitudinal axis and angulating to ~90°.
- If negative and clinical suspicion repeat daily for 3 days.
- If 2° infection saline lavage or consider antibiotics inactive against *T. pallidum* to clear contaminants (e.g. co-trimoxazole, quinolones).

Serology (all stages—see Table 6.1)

Positive serology usually found ~4 weeks after infection but may take up to 3 months to develop. Negative in up to 15% of those with 1° chancre. Similar response with endemic treponematoses (see p. 224).

- *Non-specific*

Cardiolipin antigen tests (reagin): e.g. Venereal Disease Research Laboratory (VDRL) slide test, rapid plasma reagin test. Inexpensive, readily quantifiable (useful in assessing serial titres), biological false positives, poor sensitivity in late syphilis. Usually positive 4 weeks after infection. Prozone phenomenon (false negative results from strongly positive samples due to blocking antibodies) is excluded by specimen dilution.

- *Specific for anti-treponemal antibodies*
  - Agglutination: *T. pallidum* (TP) haemagglutination assay (TPHA) also known as MHA-TP (microhaemagglutination assay for TP) and TP particle agglutination (TPPA). Widely available for screening and confirmation.
  - Enzyme immunoassay (EIA): simple, can be automated, widely used for screening and confirmation.
  - Fluorescent treponemal antibody absorbed (FTA abs) test: historical confirmatory test.
  - Specific antitreponemal immunoglobulin M (IgM) detection (EIA or FTA abs): usually first serological response. Important in diagnosing early congenital syphilis.

Table 6.1 Syphilis—serological response

Stage	VDRL	TPPA/TPHA	EIA	IgM
1°	Positive (60–90%)	Positive (90–100%)	Positive (90%)	Positive
	Usual titre Neat—1:16	Usual titre; 80–320		
2°	Positive*	Positive	Positive	Positive
	Usual titre 1:32–1:256	High titres (about 5120)		
Early latent	Positive*	Positive	Positive	Usually positive
	Usual titre 1:16–1:64	Titres still usually high		
Late syphilis	Positive (50–65%)	Positive	Positive	Usually negative
	Usual titre Neat—1:16 but often high if active.	Low titres (80–640) unless active syphilis		
Old treated syphilis†	Usually negative or very low titre	Usually positive	Usually positive	Negative (unless recently treated early syphilis)
Congenital syphilis	The demonstration of IgM is important as it does not cross the placenta and usually represents active infection. May take up to 3 months to appear.			

* Excluding possible prozone phenomenon.
† Provided there has been initial seroconversion

Biological false positive reactions (cardiolipin tests) occur in <1% of the population

- Acute (disappear within 6 months)—usually <30 years of age
  - Acute febrile illnesses (e.g. infectious mononucleosis, viral hepatitis).
  - Vaccination.
  - Pregnancy.
- Chronic (persist beyond 6 months)—usually >30 years of age
  - Chronic infections (e.g. leprosy).
  - Autoimmune conditions (e.g. lupus erythematosis).
  - Drug addiction.

Diagnosis—additional investigations

Other direct diagnostic tests which may be available in early syphilis

- Direct fluorescent antibody stain (of acetone fixed smears).
- Polymerase chain reaction (95% sensitive, 99% specific for 1° syphilis and 80% sensitive, 99% specific for 2° syphilis).

Cerebrospinal fluid: suspected or increased risk of neurosyphilis (acquired and congenital)

- ↑ white cell count $>5\times10^6$/L
- ↑ protein >0.4g/L
- Positive treponemal antibody tests, especially cardiolipin.
- TPHA index >70.

TPHA index ≈ CSF TPHA titre ÷ albumin quotient (CSF albumin × 10^3 ÷ serum albumin)

Biopsy and histology

Important to exclude malignancy in suspected oral gummata.

X-ray

- Cardiovascular: aortic dilatation with linear 'egg shell' calcification.
- Tabes dorsalis: neuropathic joints (bone destruction and osteophyte formation).
- Bone gummata: osteomyelitic lesions sometimes hidden by reactive osteosclerosis; periosteal thickening.
- Early congenital: periostitis (new bone formation), metaphyseal calcification, dactylitis (spindle-shaped finger swelling).

Computerised tomography angiography

Cardiovascular syphilis (level of ventricular reflux).

Ophthalmic slit lamp examination

If eye pathology suspected.

Ultrasonography

For intrauterine congenital syphilis

- hepatomegaly
- splenomegaly
- placentomegaly
- scalp oedema
- polyhydramnios.

Syphilis management—early and late

Treatment principles

Optimal treponemal antibody sensitivity occurs during bacterial division (every 33 hours). Penicillin (1st line treatment) levels must be >0.018mg/L for 7–10 days (early syphilis) and 14–21 days (late syphilis). Desensitization should be considered as an option in those with penicillin allergy. Antibiotic free time or suboptimal levels should not exceed 24–30 hours.

Early syphilis

1st line

- Intra muscular (IM) procaine penicillin G 600–750mg daily for 10 days.
- Benzathine penicillin 2.4g IM once (USA—Centers for Disease Control (CDC) guidelines) or twice (UK guidelines), two doses a week apart.
- Oral doxycycline 100mg twice daily for 14 days.

2nd line

- IM ceftriaxone 500mg daily for 10 days (if no penicillin anaphylaxis).
- Oral erythromycin 500mg 4 times a day for 14 days (but less CSF and placental penetration than other treatments).
- Oral amoxicillin 500mg with oral probenecid 500mg each 4 times a day for 14 days.
- IV penicillin G, 6g every 6 hours until total dose is 54g.
- Oral azithromycin 500mg daily for 10 days. ▶ Resistant cases have been reported from the USA and Ireland.

▶ If neurological or ophthalmic involvement treat as for neurosyphilis.

Late latent, cardiovascular gummatous, and syphilis (neurosyphilis excluded)

- IM procaine penicillin G 600–750mg daily for 17 days.
- IM benzathine penicillin 2.4g weekly for 3 doses.
- Oral doxycycline 200mg twice daily for 28 days.

Neurosyphilis

Higher doses and longer duration of treatment recommended.

- IM procaine penicillin G 2g daily with oral probenecid 500mg 4 times a day for 17 days.
- Oral doxycycline 200mg twice daily for 28 days.
- Oral amoxicillin 2g 3 times a day with oral probenecid 500mg 4 times a day each for 28 days.
- IV/IM ceftriaxone—limited data but good CSF penetration.

Steroids are considered with antibiotics in the following situations

- Interstitial keratitis—0.1% betamethasone eye drops.
- Optic atrophy—oral prednisolone.
- Nerve deafness—oral prednisolone.
- Cardiovascular syphilis or neurosyphilis associated with optic neuritis—oral prednisolone 10–20mg 3 times a day for 3 days starting 1 day prior to antibiotics (to cover a possible Jarisch–Herxheimer reaction).

Jarisch–Herxheimer reaction

Non-specific acute febrile illness associated with the start of antibiotic treatment, especially 2° (about 75%) and 1° syphilis (about 50%), developing in 4 hours and resolving within 24 hours.
Features: myalgia, rigors/chills, flush/fever/hypotension/deterioration of clinical lesions (therapeutic paradox), then resolution.
Management: warn and reassure, bed rest, aspirin/paracetamol.
Special care required: optic neuritis, uveitis, nerve deafness (severe deterioration—see steroids), and pregnancy.

Syphilis management—review, partners, pregnancy, and congenital infection

Review

- Early syphilis: serological review monthly for 3 months, then at 6 months and 1 year.
- Late syphilis: serological review 6 monthly until cardiolipin antibody tests are serofixed.
- Neurosyphilis: 6 monthly CSF cell count until normal.

Consider re-infection or relapse if cardiolipin antibody titres ↑ 4-fold, fail to ↓ 4-fold if initially high (>1:32), or clinical evidence of infection.
If HIV co-infection maintain annual serological review for life.

Partner notification and contact management

- 1°: all sexual partners within previous 3 months.
- 2° and early latent: consider all sexual contacts within previous 2 years.

Maintain under serological review for 3 months from last sexual risk.

- Late syphilis: as index case is not sexually infectious at diagnosis an estimate of when the infection was acquired should be made (e.g. from previous negative serology) and contacts from within 2 years of this time notified.

Epidemiological treatment

Consider in contacts of early syphilis if full surveillance is impossible

- IM benzathine penicillin 2.4g (single dose).
- Oral doxycycline 100mg twice daily for 14 days.

Pregnancy

Penicillin in standard dosage. In early syphilis, Jarisch–Herxheimer reaction may cause uterine contractions, fetal distress, and preterm labour especially if the fetus is infected. Ultrasonography before treatment in late 2nd or 3rd trimester is advisable with hospitalization for fetal and maternal monitoring during the first 24 hours if the fetus has stigmata of congenital syphilis. If penicillin cannot be used then treat with erythromycin or azithromycin as detailed above but neonates should be treated at birth. Serological review of the mother after treatment should include repeat tests in the 3rd trimester and at term.

Child

Serology should be checked at birth, including IgM, which indicates neonatal infection as it cannot cross the placenta. Repeat 3 and 6 months after birth. Reagin tests should be negative at 6 months but passively transferred maternal anti-treponemal antibodies may persist for 15 months. A positive antibody test at 18 months indicates congenital syphilis. Neonatal treatment should be provided for those:

- with clinical or serological evidence of infection
- whose mother:
  - has untreated syphilis

- has possible re-infection or lacks serological evidence of response
- received late treatment (within 1 month of delivery)
- was not treated with penicillin.

Serology should be repeated every 2 to 3 months to ensure a satisfactory response to treatment (4-fold ↓ in reagin test titre).

Paediatric treatment regimens

- Intravenous benzyl penicillin 60–90mg (100,000–150,000U) per kg body weight daily in divided doses of 30mg (50,000U) 12 hourly for first 7 days, then 8 hourly for 10 days.
- IM procaine penicillin G 50mg (50,000U) per kg body weight daily for 10–14 days.
- If penicillin allergy, consider desensitization.

Co-infection with HIV

- Temporary ↓ of CD4 count and ↑ viral load and shedding with new syphilis infection.
- ↑ risk of HIV acquisition with infectious syphilis.
- Meningitis, meningovasculitis, and ocular disease more common if treponemal CNS infection although this, in itself, is not more likely.
- ↑ risk of ulcerating lesions in 2° syphilis.
- More rapid progression to gummatous syphilis.
- Syphilis serological response is usually normal but rarely atypical reactions arise.
- Treatment 💣
  - UK guidelines recommend daily procaine penicillin G as 1st line treatment for 17–21 days although they recognize benzathine penicillin regimens, providing follow-up is adequate. USA (CDC) guidelines recommend benzathine penicillin although they provide option of extending duration of treatment to weekly injections for 3 doses. 2nd line oral doxycycline and amoxicillin/probenecid are suboptimal, azithromycin unproven and erythromycin not recommended.
  - Follow-up after treatment should be for life.

Chapter 7

Gonorrhoea

Introduction

Gonorrhoea—literally 'flow of seed' as named by Galen, Greek physician, in 2nd century AD—has probably been known to be sexually transmitted for several millennia as shown by references in the Old Testament (Leviticus, chapter XV) and attribution of 'strangury' to 'pleasures of Venus' by Hippocrates.

Aetiology: *Neisseria gonorrhoeae*

A Gram-negative kidney shaped coccus of about 1μm in diameter; appears in pairs, diplococci, with concave aspects facing each other typically inside polymorphonuclear leucocytes (PMNLs). Fastidious growth requirements: temperature of 35–37°C, pH of 6.5–7.5, atmosphere of 5–7% carbon dioxide, and selective and enriched culture media (e.g. Thayer–Martin or Modified New York City) supplemented with iron, essential amino acids, glucose, and antimicrobials to inhibit other organisms

Humans are the only natural host. Primarily infects the columnar epithelium of lower genital tract, rectum, pharynx, and conjunctiva with transluminal spread to epididymis and prostate in ♂ and endometrium and pelvic organs in ♀ with occasional haematogenous dissemination.

Epidemiology and transmission

WHO estimates 62 million cases annually worldwide. In the UK the incidence peaked in the late 1960s and early 1970s. This was followed by a marked fall between 1985 and 1995 coinciding with the AIDS awareness campaign. However, since 1997 there has been a steady upward trend.

Highest incidence in the following: young people, urban dwellers, socio-economically deprived persons, migrants, and certain ethnic minorities. Rates of gonorrhoea are regarded as surrogate markers of unsafe sexual behaviour. An episode of gonorrhoea does not confer immunity as outer membrane proteins vary. Re-infection is common.

Closely associated with other STIs especially *Chlamydia trachomatis*, (up to 40% of ♀ and 25% of ♂ with gonorrhoea).

Sexual and non-sexual transmission

Anogenital and pharyngeal infections: almost exclusively sexually transmitted. Although recoverable from laboratory, suspensions left on surfaces, such as toilet seats for up to 24 hours, loses viability on drying and evidence of transmission from toilet seats is contentious. Fomite transmission is very unusual but anecdotal cases have been reported following the shared use of a portable male urinal and inflatable sex doll.

Adult conjunctivitis: often associated with anogenital infection due to autoinoculation but non-sexual transmission is possible as reported in sporadic epidemics and isolated cases attributed to poor hygiene, accidental inoculation or irrigation with urine (folk remedy). Flies have been implicated as vectors responsible for an outbreak in Australia.

Neonatal infection: vertical transmission due to exposure in birth canal following rupture of membranes.

Infectivity

- ♂ to ♀ infection after one episode of sex—60–80%. Risk reduced by about 40% by use of condom.
- ♀ to ♂ infection after one episode of sex—20%. Risk reduced by up to 75% by use of condom.
- Pharynx to urethra—26% of partners.
- Vertical transmission—up to 30%.

Spontaneous clearance

Pharyngeal infection—almost 100% in 12 weeks.
Anogenital and conjunctival infections—no data available.

Clinical features

Sites of infection

Commonly identifiable at several different sites

	Heterosexual ♂ (%)	Homosexual ♂ (%)	♀ (%)
Urethra	>90	60–70	65–75
Cervix	—	—	80–90
Pharynx ± other site(s)	3–10	10–30	5–15
Pharynx only	<5	10–15	<5
Rectum ± other site(s)	—	25–50	25–40
Rectum only	—	20–40	5

Male genital infection

Symptoms

- Incubation period: 5–8 days; range 1–14.
- Urethral discharge in 80% (typically profuse and yellow/green/white) and/or dysuria in 50%. May be scanty and mucoid initially but becomes profuse and purulent within 24 hours. Asymptomatic in 5–10%.

Signs

- Mucopurulent or purulent urethral discharge, typically profuse but if scanty can be elicited by urethral massage.
- Erythema of the urethral meatus sometimes with oedema.
- Urine 'threads'—plugs of pus from urethral (Littré's) glands in first passed 20mL urine indicating anterior urethritis.

Female genital infection

Symptoms

- Asymptomatic 50–70% (>50% are usually seen as contacts).
- Symptoms when present appear within 10 days of infection.
- ↑ vaginal discharge in up to 50% (often related to co-infection).
- Lower abdominal pain in up to 25%.
- Dysuria without frequency ~12%.
- Intermenstrual bleeding or menorrhagia (unusual).

Signs

- Commonly, no abnormal findings.
- Cervix: Mucopurulent discharge and easily induced bleeding (<50%).
- Pelvic/lower abdominal tenderness (<5%).

Extragenital infections in ♂ and ♀

Rectal infection

In homosexual ♂

In the UK ↓ between 1985–95 (following AIDS awareness campaign) but has since ↑. Usually asymptomatic (~90%) but may cause anal discharge, pain, discomfort or pruritus, and less frequently rectal bleeding, tenesmus, and constipation. Proctoscopy may show mucoid or purulent discharge, erythema, oedema, and friability.

In ♀

An estimated 10% (possibly more) may be due to anal sexual intercourse. The positive correlation with duration of cervical infection suggests tracking of infected material into the anal canal as the main cause. Usually asymptomatic but symptoms and signs as in ♂.

Pharyngeal infection

Asymptomatic in >90%. Occasional mild pharyngitis and/or cervical lymphadenopathy. Almost 100% spontaneous clearance within 12 weeks but significant association with disseminated gonococcal infection.

Conjunctival infection

Adult infection, which is uncommon, presents with purulent discharge and inflammation affecting one or both eyes. If untreated, complications such as keratitis and pan-ophthalmitis, can lead to blindness.

Prepubertal children

In girls the vulval and vaginal epithelium are vulnerable to infection. Although theoretically infection may be acquired accidentally from infected secretions especially with poor sanitation and hygiene, gonorrhoea is a strong indicator of sexual abuse. It usually presents as a purulent, oedematous vulvo-vaginitis.

Gonococcal urethritis in boys, or pharyngeal and rectal infection in both sexes, are almost always the result of sexual abuse.

Complications

In ♂

- Infection of the median raphe—linear erythematous swelling.
- Tysonitis—painful swelling of parafrenal gland.
- Meatal paraurethral gland abscess.
- Periurethral cellulitis and abscess—inflammation of Littré's glands with duct obstruction produces small cysts and abscesses causing tender swelling in fossa navicularis or bulb. Urine flow may be restricted. Painful erections ± ventral angulation if corpus spongiosum is affected.
- Urethral strictures and fistulae—sequelae of periurethral abscess in untreated infection.
- Cowperitis and abscess—Cowper's (bulbo-urethral) glands at the base of the prostate are affected causing fever, pain in perineum, particularly on defecation and urinary frequency or retention. Abscesses usually point to one side of the perineum or are palpable rectally.
- Prostatitis and seminal vesiculitis—acute features include: fever, malaise, perineal discomfort, tenesmus, suprapubic pain, urgency of micturition or retention, haematuria, and painful erections. A tender swollen prostate on rectal examination. Chronic prostatitis may develop.
- Epididymitis (<1%)— see p. 162.

In ♀

- Inflammation of paraurethral—Skene's—glands.
- Bartholinitis ± Bartholin's abscess: single or bilateral. Vulval pain and erythema with tender cystic swelling of the posterior half of labium majora. Pus may be seen or expressed from the duct orifice.
- Pelvic inflammatory disease (PID)—may occur in 10–20% of untreated infections. See p. 144.

Systemic

Perihepatitis (Fitz–Hugh Curtis syndrome)

Usually found in ♀ with associated PID, suggesting intra-abdominal spread, but also rarely reported in ♂ implicating lymphatic or haematogenous dissemination. See p. 147.

Disseminated gonococcal infection (DGI)

Occurs in <1% with mucosal infection.

- Host factors
  - 4 fold ↑ in ♀ (especially during or just after menstruation or in pregnancy particularly with pharyngeal infection).
  - Complement deficiency predisposing to recurrent episodes in <10% with DGI.
- Bacterial factors
  - Serogroup IA-1(WI).
  - Auxotype AHU$^-$ (arginine, hypoxanthine, and uracil dependent).
  - Complement resistance.
  - Penicillin sensitivity and vancomycin susceptibility but these vary over time and penicillin resistant strains now play a significant role.

Clinical features

The preceding mucosal infection tends to be asymptomatic. Usual presentation: mild fever, skin rash, and arthralgia ± arthritis.

- Skin (gonococcal dermatitis) in 67%—initial macules develop into papules, vesicles with petechiae then into typical necrotic pustules surrounded by erythema. Usually at extremities (especially hands).
- Skeletal—tenosynovitis (in ~33%) producing migratory arthralgia mostly wrists, fingers, toes, and ankles. Arthritis (single joint), in ~50%, with effusion typically involving the knee, wrist, or metacarpo-phalangeal joints.
- Other sites (rare)
  - Heart—endocarditis in 1–3% leading to aortic incompetence and cardiac failure. Also pericarditis and myocarditis.
  - Hepatitis.
  - Meningitis, similar to meningococcal (very rare).

Pregnancy and the neonate

In pregnancy the proportion of pharyngeal infection is ↑ by 15–35%, presumably due to ↑ in oral sex. Genital infection is less likely to be complicated by PID (because of thickening of cervical mucus) but cases of salpingitis have been reported in the 1st trimester.

Adverse pregnancy outcomes

- Infection of chorio-amnion can cause septic abortion but there is no consistent evidence for an ↑ risk.
- Preterm delivery and low birth weight ↑ by 3- to 6-fold.
- Premature rupture of membrane (PROM) is more frequent.
- Postpartum/intrapartum or postabortal endometritis and pyrexia illness are ↑ (3-fold) and occur in ~42% with gonorrhoea.
- Some studies suggest that risk of DGI is ↑, reflecting ↑ pharyngeal infection.

Screening in pregnancy advisable in PROM, septic abortion, intra/postpartum fever or those considered to be at risk.

Neonatal gonococcal infection

Occurs because of exposure in birth canal during labour.

Gonococcal ophthalmia neonatorum

A notifiable disease in the UK, defined as conjunctivitis with a purulent discharge in an infant arising within 21 days of birth. Occurs in 30–40% of those exposed with ↑ risk if PROM or preterm delivery. Typically develops within 2–5 days of delivery and presents with oedema of the conjunctiva and eyelids with profuse discharge. Without treatment infection may extend to sub-conjunctival connective tissue and the cornea leading to ulceration. If ulcers perforate anterior synechiae formation or panophthalmitis may follow, which can result in blindness.

The rate of infection in at-risk infants is ↓ to 2–5% by prophylaxis (1% silver nitrate solution—'Crede prophylaxis'; 1% tetracycline or 0.5% erythromycin ointment) applied to the eyes soon after birth.

Gonococcal arthritis

Associated with vulvo-vaginitis, proctitis, or ophthalmia neonatorum.

Usually polyarticular presenting as pseudoparalysis. Rarely progressive. Skin lesions not usual.

Scalp abscess

Follows trauma to scalp e.g. with intrauterine fetal monitoring.

Other neonatal gonococcal infection

- Pharyngeal infection in ~33% with ophthalmia neonatorum. Rhinitis may be associated.
- Vaginitis, urethritis, and anorectal infection.
- Neonatal sepsis without arthritis particularly in preterm infants. *N. gonorrhoeae* is recoverable from nasogastric aspirate or blood. Rarely complicated by meningitis.

Frequently asked questions

How long can I have had gonorrhoea for?

In ♂ urethral symptoms usually appear within 10 days of exposure to gonorrhoea although 5–10% are asymptomatic when diagnosed. Symptoms are much less common with rectal and throat infection. Up to 70% of ♀ diagnosed with gonorrhoea are asymptomatic. Therefore although most people are probably diagnosed shortly after being infected it is possible that it may have been present for weeks or months.

Can it be cured?

Yes, gonorrhoea can be cured by antibiotics. When swabs are taken for gonorrhoea culture, the laboratory also tests for antibiotic sensitivities, so that the appropriate antibiotic is identified. It is recommended that, while awaiting these results, an antibiotic be used to which >95% of the local stains of *N. gonorrhoeae* are sensitive.

Will it have done any damage?

In ♀: PID may occur in 10–20% of untreated cases of gonorrhoea. Infertility may occur as a result of PID.

In ♂: urethral strictures and fistulae are sequelae of periurethral abscesses in untreated gonorrhoea and it may also cause epididymitis.

Do I need a test of cure?

No. Although this was a recommended practice, audit studies have shown that it is unnecessary, provided that the isolate is fully sensitive to the antibiotic administered, the patient has taken all of their medication correctly and has not been re-exposed to the infection.

Can I have caught this from a toilet seat?

Not normally. However in pre-pubertal girls the vulvo-vaginal skin is vulnerable to *N. gonorrhoeae* and a report has alleged acquisition of gonorrhoea from a dirty toilet seat in an aeroplane by an 8-year-old girl.

I'm pregnant, can it harm my baby?

There is a risk of neonatal infection due to exposure in the birth canal during labour. Gonococcal ophthalmia neonatorum is acquired by 30–40% of infants exposed to *N. gonorrhoeae.*

Without treatment there are ↑ risks of preterm delivery, low birth weight, premature rupture of membranes, and postpartum/post-abortion endometritis.

Diagnosis

Screening

- Genital—♂ urethra, ♀ cervix and urethra.
- Pharynx—all homosexual ♂ and heterosexuals with symptoms of gonorrhoea elsewhere or history of contact.
- Rectum—all homosexual ♂ (advised as ~20% with rectal infection deny receptive anal intercourse) and ♀ with symptoms, gonorrhoea elsewhere or history of contact

►Sensitivity of cervical culture alone is 75–85%. A single set of tests from the urethra, cervix, rectum, and pharynx ↑ this to >95%.

- Conjunctivitis: include potential 1° infection sites.
- DGI
  - from potential 1° infection sites;
  - material from skin lesions and joint aspirate;
  - blood culture.

Culture of joint fluid and skin lesions is insensitive therefore nucleic acid amplification test (NAAT) is recommended.

Microscopy

Microscopy (1000x) of Gram-stained genital specimens shows *N. gonorrhoeae* as Gram-negative diplococci within PMNLs (Plate 6). Smear sensitivity (compared with culture):

- in ♂: urethra 90–95% (symptomatic) and 50–75% (asymptomatic);
- in ♀: cervix 23–65% and urethra 20%;
- rectum: blind swab 40%; using proctoscope 70–80%.

Microscopy is not appropriate for pharyngeal specimens as other Neisserial commensals are commonly seen. Conjunctival specimens are suitable for Gram-staining and microscopy.

Laboratory detection of *N. gonorrhoeae*

Culture—isolation and identification of N. gonorrhoeae

Dependent on good specimen collection and efficient transport to the laboratory. ► Caution with lubricants during examination, as they may inhibit the growth of *N. gonorrhoeae*.

Specimens for culture may be:

- directly inoculated onto culture medium and incubated;
- transported in a non-nutrient medium (e.g. Amies, Stuart), or a carbon dioxide producing culture medium.

Transport media should be kept at ≤4°C after inoculation (check product information or with local laboratory). Provided that the material in transport medium is processed within 48 hours, there is only ~5% loss in sensitivity compared with direct inoculation.

The culture medium is examined at 24 and 48 hours for growth. Presumptive identification is by positive cytochrome oxidase reaction and microscopy. Definitive identification by a combination of further tests, e.g. carbohydrate utilization (*N. gonorrhoeae* utilizes glucose only), monoclonal antibody test (e.g. Phadebact), and enzyme substrate degradation.

Molecular detection

NAATs are ~100% sensitive for genital, rectal, and pharyngeal specimens compared directly with culture (75–85% endocervix, <60% rectum, <50% pharynx) but cannot identify antibiotic sensitivities. They are suitable for urine and vulval samples but are unlicensed for rectal and pharyngeal specimens. False positive reactions may ↓ positive predictive value to <90%.

Typing

Serotyping, auxotyping, opa-typing, and plasmid analysis are not applicable to routine clinical practice but are useful in monitoring the epidemiology of the infection and the identification of transmission chains.

Antibiotic sensitivity

Identifies appropriate treatment. Sensitivity predicts success in >95% with intermediate sensitivity suggesting failure in 5–15% although ↑ dosage may be effective. Resistance may be due to plasmids (circular DNA fragments independent of chromosome) or chromosomal mutations.

Management

► Advise avoidance of sexual intercourse until the patient and partner(s) have completed treatment and resolution has been established. Screen for *C. trachomatis* using a sensitive assay (NAAT) or provide epidemiological treatment. Treatment before antibiotic sensitivity is known should be with an antibiotic to which >95% of local strains are sensitive.

Uncomplicated genital and rectal infections (All single doses)

- Recommended
  - Ceftriaxone 250mg intramuscularly (IM)
  - Cefixime 400mg oral
  - Spectinomycin 2g IM.
- Alternative (if regional prevalence of resistance <5%)
  - Ciprofloxacin 500mg oral
  - Ofloxacin 400mg oral
  - Ampicillin 2g or 3g plus probenecid 1g oral.

Complicated genital infection (See p. 150, p. 168)

Pharyngeal infection (All single doses)

- Ceftriaxone 250mg IM
- Ciprofloxacin 500mg oral
- Ofloxacin 400mg oral.

Pregnancy and breastfeeding (All single doses)

Quinolone and tetracycline antimicrobials are contraindicated.

- Ceftriaxone 250mg IM
- Cefotaxime 500mg IM
- Ampicillin 2g or 3g plus probenecid 1g oral (providing local prevalence of penicillin resistant *N. gonorrhoeae* <5%);
- Spectinomycin 2g IM.

Adult gonococcal conjunctivitis

Ceftriaxone 1g IM as a single dose (limited evidence-base).

Disseminated gonococcal infection

Hospital admission is recommended. Assess for endocarditis/meningitis.

- A parenteral antibiotic is necessary initially. Examples:
  - Ceftriaxone or cefotaxime or ceftizoxime 1g IM 8 hourly
  - Ciprofloxacin or ofloxacin 400mg IV 12 hourly
  - Spectinomycin 2g IM 12 hourly.
- The parenteral antibiotic should be continued for 24–48 hours until improvement, and then replaced with oral cefixime 400mg, ciprofloxacin 500mg, or ofloxacin 400mg twice daily for 7 days.

Other situations

- Gonococcal meningitis and endocarditis: Intravenous antibiotic for at least 2 and 4 weeks, respectively.
- Ophthalmia neonatorum: Single dose of ceftriaxone 25–50mg/kg up to a maximum of 125mg.
- Neonatal sepsis, scalp abscess, meningitis, and arthritis: ceftriaxone 25–50mg/kg daily IV or IM for 7–14 days.
- Neonatal prophylaxis: If mother is not treated before delivery a single dose of ceftriaxone 25–50mg/kg to a maximum of 125mg.
- Prepubertal infection
  - Weight >45kg—adult regimens.
  - Weight <45kg—ceftriaxone 125mg IM (single dose).

Partner notification

Partner notification is essential. Contact tracing period:

- ♂ symptomatic urethral infection—2 weeks prior to onset of symptoms or until last sexual partner, if longer.
- other—3 months prior to diagnosis or until the last sexual partner.

Epidemiological treatment and, ideally, screening should be offered to sexual partners. Similar principles should apply to the mother of a neonate with gonococcal infection and her sex partner/s.

Follow-up

Tests of cure are unnecessary, provided the isolate is sensitive to the antibiotic prescribed and the patient has adhered fully to the treatment and advice provided. If required, culture should be delayed for at least 72 hours and NAAT at least 2 weeks after treatment.

HIV infection

Gonorrhoea facilitates HIV transmission, producing ↑ in detectable virus in genital secretions; this is reversed following antibiotic treatment.

Chapter 8

Chlamydia trachomatis infections

Introduction

Although recognized since antiquity (e.g. description of trachoma in Egyptian papyri) the discovery of *Chlamydia trachomatis* as a cause of genital tract and ocular infections was only made in the early part of the 20th century.

Aetiology

C. trachomatis is a bacterial species within the genus *Chlamydia* (Table 8.1). Divided into four biovars—lymphogranuloma venereum (LGV), trachoma, murine, and swine—subdivided into several serovars based on the major outer membrane protein (MOMP) antigens. Serovars D to K of the trachoma biovar are sexually transmissible and 'chlamydial infection' commonly refers to infection with this group. Genotyping based on MOMP genes increasingly refines classification of the species and is a useful research tool.

An obligate intracellular pathogen depending entirely on host cell adenosine triphosphate for its energy. Two distinct structures appear during its life cycle of 48–72 hours:

- elementary body (0.35µm). Infectious form, attaches to and enters host cells (columnar and pseudostratified columnar), transforming after 6–9 hours into a:
- reticulate body (1µm). Non-infective replicative phase within intracellular vacuoles (endosomes). These fuse into an inclusion where reticulate bodies multiply for 24–48 hours. Maturation back into elementary bodies is followed by their release.

Epidemiology and transmission

The World Health Organization estimated the annual worldwide incidence of new infections to be 92 million in 1999. Genital chlamydial infection is the most common STI in the UK with the highest incidence amongst ♀ in the 16–19 age group and ♂ aged 20–24. Factors associated with ↑ prevalence of chlamydial infection include being unmarried, ↑ number of sexual partners, ethnic minority status, inconsistent, or non use of barrier methods of contraception and use of oral contraceptive pill. Prevalence of the infection in various settings is shown in Table 8.2.

- Transmissibility of the infection after a single act of unprotected penetrative sexual intercourse is estimated to be ~10% for both sexes. Correct use of condoms reduces the risk by ~40%.
- Spontaneous bacterial clearance is estimated to occur in ~20–28% within 3 months and 50% by 15 months. Persistence for up to 6 years has been reported and is believed to be longer in ♀ than ♂.

Table 8.1 *C. trachomatis* and related species

Species	Biovar	Serovar	Natural host	Human disease
C. pecorum	—	Multiple	Sheep, cattle, swine	None
C. psittaci	—	Multiple	Birds, lower mammals	Psittacoss
C. pneumoniae	—	TWAR	Human	Respiratory disease
C. trachomatis	LGV	L1, L2, L3	Human (infects macrophages)	Lymphogranuloma venereum
	Trachoma	A, B, Ba, C	Human	Hyperendemic trachoma
		D–K	Human (infects squamocolumnar cells)	Conjunctivitis, non-gonococcal urethritis, cervicitis, salpingitis, proctitis, epidydymitis, pneumonia of newborn
	Murine	—	Mouse	None
	Swine	—	Swine	None

Table 8.2 Mean prevalence of chlamydial infection in ♀ in different settings*

Survey population	Prevalence %				
	Overall	**<20 years**	**20–24 years**	**25–29 years**	**>30 years**
General population	1.6	3.8	2.7	2.2	0.9
General Practice	7.1	8.6	5.9	2.9	1.1
Family planning	8.1	10	7.4	3.8	1.5
Ante-natal clinic	8.5	13.5	6.5	7.2	0.1
Termination service	8.5	13.5	9.7	2	1.2
Youth clinic	12.2	12.3	10	—	—
GUM clinic	12.7	17.3	12.4	4.9	5.1

* UK data based on a meta-analysis published in 2004.

Source: Table 4, p. 360 of E J Adams, A Charlett, W J Edmunds, and G Hughes (2004). *Chlamydia trachomatis* in the United Kingdom: a systematic review and analysis of prevalence studies. *Sex Transm Infect.* **80**(5): 354–62. Reproduced with permission from the BMJ Publishing Group.

Clinical features

Sites of infection

- ♂: Urethra [35–50% of non-gonococcal urethritis (NGU)]; epididymis; prostate (inconclusive evidence).
- ♀: Cervix (75–85%); Urethra (50–60% overall, 15–20% urethra only); Bartholin's gland; endometrium; fallopian tubes; vagina if prepubertal.
- ♂ and ♀ : Conjunctiva; rectum (8–10% in homosexual ♂); pharynx (1–2%); hepatic capsule; synovium; rarely endocardium and meninges.

Male genital infection

Symptoms

- Incubation period: 7–21 days.
- Urethral discharge and/or dysuria in ~50%. Remainder asymptomatic.

Signs

~60% of ♂ have signs.

- Usually mild to moderate opaque or clear urethral discharge.
- Sometimes oedema and erythema of the urethral meatus.
- Often urine 'threads'—plugs of pus from urethral (Littré's) glands in first passed 20mL urine indicating anterior urethritis.

Female genital infection

Symptoms

- Asymptomatic in up to 80%.
- Symptoms include
  - Increased vaginal discharge
  - Dysuria without frequency
  - Intermenstrual bleeding and/or menorrhagia
  - Postcoital bleeding
  - Low abdominal pain.

Signs

- Usually no abnormal findings.
- Cervix: Mucopurulent cervicitis (MPC)—mucopurulent discharge and/or oedema, congestion and friability (easily induced bleeding), present in about a third including those asymptomatic.
- Incidental finding on colposcopy of 'cobblestone' appearance of the cervix due to raised lymphoid follicles.
- Cervical ectopy is positively correlated with chlamydial infection.

Extragenital infections in ♂ and ♀

Rectal infection

In homosexual ♂

- Attending GUM clinics:
  - up to 15% of those with proctitis (consider also LGV—see p. 218)
  - up to 10% on routine screening (67% without urethral infection).
- Usually asymptomatic (>60%) but may cause anal discharge, pain, discomfort, or pruritus, and less frequently rectal bleeding, severe anal pain, tenesmus, and constipation with overt proctitis.

- Occasionally external anal erythema or discharge. Proctoscopy may show mucoid or purulent discharge, erythema, oedema, or friability in those who are symptomatic.
- 'Cobblestone' appearance if magnified with a colposcope.

In ♀

- Attending GUM clinics—up to 5% (may occur without urogenital infection).
- Usually asymptomatic but symptoms and signs as with ♂.

Pharyngeal infection

- Limited data—♂ (including homosexual) <1% and ♀ <3%.
- Usually asymptomatic but mild pharyngeal symptoms may be reported.

Conjunctival infection

- Concomitant anogenital infection in 60–70%.
- Partners: ~50% ♀ and ~80% ♂ have chlamydial or non-specific genital infection.

Unilateral or bilateral follicular conjunctivitis presenting 1–2 weeks after exposure with conjunctival irritation, discharge ± photophobia/periorbital pain. Signs include conjunctival injection ± chemosis and ulceration ('Herber's pits') in severe cases and hyperaemia with follicles ½–1mm in diameter ± palpebral conjunctival oedema. May result in conjunctival scarring. Epithelial keratitis (unusual) does not lead to corneal scarring.

Prepubertal children

In girls the vulval and vaginal epithelium are vulnerable to infection. Urethral, pharyngeal, and rectal infections may also occur. Prepubertal infection is a strong indicator of sexual abuse. ► However, perinatal *C. trachomatis* infection may persist for at least three years following delivery.

Complications

Local

In ♂

- Prostatitis and seminal vesiculitis—the role of chlamydial infection is not well established.
- Epididymitis—(see p. 162).

In ♀

- Bartholinitis ± Bartholin's abscess—one or both sides. Pain in vulva with tender cystic swelling of the posterior half of labia majora with erythema; pus may exude or be expressed from the duct orifice.
- Endometritis—may cause irregular vaginal bleeding.
- Pelvic inflammatory disease (PID) and sequlae—may occur in about 10–30% of untreated infections.
- Cervical neoplasia—epidemiological studies show a correlation with previous chlamydial infection.

Systemic

- Perihepatitis (Fitz–Hugh Curtis syndrome)—usually found in ♀ with associated PID suggesting intra-abdominal spread but also rarely reported in ♂ implicating lymphatic or haematogenous dissemination.
- Sexually acquired reactive arthritis (SARA) or Reiter's syndrome—polyarthritis affecting mostly weight bearing joints usually preceded by urethritis and conjunctivitis in <1% of chlamydial infections.

Pregnancy and the neonate

The infection rate in pregnancy varies between 2–30%. Genital infection is less likely to be complicated by PID (because of thick cervical mucus) but cases of salpingitis have been reported in the first trimester.

Adverse pregnancy outcomes of untreated chlamydial infection

- Chlamydial infection in pregnancy may be associated with preterm delivery and low birth weight.
- Premature rupture of membrane (PROM) more frequent.
- *C. trachomatis* has been isolated from amniotic fluid.
- Intrapartum pyrexia and late postpartum endometritis ↑ by 20–25%.
- Postabortal PID.

Neonatal chlamydial infection

Occurs because of exposure in birth canal during labour.

- Chlamydial ophthalmia neonatorum
  - 30–50% of exposed infants acquire chlamydial conjunctivitis, ↓ to 1–2% if mother treated before delivery.
  - Incubation period 5–14 days (from delivery or PROM) but can be up to 2 months.
  - Conjunctivitis—mild (scant mucoid discharge) to severe (profuse discharge). Bilateral involvement in 67%. Corneal scarring rare.

- Respiratory tract infection
  - The nasopharynx is the most frequent site of neonatal infection (70–80% of infected infants) where it is usually asymptomatic.
  - 30% with nasopharyngeal infection develop apyrexial pneumonia at 4–12 weeks of age with cough, tachypnoea, and crepitations on auscultation. Apnoeic episodes may occur. Long term outcome includes impaired lung function and obstructive pulmonary disease.
  - Investigations show hyperinflation on radiography, peripheral eosinophilia, and ↑ serum immunoglobulins.
- Others
  - Otitis media—complicating nasopharyngeal infection, may become chronic if not treated early.
  - Vaginal and rectal infection—in 10–15% of exposed infants. Usually asymptomatic and may persist for at least 3 years.

Frequently asked questions

How long could I have had chlamydia for?

Up to 80% of ♀ and 50% of ♂ infected with chlamydia are asymptomatic. It is therefore possible to be infected for months and in some cases years before it is diagnosed.

Could I have caught if from a toilet seat?

No. There is no evidence for this.

Does my partner need to be seen?

Yes there is a very high chance of infection. Screening for STIs is recommended and treatment to cover chlamydial infection should be taken.

Although my partner has not been treated since I finished my treatment we have been using condoms. This is OK, isn't it?

No. Condoms only reduce the risk of infection, not eliminate it. Your partner needs treatment and you need to be retreated.

How have I caught chlamydia when my only ever partner has tested negative?

Although now very reliable, tests for chlamydia are not 100% sensitive and therefore infection may be missed, especially if EIAs are used. In addition your partner may have received antibiotics for something else or the infection may have cleared spontaneously. Despite conflicting results in a partnership we recommend that both are treated.

Will it have affected my fertility?

Chlamydial infection is extremely common and it does not appear to impair fertility in most people who are treated properly. Untreated chlamydia can lead to PID either symptomatic or silent episodes which is associated with infertility.

Can you test my fertility?

Fertility is not assessed at a GUM clinic. 90% of couples will conceive within 12 months of trying with regular intercourse. Couples who do not conceive within 12 months may undergo infertility investigations. If a ♀ has a history of chlamydia and/or PID she may be offered investigations to check her fallopian tubes.

Diagnosis

Investigations

1° analysis—initial investigations in the clinic

Anogenital specimens

Light microscopy (1000x) of Gram-stained smears does not show *C. trachomatis* but can demonstrate polymorphonuclear leucocytes (PMNL) which may indicate chlamydial infection in the appropriate clinical context.

- Urethral in ♂: ≥5 PMNL/high power field (HPF) in the absence of Gram-negative intracellular diplococci = NGU.
- Cervical: ≥30 PMNL/HPF suggests cervicitis.
- Rectal: ≥1 PMNL/HPF suggests proctitis.

Urine

- ≥10 PMNL/HPF in threads from the first voided urine (FVU) in ♂.
- Sterile pyuria may be due to *C. trachomatis* infection.

Laboratory detection of *C. trachomatis*

DNA assays—nucleic acid amplification tests (NAAT) and DNA probe—are recommended as they are more accurate than cell culture or antigen detection.

Cell culture

100% specificity therefore still essential for medico-legal cases. Sensitivity ~70%. Vulnerable to invalidation by toxins in specimens. Suitable for genital and extragenital swabs but not urine. Should be maintained at 4°C and received by the laboratory within 24 hours.

Enzyme linked immunosorbent assay (EIA)

Several commercial assays available. High specificity (>95%) when combined with confirmatory test e.g. blocking antibody. Sensitivity (variable between assays) 15–94% on urine sample (less for ♀) and 60–85% for other specimens. Inexpensive—automation permits mass testing. Unsuitable for rectal swabs (interference by normal flora). Should be received by the laboratory in 3–5 days and preferably maintained at 4°C.

Direct fluorescent antibody (DFA)

Specificity 82–99% (observer dependent), sensitivity 68–100%. Unsuitable for large numbers (labour intensive). Suitable for all specimen sites. Swab rolled onto a slide and fixed. No special transport conditions.

Nucleic acid amplification tests (NAAT)

Amplification of:

- plasmid DNA, MOMP1, or ribosomal RNA genes—polymerase chain reaction (PCR).
- plasmid DNA + probe—ligase chain reaction (LCR). No longer available.
- RNA and hybridization with a labelled DNA probe—transcription mediated amplification (TMA).
- plasmid DNA—strand displacement amplification (SDA).
- MOMP1 RNA—nucleic acid sequence based amplification assay (NASBA).

High specificity (98–100%) and sensitivity e.g. LCR, PCR, and TMA with urine >95%, >85%, and 92%; cervical swabs >88%, >95%, and >92% respectively. Other NAATs have similar sensitivities. Suitable for any site including self-collected vulval and tampon samples. Not yet acceptable for medico-legal diagnosis. Currently unlicensed and non-validated for anorectal and oropharyngeal specimens. If delays >24 hours are anticipated storage at 4°C is recommended to avoid sample degradation. Manufacturers' instructions should be followed.

DNA probe

- Probe Assay Chemiluminescence Enhanced (PACE®).
- Hybrid Capture II.

Similar to cell culture in sensitivity and rarely used.

Chlamydial antibody in serum

While complicated infections (PID, epidydymitis) elicit strong antibody responses most mucosal infections do not. Microimmunoflourescent assay necessary to identify species specific antibody. Only useful in retrospective diagnosis. IgG titre of >1:64 may indicate a recent episode but does not exclude past infection. IgA may indicate active infection. IgM is useful in the diagnosis of neonatal pneumonia.

Frequently asked questions

I'm pregnant can it harm my baby?

Chlamydia in pregnancy is associated with ↑ risk of preterm delivery and low birth weight. Premature rupture of membranes is more frequent, as is intrapartum pyrexia, postpartum endometritis and postabortal PID.

Neonatal chlamydia infection is due to exposure in the birth canal during labour. 30–50% of exposed infants will develop chlamydia ophthalmic neonatorum. Treatment of the mother for chlamydia prior to delivery is associated with a decrease in incidence to 1–2%. There is a risk of respiratory tract infection in the neonate after birth canal exposure.

Do I need a test of cure?

Routine test of cure is not necessary following standard, 1st line treatment e.g. doxycycline 100mg twice daily for 7 days or azithromycin 1g single dose. If a ♀ has been treated with erythromycin, (usually in pregnancy when doxycycline is contraindicated), a test of cure is recommended 3 weeks after completion of therapy.

Management

▶Advise avoidance of sexual intercourse including with condoms until the patient and partner(s) have completed treatment and symptoms have resolved.

Uncomplicated genital and rectal infections

Recommended treatment regimens

- Doxycycline 100mg twice daily for 7 days
- Azithromycin 1g as a single dose.

Alternative regimens

- Tetracyclines
  - Deteclo 300mg twice daily for 7 days
  - Tetracycline 500mg 4 times a day for 7 days (compliance problem)
  - Minocycline 100mg once daily for 7 days.
- Macrolides
  - Erythromycin 500mg twice daily for 14 days or 500mg 4 times a day for 7 days (↑ side-effects with the latter)
  - Clarithromycin 400mg twice daily for 7 days.
- Fluroquinolones
  - Ofloxacin 200mg twice daily or 400mg once daily for 7 days
  - Levofloxacin 500mg once daily for 7 days.
- Penicillins
  - Amoxicillin—used in pregnancy (see section, Pregnancy and breastfeeding)
  - Pivampicillin 700mg twice daily for 7 days (limited evidence).
- Other antibiotics (limited efficacy or applicability)
  - Co-trimoxazole (trimethoprim 160mg + sulfamethoxazole 800mg) 1 tablet twice daily for 14 days
  - Rifampicin (rifampin) 600mg once daily for 6 days.

Complicated genital infection (See p. 150, p. 168)

Pregnancy and breastfeeding

- Erythromycin 500mg daily for 14 days or 500mg 4 times a day for 7 days.
- Amoxicillin 500mg three times day for 7 days (better tolerated than erythromycin).
- Azithromycin 1g as a single dose—restricted licence in pregnancy but available data indicate no teratogenicity or adverse pregnancy outcomes.

❶ Tetracyclines, fluroquinolones, and co-trimoxazole are contraindicated in pregnancy.

Other situations

- Adult chlamydial conjunctivitis: Treatment as for genital infection i.e. systemic treatment required.
- Ophthalmia neonatorum and infant pneumonia
  - Erythromycin 50mg/kg/day oral divided into 4 doses daily for 14 days.

- Neonatal prophylaxis: Silver nitrate drops and erythromycin and tetracycline ointments are ineffective and infants born of mothers with untreated chlamydial infection should be monitored carefully for signs of conjunctivitis. Swabs should be taken for *C. trachomatis* from everted eyelids 5–10 days after birth.
- Prepubertal infection
  - Erythromycin 50mg/kg/day (up to 1g) divided into 4 doses for 14 days

  Alternative treatments
  - Age ≥8 years—doxycycline 100mg twice daily for 7 days
  - Weight >45kg—azithromycin 1g as a single dose.

Partner notification

Partner notification is essential. Contact tracing period:

- Symptomatic ♂—4 weeks prior to onset of symptoms or until last sexual partner.
- ♀ and asymptomatic ♂—6 months prior to presentation or until the last sexual partner.

Similar principles should apply to the mother of a neonate with chlamydial infection and her sex partner/s.

Follow-up

Need not necessarily be through re-attendance at the clinic. The objectives of follow-up are to assess management compliance, resolution of any symptoms and partner notification. A test of cure is only recommended if not treated with doxycycline or azithromycin or symptoms persist. Repeat treatment if risk of re-infection with untreated partner.

NAAT testing, if required, should be delayed until at least 3 weeks after the end of the treatment.

HIV infection

Chlamydial infection facilitates HIV transmission, producing ↑ in detectable virus in urethral/cervical secretions when infection is present; this is reversed following antibiotic treatment.

Chapter 9

Non-chlamydial non-specific genital infection

Introduction

Non-specific genital infection (NSGI) refers to ♂ urethritis in the absence of gonorrhoea (non-gonococcal or non-specific urethritis—NGU or NSU) and the equivalent but less well-defined condition in ♀, mucopurulent cervicitis (MPC). *Chlamydia trachomatis* is the cause in 30–50% of NGU and 25–45% of MPC. Non-chlamydial NSGI has been attributed to several causes supported by variable evidence.

Aetiology

Non-chlamydial NGU

Microorganisms

- *Mycoplasma genitalium*—up to 20% of NGU.
- *Ureaplasma urealyticum*—association with non-chlamydial NGU in up to 52% (similar prevalence in the absence of NGU). Serovar 4 more likely to play a role in NGU.
- Bacterial vaginosis (BV)—30% of ♂ with NGU have ♀ partners with BV which may be implicated in an undetermined proportion.
- Bacteria causing urinary tract infections (UTIs)—up to 6% of NGU seen in GUM clinic is due to UTI. Coliform bacteria may be associated with NGU in ♂ practising insertive anal sex.
- *Trichomonas vaginalis*—up to 15% of NGU in high prevalence areas.
- Herpes simplex virus (HSV)—up to 2% of NGU without external genital ulcers. 30% of primary genital HSV episodes in ♂ include NGU.
- Adenovirus—types 8, 19, and 37 (subgenus D) isolated from 0.4% of ♂ attending GUM clinics. 75% of isolates associated with NGU, often with conjunctivitis, pharyngitis, and constitutional symptoms. Transmission probably by oral sex.

The following organisms show a possible or occasional causal role:

- *Neisseria meningitidis*
- *Candida* species (rarely). If present usually associated with balanitis (possible reaction to partner's candidal infection)
- *Haemophilus influenzae and parainfluenzae*
- *Staphylococcus saprophyticus*
- *Corynebacterium genitalium*
- *Bacteroides urealyticus*
- *Mycobacterium tuberculosis.*

Non-microbial

- Congenital anomalies e.g. urethral stricture
- Physical irritation—trauma related to sex, manipulation or foreign body e.g. urinary catheter
- Chemical irritation
- Reactive urethritis e.g. reactive arthritis, allergens
- Stevens–Johnson syndrome.

Non-gonococcal, non-chlamydial MPC

- *M. genitalium* implicated in up to 10%.
- HSV infection.
- Possibly other as yet unidentified causes.

Mycoplasma genitalium

- A bacterium:
  - discovered in 1980 in the urethra of 2 ♂ with NGU
  - classified as belonging to the family Mycoplasmateles
  - 1 of 14 mycoplasmas of human origin
  - long flask shape with a narrow, terminal rod binding to eukaryotic cells
  - fastidious and slow growing (difficult to isolate)
  - forms fried egg-like colonies within agar medium incubated in nitrogen and 5% carbon dioxide
  - genome—580kb, smallest of any self-replicating bacterium.
- Urogenital tract—preferred site of colonization where it may invade epithelial cells.
- Sexual transmission—causal role in NGU/MPC and possibly pelvic inflammatory disease (PID)/epididymitis. Identified in:
  - 18–45% of non-chlamydial NGU
  - up to 10% of MPC
  - 16% of endometritis.
- Sensitive to tetracyclines (except when the *tetM* gene is present), macrolides, ketolides, and flouroquinolones and resistant to penicillins, sulfonamides, and rifampicin. Antibiotics only suppress growth and a competent immune system is necessary for eradication.

Clinical features

Male—NGU

Symptoms	Signs
• Urethral discharge • Dysuria • Penile irritation • None (asymptomatic)	• Urethral discharge—varying amounts, clear to yellow, spontaneous, or expressed • None (subclinical)

Up to 20% of ♂ with observable discharge have no symptoms. NGU without symptoms and signs (in ~25%) is less likely to be due to *C. trachomatis* or *M. genitalium*.

Female—MPC

Usually asymptomatic, but if severe may cause vaginal discharge and vulval irritation. Dysuria unusual.

Cervix appears inflamed, oedematous, and friable with an overlying mucopurulent discharge.

Complications

Epididymo-orchitis See p. 162.
Sexually acquired reactive arthritis See p. 172.
Pelvic inflammatory disease See p. 144.

Diagnosis

NGU

Urethral specimen, using a 5mm plastic loop or cotton-tipped swab (better quality if bladder not emptied in preceding 3 hours). If no urethral material check first voided urine (FVU).

Urethritis diagnosed by high power (1000x) microscopy of Gram-stained material:

- ≥5 polymorphonuclear leucocytes (PMNL)/field of urethral smear
- ≥10 PMNL/field of threads or deposits from FVU.

Symptomatic ♂ without evidence of urethritis may be re-assessed after retaining urine overnight (or for at least 3 hours).

MPC

No clear microscopic criteria for diagnosis as the number of cervical PMNLs varies physiologically. Diagnosis based on the cervical appearance possibly supported by microscopy (>30 PMNLs/high power field).

Other investigations

- *N. gonorrhoeae* and *C. trachomatis*—as routine.
- Mid-stream sample of urine (MSSU)—positive dipstick for leucocyte esterase, nitrites, and blood suggests UTI. Confirm with microscopy and culture.
- *M. genitalium*—culture difficult and not readily available. Polymerase chain reaction ↑ sensitivity but not yet available for routine use.

Management

► Advise avoidance of sexual intercourse, including with condoms, until the patient and partner(s) have completed treatment and symptoms have resolved. Discourage repeated self-examination and advise that other factors (e.g. spicy food) may aggravate or prolong symptoms. The standard anti-chlamydial regimens are generally effective against non-chlamydial NSGI (except if 2° to UTI/coliforms).

Recommended treatment regimens

- Doxycycline 100mg twice daily for 7 days
- Azithromycin 1g—single dose.

Alternative regimens

Tetracyclines

- Deteclo 300mg twice daily for 7 days
- Tetracycline 500mg 4 times a day for 7 days
- Minocycline 100mg once daily for 7 days.

Macrolides

- Erythromycin 500mg twice daily for 14 days
- Clarithromycin 400mg twice daily for 7 days.

Fluroquinolones

- Ofloxacin 200mg twice daily or 400mg once daily for 7 days.

Complicated genital infection See p. 150, p. 168

Epidemiological treatment regimens

As for uncomplicated infection.

Partner notification

Assessment of sexual partners may reveal possible causes (e.g. trichomoniasis) which could affect the overall management. Epidemiological treatment of the sexual partners of ♂ with chlamydia negative NGU may ↓ recurrence and a possibly↓ ♀ morbidity. Suggested 'look back' periods: 4 weeks for symptomatic ♂, up to 6 months for asymptomatic ♂.

Similarly, sexual partners of ♀ with MPC should be offered epidemiological treatment and routine screening for STIs.

Follow-up

May be by telephone to ensure management compliance, resolution of symptoms, and partner notification. If symptoms or signs persist/recur repeat urethral smear/FVU specimen. Repeat treatment if risk of re-infection.

Persistent, relapsing, and chronic NGU

- Persistent NGU = continuing despite treatment of initial episode
- Relapsing NGU = recurrence following resolution of initial episode.
- Chronic NGU = persistent or relapsing NGU ≥30 days post-treatment.

All without a risk of re-infection.

Persistent or relapsing NGU occurs in 20–60% of ♂ treated for acute NGU and half of these may become chronic with *U. urealyticum* and *M. genitalium* of possible importance. A continuing inflammatory response following eradication of active chlamydial infection has also been suggested. In this situation there is no ↑ risk of PID in ♀ partners.

Recommended treatment regimen

- Erythromycin 500mg 4 times a day for 2 weeks *plus* metronidazole 400mg twice a day for 5 days.
- Repeat epidemiological treatment of partner using erythromycin if doxycycline used initially.

Continuing symptoms

Microscopic urethritis with no signs or symptoms after two courses of treatment is of little clinical significance. Further retreatment of sexual partners is not beneficial. Limited evidence on how best to manage patients who either remain symptomatic or have frequent relapses following a 2nd course of treatment. Consider:

- Erythromycin 500mg 4 times daily for 3 weeks.
- Urological investigations—usually normal unless the patient has urinary flow problems.
- Chronic abacterial prostatitis.
- Psychosexual causes.

HIV infection

M. genitalium may enhance transmission of HIV. Impaired immune function hampers its eradication (detection rate in urethra—56% with AIDS compared to 12% HIV without AIDS).

Chapter 10

Pelvic inflammatory disease

Introduction

Pelvic inflammatory disease (PID) refers to inflammation of upper female genital tract (endometrium, fallopian tubes, and ovaries) and supporting structures (parametrium and pelvic peritoneum). Usually a result of infection:

- ascending from the endocervix
- less commonly—spread from other abdominal organs e.g. appendicitis or disseminated by blood.

Endometritis and endosalpingitis produce a purulent exudate that may escape into the rectovaginal pouch resulting in a pelvic abscess. Inflammation may spread to the ovaries (oophoritis), parametrium, and pelvic peritoneum (peritonitis).

Aetiology

Sexually transmitted infections

- *Neisseria gonorrhoeae* in 5–75%[1]. Produces complement mediated necrosis of ciliated epithelial cells.
- *Chlamydia trachomatis* in 5–45%[1]. Induces Th-2 type immune response damaging tubal epithelium.

PID in 10–30% of untreated cervical chlamydial and gonococcal infections.

Other microorganisms

- Bacterial vaginosis (BV) associated organisms (anaerobic bacilli e.g. *Prevotella* and *Bacteroides* spp., anaerobic cocci e.g. *Peptosreptococcus* spp., *Gardenerella vaginalis*, *Mycoplasma hominis*, α and non-haemolytic streptococci). Recovered from fallopian tubes in up to 20% of ♀ with PID and 80% of endometrial samples in plasma cell endometritis (accompanying PID in ascending infection).

  Statistically significant association between BV and PID. Sialidase activity of *Prevotella* and *Bacteroides* spp., weakening cervical mucous barrier, possibly promotes ascending infection.
- Other organisms have also been recovered from the fallopian tubes (Viridans group streptococci, Group A–D streptococci, *Escherichia coli*, *Bacteroides fragilis*, and coagulase –ve staphylococci).
- *Mycoplasma genitalium*—cervical infection in ~15% ♀ with PID. Experimental evidence for PID in chimpanzees.
- *Actinomyces israelii* and related species—occasionally cause a chronic pelvic abscess (<1 in 3000 cases of PID and 3% of all human actinomyces infections) usually in association with plastic intrauterine devices (IUDs) and anaerobic co-infection.
- *Mycobacterium tuberculosis*—haematogenously disseminated, an important cause in areas of high prevalence.
- *Salmonella* spp.—rarely as a result of abdominal spread from an intestinal focus of infection in typhoid and paratyphoid.

1 Worldwide data—wide ranges relate to variable infection rates and availability of reliable tests.

Factors facilitating ascending infection

- Physiological
    - Uterine contractions—↑ in the follicular phase until ovulation.
    - Loss of cervical mucus plug (formed in the luteal phase) and retrograde flow during menstruation.
    - Possible carriage of bacteria by spermatozoa.
- Latrogenic
    - Uterine instrumentation.

Epidemiology

Estimated annual incidence in industrialized countries ~1 in 1000 in ♀ aged 15–34 years (1.5–2/1000 if 15–24) with wide geographical and temporal variations. Sexual transmission is the major aetiological factor.

Factors increasing risk

- Young age—peak incidence in age group 15–24.
- Multiple partners.
- New partner within previous 3 months.
- Frequency of sexual intercourse.
- Past history of STI (patient or partner).
- Past history of PID.
- Uterine instrumentation
    - Termination of pregnancy.
    - Insertion of IUD within the previous 6 weeks. Not a high risk alone (overall incidence of PID only 0.15%) but concomitant cervical chlamydial/gonococcal infection ↑ risk to 3–5%.
    - Hysterosalpingography/hysteroscopy.
    - Endometrial biopsy, curettage, and ablation.
    - *In vitro* fertilization procedure.
- Post-partum endometritis.
- Vaginal douching.
- Cigarette smoking.

Factors reducing risk

- Hormonal contraception especially progesterone-only preparations (production of a 'luteal-type' cervical mucus plug and reduction in the tubal inflammatory response).
- Consistent use of condom or diaphragm.
- Spermicide.
- Pregnancy—PID is uncommon because of thickened cervical mucus plug and is limited to the 1st trimester (protection afforded by the amniotic sac filling the uterine cavity is absent).

Clinical features

Acute PID (symptoms for <3 weeks)

Onset within 7 days of the 1st day of menstruation correlates with gonococcal/chlamydial infection. Symptoms and signs tend to be more acute/ intense in gonococcal than chlamydial PID.

Symptoms

- Lower abdominal pain, usually subacute if mild and acute if severe.
- Deep dyspareunia, common.
- Menstrual irregularity in ~40%.
- Abnormal bleeding.
- Dysmenorrhoea.
- Vaginal discharge.
- Nausea ± vomiting if severe.

Signs

- Lower abdominal tenderness with guarding, rebound if severe.
- Adnexal and cervical motion (excitation) tenderness.
- Fever (>38°C) in ~50%, more likely in severe or gonococcal PID.
- Adnexal mass in 50% of ♀ with gonococcal PID.
- Abdominal distension due to paralytic ileus if very severe (~1%).

Chronic PID ('silent PID')

May be asymptomatic and discovered only on investigation of infertility. Symptoms include constant or intermittent pain/discomfort in lower abdomen, groin or back, dyspareunia, malaise, and frequent/heavy menstrual periods. Usually no appreciable signs but thickening of tubes and/or fixed retroverted uterus may be palpable.

Complications and sequelae

Tubo-ovarian and pelvic abscess

A late complication, likely to be associated with anaerobic bacteria.

Peri-appendicitis

Direct spread of infection from the right fallopian tube to the appendiceal serosa may produce external inflammation (serositis) without mucosal involvement. Tubo-appendiceal mass develops. 2–10% of acute appendicitis in ♀ may be due to peri-appendicitis, 25–50% of which may be linked to tubal inflammation.

Infertility

Occurs in 8%, 20%, and 40% after 1, 2, and 3 episodes of PID, respectively. Due to tubal occlusion and peritubal adhesions. The more severe the episode the higher the incidence of infertility. Conflicting evidence on risk ↓ with treatment of PID.

Ectopic gestation

7-fold ↑ in risk of ectopic gestation (9% compared with 1.3% in the absence of PID). Risk ↑ directly with PID severity and number of episodes.

Chronic pelvic pain

Incidence 12%, 33%, and 66% after 1, 2, and 3 episodes of PID, respectively. Due to pelvic adhesions that form after the initial or recurrent episodes. Affects psychosocial functioning and quality of life.

Perihepatitis (Fitz–Hugh and Curtis syndrome)

Inflammation of the hepatic capsule with 'violin string' adhesions between anterior surface of liver and abdominal wall. Results from peritoneal or lymphatic spread of pelvic gonococcal/chlamydial infection. Occurs in 10–20% with PID.

► Haematogenous spread possible (case reports in ♂ with gonorrhoea).

Symptoms and signs of PID are not always present but a past history of PID or lower genital infection may be obtained. Typical presentation is acute, often severe, with right upper quadrant pain radiating to the back and shoulder tip, made worse by deep inspiration and movement. Examination demonstrates tenderness and guarding in the right upper abdominal quadrant with Murphy's sign (↑ pain on deep inspiration, examining hand just below the right costal margin). Hepatic rub may be heard on auscultation. Pyrexia in ~50%.

Differential diagnosis: acute cholecystitis, biliary colic, pleurisy, pneumonia, or pulmonary embolism.

Investigations

Routine

- Swabs for *N. gonorrhoeae* and *C. trachomatis*.
- Gram-stained smear of cervical material—may provide presumptive diagnosis of gonorrhoea. Polymorphonuclear leucocytes (PMNLs) are non-specific (positive predictive value only 17%) but useful for exclusion of PID (negative predictive value 95%).
- Peripheral blood white blood cell (WBC) count—↑ in ~50%.
- Erythrocyte sedimentation rate (ESR)—↑ in ~75%.
- C-reactive protein (CRP)—↑ in ~75% and level reflects severity.
- Chlamydial antibody—only provides retrospective or inconclusive evidence, hence of limited value in acute PID. However, in ♀ investigated for infertility antibody, especially at high level, correlates closely with frequency and severity of tubal damage and adverse pregnancy outcome. Therefore, useful as a screening test to determine the likelihood of tubal damage and need for early laparoscopy.

► Pregnancy test—urine or plasma βhCG—essential for acute pelvic pain in all ♀ of childbearing age.

- Urine analysis ± MSU if urinary tract infection is suspected.

Specialized

Endometrial histology/microbiology—sensitivity ~70%, specificity ~90%.

Pelvic imaging—abdominal ultrasound useful for detection of pelvic abscess. Transvaginal ultrasonography reported to have ~80% sensitivity and specificity (compared to laparoscopy/endometrial biopsy). May be necessary for differential diagnosis, particularly ectopic gestation.

Laparoscopy—regarded as the gold standard but not routinely performed (time/cost/complication risk). Allows:

- Diagnosis of acute PID by identifying
  - pronounced hyperaemia of tubal surface
  - oedema of tubal wall
  - sticky exudate from fimbriae.
- Collection of laboratory specimens from affected sites.
- Identification of other causes (e.g. ectopic gestation, appendicitis, endometriosis) or complications (e.g. abscess, pelvic adhesions, 'violin string adhesions' of perihepatitis).

May fail to identify endosalpingitis/endometritis in early/mild infection.

Diagnostic criteria

Main	Additional
• Low abdominal or pelvic pain • Abdominal ± rebound tenderness/ adnexal tenderness • Cervical motion (excitation) tenderness	• Temperature >38°C • ↑ CRP/ESR • WBC >10 x 10^9 • Adnexal mass • PMNLs in cervical/vaginal Gram-stained smears

The presence of all main criteria plus one of the additional is widely used for clinical diagnosis. Positive predictive value of 65–90% compared with laporoscopy. In routine clinical practice a lower threshold is often applied for prompt antibiotic treatment.

Differential diagnosis of PID

Acute/subacute

- Ectopic pregnancy—in ruptured ectopic pregnancy sudden onset of iliac fossa or hypogastric pain often associated with syncope. Vaginal spotting in early stages. Shoulder tip pain if blood tracked into abdominal cavity. Shock with intra-abdominal haemorrhage.
- Acute appendicitis—initial peri-umbilical pain later localizing to right iliac fossa with pronounced nausea and vomiting.
- Ruptured ovarian or endometriotic cyst—sudden onset of perimenstrual lower abdominal pain, usually afebrile.
- Complications of ovarian neoplasms.
- Acute pyelonephritis—pyrexia of sudden onset, rigors, loin/iliac fossa pain, urinary symptoms.
- Mesenteric lymphadenitis, inflammatory bowel disease.
- Other abdominal emergencies.

Chronic/recurrent

- Endometriosis
- Pelvic congestion syndrome
- Ovarian cysts
- Ovarian and uterine neoplasms
- Interstitial cystitis
- Urethral syndrome
- Irritable bowel syndrome
- Inflammatory bowel disease
- Previous surgery—leading to pelvic adhesions or nerve entrapment
- Myofascial pain syndrome
- Psychosocial causes—depression, previous physical and sexual abuse/trauma leading to somatization disorder.

Management

General principles

To minimize sequelae commence treatment promptly (even before definitive diagnosis). Hospital admission if:

- systemic disturbance is severe,
- surgical/gynaecological emergency cannot be excluded,
- patient is pregnant or immunocompromised,
- tubo-ovarian or pelvic abscess is detected or suspected.

Rest and adequate analgesia are important supportive measures. IUD removal is indicated if severe PID, no improvement after 72 hours of treatment, actinomyces-like organisms present or patient requests. Removal in other situations discretionary as evidence is inconsistent. Offer emergency contraception on removal if pregnancy risk within preceding 7 days.

► Advise avoidance of sexual intercourse until the patient and partner(s) have completed treatment with resolution of symptoms.

Treatment regimens

When choosing antibiotic regimen consider:

- severity and systemic disturbance—may need parenteral treatment;
- local prevalence of *N. gonorrhoeae* and antibiotic sensitivity;
- patient preference and likelihood of adherence.

Initial regimens (may need to be altered when antibiotic sensitivities are available)

Out-patient

- Ceftriaxone 250mg IM single dose followed by doxycycline 100mg oral twice daily for 14 days plus metronidazole 400mg twice daily for 7–14 days (90–95% clinical cure rate).
- Oflaxocin 400mg twice daily for 14 days plus metronidazole 400mg twice daily for 7–14 days (95% clinical cure rate).
- Doxycycline 100mg twice daily for 14 days plus metronidazole 400mg twice daily for 7–14 days (70–81% clinical cure rate). Does not cover *N. gonorrhoeae*, viridans streptococci and coliforms.

In-patient

- Cefoxitin 2g intravenously (IV) 4 times a day plus doxycycline 100mg orally (or IV if vomiting makes oral treatment intolerable) twice daily. Add metronidazole 500mg IV if pelvic or tubo-ovarian abscess develops.
- Clindamycin IV 900mg 3 times a day plus gentamicin 2mg/kg IV or IM loading dose followed by 1.5mg/kg 3 times a day.
- Ofloxacin 400mg IV infusion twice daily plus metronidazole 500mg IV 3 times a day.
- Ampicillin/sublactam IV infusion 3g 3 times a day plus doxycycline oral or IV 100mg twice daily.

Parenteral regimen is replaced after clinical improvement by one of the oral regimens and continued for a total of 14 days.

Treatment in pregnancy

Parenteral treatment advisable. Replace doxycycline with erythromycin (50mg/kg daily by continuous IV infusion).

Treatment of actinomycosis

Remove IUD. Benzyl penicillin 18–24 million units (10.8–14.4g) IV daily as infusion (or 4 hourly injections) and metronidazole 500mg IV 8 hourly. Doxycycline, erythromycin, and clindamycin are alternatives to benzylpenicillin. Change to oral regimen after clinical improvement and continue for at least 4–6 weeks. Drainage of abscess relieves bowel or urinary tract compression. Salpingo-oophorectomy and hysterectomy may be necessary.

Partner notification

♂ sexual partner/s within a 6 month period of onset of symptoms should be contacted and offered screening for STIs and epidemiological treatment for chlamydia ± gonorrhoea taking into consideration the proven or probable aetiology.

Follow-up

Review diagnosis and management after 72 hours if acute symptoms and signs do not improve. Reassess after 2–4 weeks.

HIV infection

- ↓ production of interferon-γ may ↑ susceptibility to PID.
- Tubo-ovarian abscess formation more likely if immunocompromised.
- Symptoms may be more severe but respond well with parenteral antibiotic therapy.

Chapter 11

Prostatitis

Introduction

Prostatitis affects up to 50% of ♂ (usually older age group) at some time in their lives. The majority of cases are chronic and of these probably 90–95% are abacterial. Diagnosis is largely based on symptoms as signs and objective clinical data may be inconclusive or lacking. It is therefore important to elicit symptoms of prostatic inflammation which include:

Pain

- Perineum
- Low abdomen
- Penis (especially tip)
- Testes
- Rectum
- Retropubis and upper thighs
- Low back

Urinary dysfunction

- Frequency/nocturia
- Urgency
- Incomplete voiding
- Abnormal flow
- Urethral discharge

Ejaculatory disturbance

- Pain with/after ejaculation
- Discolouration of or blood in semen

Acute bacterial prostatitis

Uncommon but clearly identifiable condition which should be considered as a complication of acute urinary tract infection (UTI), caused by urinary pathogens especially *Escherichia coli*. There may be an underlying structural abnormality of the urinary tract which should be investigated after resolution of the acute episode.

Very rarely gonorrhoea may cause acute prostatitis.

Clinical features

- Prostatitis—prostatic symptoms with a swollen, tender prostate gland
- UTI—dysuria, ↑ frequency, urgency
- Bacteraemia—pyrexia, rigors, myalgia, arthralgia
- Abscess (rare complication)—intense pain and acute urinary retention

Diagnosis

- Midstream sample of urine (MSSU),
- Blood cultures,
- Transrectal ultrasound (also useful to exclude prostatic abscess).

Management

- Mild to moderate: oral fluoroquinolone (e.g. ciprofloxacin 500mg twice daily or ofloxacin 200mg twice daily). Trimethoprim 200mg twice daily (if fluoroquinolone intolerant or allergic). All for 28 days.
- Severe: initial parenteral broad spectrum cephalosporin (e.g. cefuroxime) plus gentamicin then switch to oral regimen during convalescence.

► Prostatic massage should not be attempted as it may precipitate bacteraemia even though seminal and prostatic fluid contains polymorphonuclear leucocytes (PMNLs) and causal bacteria.

Causes of haematospermia

- Trauma (most common cause in young ♂). Generally mild, often isolated episodes. Usually self-limiting.
- Inflammation: prostatitis, seminal vesiculitis, urethritis, epididymitis.
- Obstruction/dilatation of urogenital ducts: prostatic cysts, urethral strictures, ejaculatory duct cysts, and strictures.
- Vascular abnormalities: arterio-venous malformations, venous malformations, haemangiomata.
- Systemic disorders:
  - severe hypertension
  - haematological disorders: coagulation disorders, leukaemia
  - cirrhosis.
- Drugs: e.g. warfarin.
- Tumours:
  - benign: polyps, warts, benign prostatic hyperplasia
  - malignant: carcinoma of genital tract.

Chronic prostatitis

Classification and aetiology

Chronic bacterial prostatitis (CBP)

Recurrent bacterial infection. Detection of significant numbers of pathogenic bacteria from prostatic fluid (usually urinary tract pathogens) without concomitant UTI. May be associated with prostatic calculi.

Chronic abacterial prostatitis—inflammatory (CAP-inflammatory)

This is also known as chronic non-bacterial prostatitis. Consistent presence of leucocytes in prostatic fluid but bacteria cannot be detected in significant numbers.

Chronic abacterial prostatitis—non-inflammatory (CAP-non-inflammatory)

This is also known as prostatodynia. No bacteria or leucocytes in prostatic fluid.

CAP-inflammatory and CAP-non-inflammatory are probably variants of chronic pelvic pain syndrome. Aetiology unknown although possible association with certain fastidious bacteria (e.g. *Corynebacterium* spp.) or persisting bacterial antigens. No clear evidence to support a causative role for *Chlamydia trachomatis, Ureaplasma urealyticum, Mycoplasma genitalium*, and *Mycoplasma hominis*, although their nucleotide sequences have been demonstrated in up to 10% of cases. Mechanical causes such as intra-prostatic urine reflux and bladder neck dysfunction have been postulated although data is lacking. No conclusive evidence to support an auto-immune aetiology although asymptomatic CAP-inflammatory is well recognized in sexually acquired reactive arthritis and ankylosing spondylitis.

Other rare causes

- *Mycobacterium tuberculosis* and other atypical mycobacteria—granulomatous prostatitis
- Parasites—e.g. *Trichomonas vaginalis, Schistosoma haematobium.*
- Viruses—e.g. herpes simplex virus and cytomegalovirus in immunocompromised patients. May also present acutely.
- Mycoses—e.g. coccidiodomycosis, blastomycosis, cryptococcosis, histoplasmosis, candidiasis. More common in immunosuppressed causing a granulomatous reaction.

Clinical features

Symptoms for at least 6 months, are often ill-defined, intermittent, and variable (possibly related to sexual activity) with pain typically described as aching. The most reliable diagnostic symptoms are pain at the perineum, low abdomen, penile tip, testes, and related to ejaculation. No systemic symptoms but high levels of psychological morbidity. The prostate gland usually feels normal on digital examination with variable degrees of tenderness (local, diffuse) or none. Recurrent UTIs may be associated with chronic bacterial prostatitis.

Prostatic massage procedure

Patient should not have:

- taken antibiotics within previous 4 weeks
- ejaculated within previous 48 hours
- evidence of urethritis or UTI (exclude prior to prostatic massage)

- Place patient in left lateral position and ensure that he is breathing easily through his mouth (to avoid Valsalva manoeuvre).
- With lubricated forefinger in rectum gently press on right and left lateral aspects of prostate gland in turn and move finger to the mid-line. Repeat 3–4 times.
- Press on superior aspect of prostate gland in mid-line and move finger to its lower pole. Repeat 2–3 times.
- Prostatic fluid should appear at the urethral meatus although sometimes gentle milking of the urethra is required.

If this fails the process may be repeated. However a dry massage is fairly common.

Diagnosis

Quantitative bacteriological assessment (also known as Stamey's test)

Patient should have retained urine for at least 2 hours (ideally overnight). Prepuce is retracted and glans cleaned ensuring that any cleansing agent is removed with sterile water.

Specimens

- VBU (voided bladder urine) 1—1st passed urine (5–10mL) collected. Patient should pass 100–200mL of urine which should be discarded.
- VBU2—MSSU, 5–10mL urine collected.
- EPS (expressed prostatic secretions)—after prostatic massage if material available.
- VBU3—post-prostatic massage urine sample (5–10mL).

Tests

- VBU1, VBU2, VBU3
  - Microscopy (for PMNLs).
  - Quantitative bacteriological culture.
- EPS
  - High power field (HPF) microscopy (400x) for PMNLs.
  - Culture—quantitative.
  - Specific diagnostic tests—if fastidious bacterium or other unusual organism is suspected.

Interpretation

- Inflammatory prostatitis: PMNL=>10/HPF (EPS), or if dry massage=>10/HPF in VBU3 and >VBU1 and 2.
- CBP: colony count in the EPS and VBU3 must be at least 10x >VBU1 and 2.

Caution: EPS PMNLs may be absent in cases of inflammation and infection. However, =>10/HPF found in up to 6% of healthy controls.

Other investigations

- EPS pH: level =>8 suggestive of prostatitis.
- Serum prostate specific antigen (if >45 years in view of carcinoma risk).

► However, usually elevated with prostatitis, therefore repeat assay after resolution.

- Urological (consider especially if >45 years):
  - transrectal ultrasound if cysts, abscesses, calculi suspected.
  - cystourethroscopy and excretion urography—to exclude any underlying pathology or abnormality.
  - bladder flow and urodynamic studies.
  - prostatic biopsy, rarely indicated.

Management

Chronic bacterial prostatitis

Antibiotics for 4 weeks according to antimicrobial sensitivity, preferably a fluoroquinolone (high relative concentration in prostate tissue, 2–3x serum levels): e.g. ciprofloxacin 500mg, ofloxacin 200mg, norfloxacin 400mg all twice daily.

If intolerant or allergic; doxycycline 100mg, trimethoprim 200mg both twice daily.

Chronic abacterial prostatitis—inflammatory and non-inflammatory

In view of lack of understanding and imprecision in diagnosing these conditions it is difficult to properly evaluate treatments. No therapy has been demonstrated to be absolutely effective.

- Antibiotics: although regimens as for CBP are regularly prescribed, in view of an assumed bacterial association, there is no clear evidence to support their use.
- Alpha-blocking drugs (e.g. terazosin and alfuzosin): relax the bladder neck and prostate gland but limited and inconsistent evidence of benefit.
- Non-steroidal anti-inflammatory drugs: helpful for pain relief.
- Tricyclic antidepressants: anecdotal reports of benefit which may be due to pain modulation as with other chronic pain conditions.
- Frequent ejaculation: =>2x a week—reduces prostatic congestion and may ameliorate symptoms.
- Prostatic hyperthermia (by microwave): data limited but benefit has been demonstrated meriting further investigation.

Chapter 12

Epididymitis, orchitis, epididymo-orchitis

Aetiology

Inflammation of the epididymis (epididymitis), the testicle (orchitis), or both (epididymo-orchitis) may be caused by spread of infection or less commonly other agents from:

- The urethra or bladder through the ejaculatory duct, seminal vesicle, and vas deferens.
- Distant sites through the lymphatic or blood vessels.

Genital infection

- *Chlamydia trachomatis* and/or *Neisseria gonorrhoeae* cause ~70% of acute epididymitis in sexually active ♂ aged <35 years and 5–30% in older ♂. Up to 30% of untreated urethral infections may lead to acute epididymitis, usually unilateral.
- Coliform enteric bacteria (acquired through insertive anal sex) in up to 65% of homosexual ♂ with non-gonococcal, non-chlamydial epididymitis.
- *Treponema pallidum* is a rare cause of diffuse chronic interstitial inflammation of the testis in late benign syphilis which may lead to a gumma (or atrophy).

Urinary tract infection (UTI)

- Coliform bacteria (*Escherichia coli*, *Klebsiella* spp., and *Proteus* spp.) and *Pseudomonas aeroginosa* cause up to 80% of acute epididymitis in ♀ aged ≥35. May be associated with an underlying urological abnormality e.g. obstruction, calculus, chronic bacterial prostatitis. Urethral instrumentation (e.g. catheterization) is a predisposing factor.
- *Mycobacterium tuberculosis* associated with renal, prostatic, or seminal vesicle infection is an uncommon cause with usually insidious, occasionally acute onset. 75% of ♂ with renal tuberculosis have associated epididymitis, 65% of which is bilateral.

Other microorganisms

- *Mycobacterium leprae* commonly involves the testes ± the epididymes causing atrophy.
- Mumps: epididymo-orchitis in 20% of cases in adults, ~16% bilateral.
- *Brucella* spp. (*Br. melitensis* 5× more than *Br. abortus*) may cause orchitis in 5–18% of cases (epididymitis less evident).
- Coxsackie virus B infections may include orchitis in up to a third of cases.
- Systemic fungal and yeast infections e.g. cryptococcosis, histoplasmosis, coccidioidomycosis, and blastomycosis may produce orchitis.
- Filarial organisms, *Wuchereria bancrofti* and *pacifica* and less commonly *Brugia malayi*. If present in inguinal lymph nodes may cause chronic allergic lymphangitis of the spermatic cord and testis. This produces chronic epididymitis and orchitis with profuse effusion within the tunica vaginalis leading to scrotal oedema and elephantiasis.
- *Streptococcus pneumoniae*, *Nocardia* spp., *Haemophilus parainfluenzae*, *B. Salmonella* spp., *Neisseria meningitidis*, *Schistosoma haematobium*, and cytomegalovirus have been reported as probable causes.

Non-infective causes

- Spermatic granuloma: extravasation of spermatozoa into adjacent tissue inducing auto-immune granulomatous epididymitis (a cellular reaction) leading to fibrosis.
- Granulomatous orchitis: idiopathic or 2° to systemic granulomatous disorders.
- Behçet's disease: epididymo-orchitis in up to 20% of ♂.
- Amiodarone: side-effect in up to 11% of ♂. Causes lymphocytic infiltration and fibrosis, usually bilateral.
- Sarcoidosis: may rarely cause non-caseating granulomatous epididymo-orchitis.
- Idiopathic lymphocytic orchitis.

Clinical features

Acute

- Typically unilateral scrotal pain and swelling.
- Pyrexia may be present.
- If sexually acquired probable urethritis, often asymptomatic.
- Scrotal erythema.
- Tenderness and palpable swelling of the epididymis.
- Development of oedema and formation of a hydrocele may lead to a grossly enlarged scrotum.
- Haematospermia (rarely).
- In mumps orchitis the onset is usually within a week of parotid enlargement but sometimes follows resolution of parotitis.

Chronic

Symptoms are of >3 months duration. Pain is of variable intensity. Epididymial and testicular swelling is gradual and depends on the underlying cause.

Complications

- Hydrocele: in ~10% (usually resolves with antibiotics).
- Abscess: in up to 3% of cases.
- Infarction of the testicle: in <1% (due to compression of the swollen spermatic cord at the external inguinal ring).
- Recurrence: due to lack of adequate treatment, re-infection, or chronic inflammation. High recurrence rates in homosexual ♂ (coliform infection).
- Chronic epididymitis: follows ~15% of acute episodes.
- Infertility due to:
  - occlusion of vasa deferentia (following bilateral epididymitis)
  - impaired spermatogenesis (following bilateral orchitis).

  Possibility of infertility after unilateral epididymitis ± orchitis due to sperm agglutinins (suggested but unproven).
- Chronic prostatitis (unusual).

Investigations

Gram-stain of urethral smear

May show urethritis, i.e. ≥5 polymorphonuclear cells (PMNLs)/high power field (HPF), ± Gram-negative intracellular diplococci.

Tests for *N. gonorrhoeae* and *C. trachomatis*

Urine examination

- First-voided urine (FVU): for threads containing ≥10 PMNLs/HPF (if no urethral material).

- Midstream specimen of urine (MSSU): dipstick test for leucocyte esterase, nitrites, and blood. Send to laboratory for microscopy and culture.
- Early morning urine x 3: microscopy and culture for *M. tuberculosis* if suspected.

Screening for other STIs

If sexually transmitted epididymo-orchitis is likely.

Ultrasonography

Doppler ultrasonography (stethoscope or colour-coded duplex): useful in the differential diagnosis of acute scrotal pain and swelling. Acute epididymitis/orchitis ↑ blood flow. Radionuclide scanning may provide similar information.

Real time ultrasonography: of great value in the differential diagnosis of scrotal swellings particularly when malignancy or complications of acute epididymitis, requiring surgical intervention, are suspected.

Additional investigations

- Epididymal aspiration for microbiological specimens (usually during surgical exploration).
- Magnetic resonance imaging when diagnosis is unclear despite ultrasonography.
- Further urological investigations, e.g. urethrocystoscopy and excretion urogram, if an underlying urological abnormality is likely.

Diagnosis

Age, clinical features including sexual history, urethral Gram-stain, and urine examination are important in establishing a diagnosis, supported by specialized investigations if indicated. It is essential to exclude testicular torsion in acute presentation (requires emergency surgical intervention).

In the differential diagnosis of non-acute scrotal pain and swelling clinical assessment should attempt to identify if the lesion is within the body of the testis (malignancy more likely).

Main differential diagnosis

	Testicular torsion	Epididymitis	Testicular cancer
Age range in years	Most common 12–18 Less common 18–30	Most common 19–40 Less common <18 and >40	Peak incidence 25–35. 74% in 20–49
Pain	Sudden onset. 50% report previous short episodes of pain resolving spontaneously	Onset over 24–48 hours	Typically painless but diffuse pain or dragging sensation/ache in ~30%. 5–15% present with acute pain
Urinary symptoms	90% normal urinanalysis 4% ↑ frequency	Dysuria, ↑ frequency or urgency. Urethritis (smear/FVU) or pyuria	No association
Gastro-intestinal symptoms	~33% nausea and vomiting. 20–30% abdominal pain	Nausea and vomiting if acute orchitis develops	May occur due to metastases
Pyrexia	Usually absent	May be low grade. >40°C in acute orchitis	Usually absent
Inspection and palpation	Oedema and erythema of affected side Enlarged and exquisitely tender testis, high in scrotum Transverse lie and anterior epididymis on unaffected side	Oedema and erythema of affected side. Epididymis distinguishable from tests unless very advanced or scrotum grossly enlarged	Testicle enlarged, 15% with inflammation Solid lump not separated from testis
Cremastric reflex	Absent	Present	Present
Ultrasonography	↓ blood flow	↑blood flow	Hypo-echoic mass within the testis

Causes of scrotal mass/pain

- Trauma
- Hydrocele
- Epididymo-orchitis
- Testicular torsion
- Torsion of testicular appendix (in 6–12 year old children)
- Spermatocele
- Epididymal cyst
- Varicocele
- Hernia
- Testicular tumour
  - Germ cell tumours—seminoma and malignant teratoma
  - Lymphoma and other malignancies
- Epididymal and non-testicular neoplasms
- Fournier's gangrene
- Vasculitis: Henoch–Schonlein purpura and Kawasaki disease (<15 years), Buerger's disease (adults).

Three clues to diagnosis of scrotal mass

Clinical assessment should aim to answer three important questions in diagnosing the cause of scrotal mass.

- Is the mass intrascrotal ('get above the swelling')?
  Hernia extends above the scrotum.
- Is the mass cystic?
  Cystic mass e.g. hydrocele is usually transilluminable.
- Is the mass an integral part of the testis?
  Solid testicular mass should be regarded as malignant until proven otherwise and urgent investigations should be arranged.

Management

General

- Scrotal elevation/support and analgesics (non-steroidal anti-inflammatory) are recommended.
- Avoid sexual intercourse until both patient and partner treated and follow-up complete.

Treatment

- Empirical therapy should be commenced immediately taking into consideration the likely cause and local antibiotic sensitivities, altered if necessary when laboratory results available.

Treatment regimens

- Chlamydia/gonorrhoea (suspected/confirmed):
  - doxycycline 100mg oral twice daily for 10–14 days *plus* ceftriaxone 250mg single intramuscular dose if gonorrhoea diagnosed or probable
  - ofloxacin 200mg oral twice daily for 14 days
- Coliform (suspected/confirmed):
  - ofloxacin 200mg oral twice daily for 14 days
  - ciprofloxacin 500mg oral twice daily for 10 days

Partner notification

If the cause is or likely to be sexually transmitted, sexual contacts should be offered screening and epidemiological treatment. If chlamydia found in index case or aetiology undetermined provide anti-chlamydia treatment (as for uncomplicated infection). If gonorrhoea found/probable add treatment for gonorrhoea (as for uncomplicated infection).

Follow-up

If no improvement after 3 days review diagnosis and management. Reassess if swelling and tenderness persist after antimicrobial therapy is completed (swelling may take several weeks to resolve).

HIV infection

- Case reports of poor response to standard treatment in HIV infection.
- Unusual causes (cytomegalovirus, *M. tuberculosis*, *H. influenzae*, *Nocardia asterioides*, *Candida spp.*, and *Cryptococcus neoformans*) more common.

Chapter 13

Sexually acquired reactive arthritis

Introduction

Reactive, or post-infectious, arthritis (ReA) is a seronegative, sterile inflammation of the synovial membrane initiated by an external stimulant, usually an enteric or sexually transmitted infection (STI).

When ReA is associated with both urethritis and conjunctivitis (minority of cases) it is commonly referred to as Reiter's syndrome (after Hans Reiter who described a case in 1916 preceded by dysentery).

As Reiter's syndrome may be incomplete and other clinical features may be present, the term sexually acquired ReA (SARA) is commonly used when the main component, arthritis, follows an STI. The manifestations of post-enteric ReA are similar.

Aetiology

Although an infective urethritis or enteritis commonly triggers ReA its multi-system involvement and potential for relapse/remission (similar to other seronegative spondyloarthritides) infer an underlying reactive aetiology. However, the detection of material from sexually transmitted organisms, which may provoke SARA, suggests a more direct relationship. Other infections and conditions may be associated with a ReA (e.g. rheumatic fever) but have different clinical features. In ~25% of cases no trigger can be identified.

Sexually acquired infection

SARA typically presents in ♂ 2–4 weeks after urethritis, usually nongonococcal (NGU). Although found in ♀ it is much less common and more likely to be unrecognized as it is associated with cervicitis, commonly latent. Therefore certain organisms associated with urethritis/cervicitis are linked to SARA. Their role is unclear and SARA may arise without any demonstrable infection.

NGU (and cervicitis)

<0.8% of those with NGU develop SARA.

- *Chlamydia trachomatis*—Chlamydia-like particles, seen by electron microscopy, and chlamydial DNA, using nucleic acid amplification tests (NAAT), have been identified from synovial fluid of some patients with SARA. Associated urogenital infection has been found by non-NAAT in 30–70% (no data using NAAT).

Ureaplasma urealyticum

↑ urogenital detection rate in some with SARA without evidence of chlamydial or enteric infection. *U. ureaplasma* DNA from synovial fluid has been reported in those with SARA (using NAAT).

- *Mycoplasma genitalium*—DNA found in synovial fluid (using NAAT).

Gonorrhoea

Neisseria gonorrhoeae has been implicated in up to 14–16% cases of SARA distinct from its more common association with septic arthritis.

Enteric infection (frequency of ReA ~1–4%)

- *Shigella* spp.
- *Salmonella* spp.
- *Campylobacter* spp.
- *Yersinia enterocolitica* and *pseudotuberculosis*
- *Clostridium difficile*

Other factors

Urethral or bowel trauma (e.g. catheterization, surgery). Unusual but may precipitate recurrence.

Associations

- Gender
  - SARA ~98% in ♂ (falsely high as under diagnosed in ♀)
  - Enteric ReA ~90% in ♂
- Age
  - Usually young adults
- Geography—Urethritis appears to precede ReA more commonly in the UK and USA whereas an initial dysenteric illness has been reported more frequently in studies from continental Europe.
- Human leucocyte antigen-B27 (HLA-B27) positivity. Diagnostic relevance dubious although may be associated with ↑ risk of chronicity and recurrence
  - 30–90% of those with SARA
  - 50–80% with ReA following enteric infection

  Controls
  - N. American Indians, Lapps, northern Scandinavians—26–50%
  - Most Europeans—7–10%
  - Blacks—<2%
- Genetic predisposition—May be family history of:
  - SARA
  - other seronegative spondyloarthropathy (see Box)
  - iritis.

Seronegative, HLA-B27 associated, spondyloarthropathy

- Reiter's disease
- Ankylosing spondylitis (idiopathic)
- Bowel disease
  - Ulcerative colitis
  - Crohn's disease
  - Whipple's disease
- Psoriatic arthritis

Clinical features

Usually starts within 4 weeks of 1° urogenital or enteric infection. ~10% do not have a preceding symptomatic infection.

Urogenital

Men

- Urethritis (usually NGU): discharge/dysuria in ~80% with SARA, NGU in:
  - ~70% of ♂ with post-enteric ReA
  - ~60% of cases of recurrent SARA which may be associated with a new infection or may arise spontaneously (a new infection does not necessarily trigger a recurrence).
- Chronic prostatitis in 95% of cases of SARA

Women

- Urethritis (dysuria/discharge) uncommon (short urethra)
- Cervicitis usually asymptomatic but may be visible on examination.

Bladder and upper urinary tract

Mild, sterile (by conventional culture), cystitis found in 20% although severe haemorrhagic manifestations have been reported. Glomerulonephritis and IgA nephropathy rarely associated.

Musculo-skeletal

- Arthritis: asymmetrical polyarthritis (>95%) predominantly affecting the lower limbs starting ~14 days after genital symptoms. Low back pain common (~50%) with sacroiliitis in 10%. Joints not involved simultaneously but overall severity peaks ~14 days after the onset of the arthritis. Rapid muscle wasting in relation to joints involved is common.
- Enthesitis (inflammation at insertion point of ligaments, tendons, and capsules) and tenosynovitis
  - Plantar fasciitis in ~20%, may be associated with calcaneal enthesitis
  - Achilles tendonitis in 10–15%

Contribute to painful feet and difficulty walking. Enthesitis may also be found at insertion points around the pelvis and ribs.

Ophthalmic

- Conjunctivitis: usually bilateral found in 20–50% of cases of SARA. Generally mild and self-limiting. Typically develops after the appearance of symptoms from the provoking infection and the onset of arthritis.
- Iritis: late manifestation of an initial episode or recurrence in 2–11%. Usually unilateral presenting as a painful eye with blurred vision and inflammation at the margins of the cornea. Associated with sacroiliitis.
- Episcleritis: keratitis and corneal ulceration have also been reported.

Dermatological (skin manifestations commonly occur together)

- Keratoderma blennorrhagica (KB): identical to pustular psoriasis and found in up to 33%, although may be greater as often asymptomatic. Most commonly found on the soles of the feet (often the only site involved) though other sites may be affected e.g. penis (especially if circumcised), palms, toes, scalp, scrotum, and sometimes a generalized rash. The lesions, which may exhibit the Koebner phenomenon, typically appear as hard parakeratotic nodules or soft limpet-like patches, usually brown in colour becoming pustular.

- Erythema nodosum: rarely reported
- Nails: ~10% of patients develop thickening and ridging of the nails which may progress to subungual abscess formation with shedding. Pitting is not a feature.
- Genital lesions: balanitis (often asymptomatic) is found in 20–40% and is an early finding. If circumcised the psoriatic lesions are elevated, dry and scaly (as KB). In the uncircumcised erythematous confluent patches appear circumscribed by a well-defined pale margin creating a geographical appearance and referred to as circinate balanitis. May be found in ♂ presenting with urethritis and no other clinical features. Circinate vulvitis has also been reported in ♀. Lesions usually resolve spontaneously within 4 weeks.
- Oral lesions: found in 10–16% (although under diagnosed as asymptomatic). The palate, buccal mucosa, gingiva, and tongue may show erythematous or circinate lesions and ulceration. Patchy loss of papillae can appear over the tongue (geographical tongue).

Other manifestations

- Constitutional symptoms: malaise and fever in ~10%.
- Cardiovascular system
    - Thrombophlebitis (deep leg veins) in ~3% (symptoms may resemble a ruptured knee joint capsule, a rare complication of arthritis).
    - Myocarditis—1° heart block in up to 14%.
    - Pericarditis—rare.
    - Aortitis with aortic incompetence—very rare.
- Respiratory system—pleurisy in up to 8%.
- Nervous system: <2%—meningoencephalitis, peripheral neuropathies, amyotrophic lateral sclerosis.
- Enteric—non-specific mucous enterocolitis may occasionally appear at onset of symptoms.
- Amyloidosis: very rare.

Natural history

Most initial episodes resolve within 2–6 months although they may extend to >1 year in ~35%. 15–30% may develop progressive, chronic arthritis, sacroiliitis, and dactylitis ('sausage digits'). Recurrences occur in ~50% with an annual risk of ~15%.

Without treatment urethritis and conjunctivitis usually resolve in up to 4 weeks. The dermatological manifestations also generally settle within 4 weeks although KB may persist for 2–3 months or longer.

Iritis is liable to recur, especially if associated with sacroiliitis.

Diagnosis

► Clinical: there is no simple diagnostic test for SARA and Reiter's syndrome. Diagnosis made on clinical grounds, although it may be supported by the following investigations.

- Screen for STIs or stool cultures and *Yersinia* spp. serology if enteric infection suspected.
- Full blood count
  - Normochromic, normocytic anaemia in severe cases
  - Polymorphonuclear leukocytosis in up to 30%
- Erythrocyte sedimentation rate/C-reactive protein: elevated in >90% with SARA. Level gives an indication of disease activity.
- Urinalysis: Proteinuria, microscopic haematuria, pyuria in up to 50%.
- Radiology: early SARA—no findings. In progressive disease:
  - periostitis (tibia, fibula, hands, and feet)
  - articular erosions with joint narrowing (hands, feet, posterior aspect of calcaneous)
  - periosteal reaction at sites of tendon insertion producing 'spurs', especially calcaneum (>50% of chronic cases)
  - sacroiliitis in 50% with severe chronic disease.
- Slit lamp examination: suspected iritis.
- Electrocardiography and echocardiography if suspected cardiac involvement.

► HLA-B27 testing is not advocated as it has low diagnostic predictive value.

- Negative/normal findings
  - Antistreptolysin O titre
  - Rheumatoid factor (though 4% positivity rate in normal population)
  - Antinuclear antibody test
  - Uric acid levels
  - Synovial fluid sterile with no crystals.

The commonest differential diagnosis is gonococcal arthritis, especially if SARA presents as a monoarthritis (3–7% of cases). Culture of synovial fluid is usually negative but gonorrhoea may also trigger SARA. If in doubt treatment should be given to cover disseminated gonococcal infection which, unlike SARA, should show rapid improvement.

Other causes of acute painful swollen joint(s)

- Direct infection
  - Acute septic arthritis (~80% due to Gram-positive aerobes)
  - Tuberculosis
  - Fungal infections—unusual (e.g. blastomycosis, candida species)
- Direct infection and/or reactive arthritis
  - Gonococcal arthritis (usually monoarthritis)
  - Meningococcal arthritis
  - Reaction to streptococcal infection (e.g. rheumatic fever)
  - Bacterial endocarditis
  - Syphilis
  - Viral infections (including human immunodeficiency, hepatitis B, herpes simplex and parvo viruses)
  - Lyme disease
  - Brucellosis.
- Others
  - Trauma and foreign body reaction (also exacerbation of osteoarthritis)
  - Seronegative HLA-B27 associated spondyloarthritides (see previous Box)
  - Rheumatoid arthritis and other seropositive connective tissue diseases
  - Still's disease (juvenile rheumatoid arthritis, seronegative)
  - Erythema multiforme and Stevens–Johnson syndrome
  - Reaction to drugs and vaccines
  - Behçet's disease
  - Gout/pseudogout
  - Haemachromatosis
  - Sarcoidosis
  - Haemophilia and other clotting deficiencies
  - Acute leukaemia.

Management

General

Full information on SARA and its clinical course should be provided with advice on the avoidance of future potential triggers. Partner notification (with epidemiological treatment) may be required depending on the initial provoking infection.

► Liaise with or refer to the appropriate specialty for extra-genital manifestations, especially if severe.

Antibiotics

SARA

The provoking infection in acute SARA (usually NGU) should be treated as for an uncomplicated infection (see p. 140). Treatment of the triggering infection does not appear to affect the course of any established skeletal, skin, or ophthalmic manifestations and it is unclear if such intervention before their onset is of benefit. The role of long-term antibiotics is uncertain (conflicting data).

Early treatment of urogenital infection may ↓ risk of relapsing arthritis in those with a history of ReA.

Enteric

Short-term antibiotics for the underlying enteric infection do not appear to alter the course of ReA or Reiter's syndrome. Any associated urethritis should be treated as above.

Prolonged treatment for 4–6 weeks may be of benefit for arthritis triggered by *Yersinia enterocolitica*.

Ophthalmic

- Conjunctivitis—usually no treatment required
- Iritis—mydriatics and topical steroids

Arthritis and enthesitis

- Rest, avoidance of weight bearing, passive muscle exercises to limit wasting
- Non-steroidal anti-inflammatory drugs with dosage at night to reduce morning stiffness
- Corticosteroids:
    - systemic prednisolone only rarely indicated if severe polyarthritis with other systemic symptoms
    - local injection at tendon insertion or into a severely swollen knee joint following aspiration may be of value
- Options for chronic disabling arthritis include:
    - sulfasalazine
    - methotrexate
    - azathioprine.

Skin

Manifestations are self-limiting and unless unusually severe treatment is not required. However, topical corticosteroids may be indicated for severe circinate balanitis and KB with topical calcipotriol, systemic methotrexate, and retinoids options for intractable cases.

HIV infection

Although some early reports described an association between HIV infection and SARA this has not been substantiated in more recent publications. If SARA does occur it is likely to be more severe.

Bacterial vaginosis and anaerobic balanitis

Introduction

First described as 'non-specific vaginitis' in 1955 by Gardner and Dukes with the term 'bacterial vaginosis' (BV) formally introduced in 1984.

Characterized by bacteriological imbalance of vaginal flora with overgrowth of characteristic commensal bacteria (*Gardnerella vaginalis*, anaerobic bacteria, and mycoplasmas), replacing normally predominant *Lactobacillus* spp. and producing an altered vaginal discharge.

Aetiology

Vaginal hydrogen peroxide producing lactobacilli appear to be protective as the prevalence of BV is only 4% compared to 32% in those with non-hydrogen peroxide producing organisms.

Organisms

- *G. vaginalis*—facultative anaerobic, small Gram-negative bacillus (often stains Gram-positive). Found in high concentrations (>100× normal) in up to 95% of BV but can be isolated in up to 58% of those with normal discharge
- Anaerobic bacteria in high concentrations
  - *Mobiluncus* spp.—sickle-shaped rods displaying vigorous motility, including corkscrew motion, in vaginal wet mounts. Cultured in 14–96% ♀ with BV (<6% without) and seen on microscopy in up to 77%.
    - *Mobiluncus mulieris* (long, Gram-negative)
    - *Mobiluncus curtisii* (short, Gram-variable usually stain positive)
  - *Prevotella* spp. (e.g. *P. bivia*)
  - *Prophyromonas* spp.
  - Peptostreptococci (e.g. Streptococcus intermedius)
  - *Fusobacterium* spp.
  - *Bacteroides* spp.
  - *Atopobium vaginae*—a recently discovered, metronidazole resistant, Gram-positive anaerobe, may be responsible for metronidazole treatment failure.
- Aerobic bacteria (e.g. alpha-haemolytic streptococci, coliforms)
- *Mycoplasma hominis*—found in 24–75% ♀ with BV (13–22% without BV)

Factors

- Non-white ethnicity
- Use of intrauterine device (IUD): >2×↑
- Vaginal douching
- Sexual: not considered to be sexually transmitted though following features suggest a sexual link:
  - Lower mean age of coitarche
  - New sex partner or multiple sex partners
  - Associated with *Neisseria gonorrhoeae* and *Chlamydia trachomatis*
  - BV discharge inoculated into healthy vagina can induce BV in recipient though no evidence of transmission by a single organism

- ↑ rate in lesbians (compared with heterosexuals) with ×20 ↑ if partner has BV. Apparent relationship with receptive cunnilingus but no other practices including the shared use of dildoes and anal penetration with fingers.

Against sexual transmission (heterosexual)

- Comparative study—BV found in similar proportion of virginal and sexually active adolescents (12 and 15% respectively).
- Although *G. vaginalis* is isolated in up to 80% of the urethras of ♂ sex partners of ♀ with BV their concurrent treatment does not ↓ ♀ recurrence rate.
- No association with partner being uncircumcised.

Clinical features

- Asymptomatic— ~50%.
- Vaginal discharge—symptom in 49% (20% without BV), sign in 69% (3% without BV).
  - Volume—usually moderate (varies from scanty-profuse).
  - Colour—grey in 65–85%, white in 7–30% (remainder yellowish).
  - Nature—homogeneous vaginal discharge, like 'thin flour paste' adhering to vaginal walls as a thin film). Frothy in 27–80% (1–18% normal women).
- Malodour—fishy, ammoniacal smell reported in 20–49% but probably higher as may not be volunteered due to embarrassment. (Reported in 20% without BV). Smell enhanced when vaginal pH ↑ (e.g. during menstruation and following contact with alkaline prostatic fluid after intercourse) releasing volatile amines.
- Irritation—a non-inflammatory process so absent in most cases.

Associations

- *N. gonorrhoeae* and *C. trachomatis:*
  - 3.8-fold risk of *N. gonorrhoeae* or *C. trachomatis* in ♀ with symptomatic BV
  - ↑ in ♀ with BV if ♂ partners have urethritis
- Non-specific urethritis (NSU) in ♂—possible association with BV in ♀ partner
- Trichomoniasis—bacterial overgrowth as BV but purulent

Complications

- Post-hysterectomy vaginal cuff cellulitis
- Post-abortion pelvic inflammatory disease (PID)
- Possibly contributes to spontaneous PID, especially with IUD but no data on role of BV during IUD insertion
- In pregnancy

Increased bacterial production of cytokines and prostaglandins and amniotic fluid/chorioamniotic infection leading to:

- chorioamnionitis
- low birth weight
- preterm birth (relative risk 1.5–2.3) from preterm labour and premature rupture of membranes
- 2nd trimester miscarriage (up to 3–6-fold risk)
- endometritis (pre/post delivery including caesarean section).

History of previous premature delivery increases risk of further preterm birth 7-fold with BV.

Frequently asked questions

What is bacterial vaginosis?

It is a condition caused by the overgrowth of normal vaginal bacteria causing an imbalance and an altered vaginal discharge.

Is it sexually transmitted?

It is not thought to be sexually transmitted, and so partners of ♀ with BV are not treated. Lesbian partners of ♀ with BV also have a higher incidence of BV although the reason is not clear.

Is it like thrush?

Thrush (candidiasis) is caused by a yeast, usually *Candida albicans* (90%). Bacterial vaginosis is due to an imbalance of normal vaginal flora, with a loss or reduction in lactobacilli and an overgrowth of largely anaerobic bacteria especially *Gardnerella vaginalis.*

Thrush usually causes a thick white vaginal discharge, itching, and soreness. BV is usually associated with a thin white/grey discharge and an offensive fishy smell.

Both thrush and BV are prone to recur.

Is it treated with anti-thrush preparations?

No. Thrush is treated with topical (pessaries/creams) or oral azoles. BV is treated with metronidazole or clindamycin either topically or orally.

Can my partner catch it from me?

It is not sexually transmitted. ♂ may occasionally develop balanitis with bacteria similar to those found with BV but it does not appear to be related to intercourse with a partner who has BV. However, the increased incidence of BV in lesbian couples suggests a sexual link.

Does my partner need treatment?

No. BV is not sexually transmitted.

Will I ever get rid of it?

Overall cure rate is 95%. Recurrence rate is about 15–30% with majority recurring within 3 months of treatment.

Diagnosis

- Gram-stain

Simple, fast, and accurate way to diagnose BV. Typical appearance is substantial reduction or absence of lactobacilli (Gram +ve rods) replaced by small Gram-variable bacilli (*G. vaginalis*) adhering to shed epithelial ('clue') cells without polymorphs (Plate 7). Other small Gram-negative bacilli (e.g. *Bacteroides* spp.), Gram-positive cocci (e.g. peptostreptococci), Gram-variable sickle-shaped rods (*Mobilincus* spp.) may be found. The latter are seen more easily as motile organisms on a wet mount which may also show long, thin pointed rods (fusiform bacilli).

  - *Hay/Ison Gram-stain method*

Simple qualitative method grading smears as—grade 0, epithelial cells/no bacteria; grade I, (normal) lactobacilli only; grade II, (intermediate) reduced lactobacilli/mixed bacteria; grade III, (BV) mixed bacteria with few or absent lactobacilli; grade IV, epithelial cells covered with Gram +ve cocci only.

  - *Nugent Gram-stain method*

Although sensitive this is too complex and time-consuming for routine clinical use. Based on the quantitative scoring of *Lactobacillus*, *G. vaginalis*, *Bacteroides* morphotypes, and *Mobiluncus* spp. on a Gram-stained vaginal smear. High scores (>6) equate to BV, medium scores (4–6) intermediate and 0–3 normal.

- Amsel criteria (regarded as 'gold standard' for research)

3 of 4 criteria to be fulfilled:

  - characteristic discharge
  - positive amine ('sniff' or 'whiff') test. Drop of 10% potassium hydroxide on vaginal fluid releases 'fishy' smelling amines (avoid semen which may give false positive result). No longer recommended for safety reasons.
  - pH >4.5 (avoiding cervical mucus [pH 7.0], blood, and seminal fluid)
  - vaginal 'clue' cells on wet-mount microscopy.

- Detection of amines in vaginal fluid by chromatography, biochemical assays or electronically (the 'electronic nose'). Not generally available for routine clinical use.

Diagnostic methods

	Sensitivity (%)	Specificity (%)
Amsel criteria: atypical discharge	52–69	78–97
pH > 4.5*	97	53
amine test*	43–80	99
clue cells	80–90	94
Nugent Gram-stain method†	86–89	83–96
Hay/Ison Gram-stain method†	94	93
Detection of amines in vaginal fluid†	79–87	76–95

* Providing sample not contaminated with blood or seminal fluid.
† Compared with Amsel criteria (on premise they are most accurate method for diagnosing BV).

Frequently asked questions

Can I prevent it from coming back?

♀ who suffer from recurrent BV can be treated with episodic, anticipatory, or cyclical metronidazole or clindamycin. As BV is associated with a high vaginal pH it is advisable to try to keep it low to prevent recurrences. This can be done by decreasing menstruation e.g. with depo-provera or using acetic acid vaginal jelly. If a ♀ has an IUD and suffers from recurrent or persistent BV it may be advisable to remove the IUD and to try another method of contraception.

Is it the cause of my abdominal pain?

Usually not on its own. However, BV is associated with PID especially when there is an IUD *in situ*. BV is also associated with post-abortion PID and post-hysterectomy vaginal cuff cellulitis.

Is it harmful in pregnancy?

BV is associated with an increased risk of preterm delivery. It is therefore recommended that ♀ with a history of a preterm delivery are screened for BV during pregnancy and treated if positive. It is not recommended that all pregnant ♀ are screened for BV, however, if a pregnant ♀ is found to have BV during routine testing e.g. for a symptomatic discharge, she should be treated. Meta analysis has shown that metronidazole is safe in pregnancy at all trimesters, though large doses are best avoided.

Management

Variations in vaginal bacterial flora are common and BV type features are often transient and self-limiting. Treatment is recommended for those with symptoms or clear signs of BV but generally not for asymptomatic BV or *G. vaginalis* colonization. Overall cure rates are ~95%.

- Metronidazole
  - Oral—400–500mg twice daily for 5–7 days; 2g as a single dose.
  - Intravaginal—0.75% gel 5g once daily for 5 days.
- Clindamycin
  - Oral—300mg twice daily for 7 days.
  - Intravaginal—2% cream 5g once daily for 7 days; 100mg ovule once daily for 3 days.
  - Tinidazole—2g oral as a single dose.

No indication for the epidemiological treatment of sexual partners.

In pregnancy

Caution is advised in the use of metronidazole during pregnancy and breast feeding with high-dose regimens avoided. However, meta-analyses have shown no evidence linking birth defects to the use of metronidazole in early pregnancy.

- Symptomatic ♀ should be treated (as if non-pregnant)
- ♀ with previous preterm birth or 2nd trimester miscarriage should be screened and treated systemically if found to have BV early in 2nd trimester. 5-day oral metronidazole treatment of choice. Review 1 month after treatment
- Clindamycin (both topical and oral) provided to asymptomatic pregnant ♀ with BV or an intermediate bacterial flora at 12–22 weeks' gestation has been shown to ↓ late miscarriage and spontaneous preterm birth rates (by up to 50%)

Persisting or recurrent BV

Eliminate possible factors that may influence the microbiological flora (e.g. douching, shampoos, spermicides, etc.).

Lack of evidence but consider the following:

- persistent:
  - change treatment (from metronidazole to clindamycin or vice-versa)
  - consider removing IUD if *in situ*
  - oral co-amoxiclav (amoxicillin 250mg + clavulanic acid 125mg) 375mg 3 times a day for 7 days, as possibility of resistance or metronidazole de-activation by other vaginal bacteria. May also be considered initially if metronidazole and clindamycin cannot be used.
- recurrent: 15–30% recur within 3 months, with ~50% relapsing once in next 7 years (70% of these during 1st year) commonly associated with a new sexual partner.

Following initial treatment mildly abnormal microscopy or elevated pH may be found suggesting relapse rather than re-infection.

If using IUD, remove and suggest alternative contraception. Consider method which reduces or stops menstrual flow (e.g. progesterone only preparation) to maintain low pH.

Episodic, anticipatory, pulse, suppressive, or cyclical treatment, using metronidazole or clindamycin, (if recurrences fall into a pattern).

- Other approaches:
  - 3% hydrogen peroxide single vaginal wash
  - lactobacillus replacement (no clear evidence of benefit)
  - agents lowering vaginal pH (e.g. lactic or acetic acid gel)—suggested in those with normal microscopy but ↑ vaginal pH. Can also be used in other situations which raise PH such as seminal fluid or menstrual blood in the vagina.

HIV infection

Acquisition and transmission ↑ with BV 2–5-fold.

Anaerobic and *G. vaginalis* associated balanitis/balanoposthitis

♂ partners of ♀ with BV are usually asymptomatic and unlikely to develop balanitis/balanoposthitis.

G. vaginalis can be found in 31% of those with a non-candidal balanoposthitis. Usually mild but may be foul smelling in association with anaerobes, especially *Bacteroides* spp. (commonly *B. melaninogenicus*). Normally found in those with underlying phimosis and poor hygiene. An offensive subpreputial discharge may occur with 2° erosions and preputial oedema. Usually resolves with advice on hygiene and the use of saline lavage although oral metronidazole is sometimes required. Clindamycin cream 2% twice daily or oral co-amoxiclav 375mg 3× a day for 1 week may also be used.

Chapter 15

Trichomoniasis

Introduction

Trichomonas vaginalis first described by Donné in 1836.

Aetiology

Flagellated protozoan of the order Trichomonadida parasitic to the human genitourinary tract. *T. vaginalis* (TV) is usually oval, measures up to 15μm in length *in vivo* (the size of a leucocyte). Propelled by four anterior flagella arising from an anterior kinetosomal complex. An additional 5th flagellum is attached to an undulating membrane that extends halfway down the organism and an axostyle projects from the end of the body. Trichomonads lack mitochondria but contain hydrogenosomes, large cytoplasmic granules involved in catabolism (Fig. 15.1 and Plate 8). Grows in a moist environment, at 35–37°C and a pH between 4.9 and 7.5. Multiplication is by mitosis occurring optimally every 8–12 hours and cysts are not produced.

Epidemiology and transmission

Common worldwide but steady decline in developed countries over the past 20 years. Reason unclear but may relate to standard cervical cytology screening which can also detect TV. Almost exclusively sexually transmitted from infected genital secretions.
The parasite can be found:
♀: vagina, cervix, urethra, bladder, and the ducts of Bartholin's and Skene's (periutheral) glands.
♂: anterior urethra, subpreputial sac, glans penis, prostate, epididymis, and semen.

Sexual transmission

- Most commonly found in ♀ during the most sexually active years (16–35 years) and in those more sexually active.
- Recognized association with other STIs (e.g. gonorrhoea).
- High rate of re-infection unless ♂ partners are treated (up to 70% carry the parasite).

Detection rates in ♂ contacts of infected ♀:

- sex within previous: 48 hours—70%, 5 days—40%,
- after 14 days—33%, 21 days—12%.

Detection rates in ♀ contacts of infected ♂: 67–100%.
♀ to ♀ sexual transmission is well recognized and may relate to the shared use of sex toys.

Non-sexual transmission

Protozoa may survive up to 45 minutes on toilet seats and for several hours in moist washclothes although transmission unlikely.

- Direct ♀ to ♀ transmission related to poor hygiene has been suggested but lacks evidence.
- Neonatal vulvo-vaginitis arising from infection acquired at delivery may arise but is rare (5% of those born to mothers with TV).

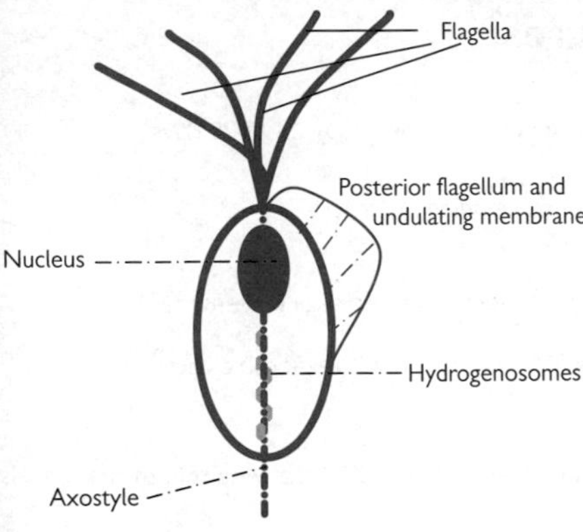

Fig. 15.1 *Trichomonas vaginalis*

Frequently asked questions

Is it always sexually transmitted?

Generally yes, although it has been suggested that transmission could occur through moist flannels which are shared.

How long has it been present?

Symptoms usually develop within 1 month of acquiring infection although up to 50% of ♀ are diagnosed without symptoms.

Does my boyfriend require treatment?

Yes. ♂ commonly carry *T. vaginalis* without any symptoms. Unless he is treated there is a high rate of re-infection.

Clinical features

Women

Incubation period (before symptoms develop)—4 to 28 days.

Symptoms

- 20–50% asymptomatic (depending on criteria)
- Vaginal discharge—56%
- Dysuria—18%
- Low abdominal pain (probably related to vaginitis)—up to 12%
- Vulval discomfort
- Vaginal malodour— ~50%, associated with anaerobic bacterial overgrowth.

Signs

- Frothy yellow vaginal discharge in 10–30%, otherwise thin/thick, scanty/profuse
- Vulvovaginitis
- 'Strawberry cervix' (colpitis macularis)—small punctate cervical haemorrhages with ulceration found in 2–5%
- Urethritis— ~25%
- No signs—5–15%
- Isolated case reports of detection from fallopian tubes (in salpingitis) and peritoneal fluid.

Complications

- Independent association in pregnancy with premature rupture of the membranes, preterm delivery and low birth weight.
- Association with cervical carcinoma but uncontrolled for other genital pathogens (e.g. human papilloma virus) therefore no proven causal relationship.

Spontaneous resolution occurs in 20–25%.

Men

- ~50% asymptomatic.
- Commonest feature: small to moderate urethral discharge—non-gonococcal urethritis (NGU). Trichomonal infection may be the cause in up to 15% of cases in high prevalent areas.
- Balanoposthitis: 4–11% (rarely with 2° ulceration).
- Prostatitis, epididymitis, cystitis alleged but probably due to other associated infection.
- Isolated case reports associated with penile ulceration and median raphe suppuration.

Diagnosis

Direct microscopy

Vaginal discharge examined as an isotonic saline suspension by dark ground or phase contrast microscopy. Readily recognizable motile protozoa propelled by flagella and undulating membrane but must be examined immediately otherwise 20% failure within 10 minutes (Fig. 15.1 and Plate 8). ♂ urethral discharge and subpreputial material can be examined in a similar fashion. Alternatively dried smears can be stained with acridine orange and viewed using fluorescent microscopy. This is more sensitive than using wet preparations.

In ♀ the overall sensitivity of microscopy ranges from 40 to 80% but in ♂ is only ~30%.

Culture

As well as vaginal, urethral, and subpreputial samples, a centrifuged deposit of 1st morning urine can also be tested by culture (especially useful for ♂). Ideally specimens should be placed in culture medium, e.g. Feinberg–Whittington. Otherwise forward in transport medium e.g. Amies' or Stuart's and inoculate in growth medium within 24 hours. Culture under partial or complete anaerobic conditions.

In ♀ the sensitivity of culture is ~95% and in ♂ 60–80% for urethral and urine samples but ↑ when combined.

Latex agglutination

Eluate prepared by agitating vaginal swab in phosphate buffered saline. One drop of material mixed with a drop of test latex on a black slide and rocked for 2 minutes. Agglutination of the test, but not control latex indicates TV antigen. Limited data but sensitivity ~99%, specificity ~92%.

Papanicolaou-stained cervical smears

TV is sometimes reported on cervical cytology. Although reasonably sensitive (60–80%) specificity varies and may be only ~70% so positive cases should be confirmed by microscopy or culture.

Polymerase chain reaction (PCR)

PCR tests are undergoing development with variable results although sensitivities and specificities up to 97% and 98% have been reported. Currently these are not available for routine use.

Management

- ►Sexual partners should be treated simultaneously and sexual intercourse avoided until treatment has been completed.
- If ♂ contacts present with NGU it is reasonable to treat initially as TV infection and review after treatment.
- Screening for other STIs for patients and their contacts is advised.
- Treatment should be systemic in view of the high rates of urethral and periurethral gland involvement.

Treatment

Oral metronidazole: 400–500mg twice daily for 5–7 days or 2g, 1 dose. The only effective agents are the 5-nitroimidazoles (overall cure rates ~95%) with metronidazole the most extensively used. If allergy reported consider metronidazole desensitisation (see Table 15.1 for schedule). Single dose has the advantage of ↑ adherence but has ↓ cure rate (by 6–12%), especially if partner(s) not treated simultaneously. Patients should be advised to avoid alcohol while taking treatment and for 48 hours thereafter because of a possible disulfiram-like (antabuse) reaction.

Although caution is advised in the use of metronidazole during pregnancy the manufacturers only warn against high-dose regimens (see p. 190).

Alternative 5-nitroimidazoles include tinidazole (2g orally as a single treatment)—have a longer half-life than metronidazole.

Treatment failure

- Non-adherence, re-infection, poor absorption (unusual).
- Low plasma zinc (unusual)—provide oral zinc supplement.
- 5-nitroimidazoles de-activation by vaginal bacteria. Both aerobes and anaerobes including β-haemolytic streptococci are implicated. If suspected treat with amoxicillin or erythromycin in addition to 5-nitroimidazole.
- Resistance (usually but not always to all 5-nitroimidazoles). Testing should be under aerobic conditions, but is not readily available, however, data suggests that repeat treatment failures are invariably resistant. There are no reliable alternatives to 5-nitroimidazoles.

Treatment options to consider in resistant cases

- Enhanced oral metronidazole: e.g. 400mg 3 times daily for 7–10 days or 2g daily for 3–5 days with oral amoxicillin 250mg 3 times daily, or oral erythromycin 250mg 4 times daily, both for 5–7 days.
- Other azole products e.g. tinidazole up to 2g twice daily, (+/– vaginal tinidazole tablets) +/– amoxicillin/erythromycin +/– clotrimazole 500mg pessary daily, all for 14 days.
- High dose oral or intravenous metronidazole (up to 3–3.5g per day for up to 14 days.) +/– amoxicillin/erythromycin for 14 days +/– clotrimazole 500mg pessary daily for 14 days.
- High dose oral metronidazole with intravaginal metronidazole 1g daily for ≥7 days, or metronidazole rectal suppository 1g daily for ≥7 days, or vaginal douches—zinc sulphate 1% or 3% acetic acid.
- 6% nonoxynol-9 pessaries (prolonged treatment for up to 7 months)

- Acetarsol pessaries 500mg daily for 10–14 days.
- Paromomycin sulfate pessaries 250mg once or twice daily for 14 days.

Table 15.1 Desensitisation schedule for metronidazolea

Dose	Metronidazole	Contained in amount
5μg IV	5μg/mL	1mL
15μg IV	5μg/mL	3mL
50μg IV	50μg/mL	1mL
150μg IV	50μg/mL	3mL
500μg IV	500μg/mL	1mL
1.5mg IV	500μg/mL	3mL
5mg IV	5mg/mL	1mL
15mg IV	5mg/mL	3mL
30mg IV	5mg/mL	6mL
60mg IV	5mg/mL	12mL
125mg IV	5mg/mL	25mL
250mg Oral	One 250mg tablet	—
500mg Oral	One 500mg tablet	—
2g Oral	Four 500mg tablets	—

Require continuous surveillance with emergency resuscitation available.
Intravenous increments are administered at 15–20 min intervals with oral doses given 1 hour apart.

Source: Reprinted from Pearlman *et al. Am J Obstet Gynecol*, **174**, 934–6 (1996). With permission from Elsevier.

Trichomoniasis and HIV infection

HIV acquisition is associated with TV, probably related to genital inflammation

Chapter 16

Genital candidiasis

Introduction

Also referred to as candidosis, moniliasis, or thrush. This is considered as pathogenic activity by commensal yeasts in individuals with reduced local or systemic resistance. Association with vaginitis first described in 1849 although oral thrush recognized in the 4th century BC.

Aetiology

Candida spp., especially *Candida albicans* responsible for 85–90% of infections and *Candida glabrata* 3–15%. Other yeasts rarely implicated include *C. tropicalis* (~4%), *C. parapsilosis* (~4%), *C. krusei* (~2%), *C. stellatoidea and C. gulliermondi*. Occasional cases of vaginitis reported include *Saccharomyces cerevisiae*, a yeast from the family *Cryptococcaceae* (to which *Candida* also belongs) and *C. dubliniensis*.

All pathogenic *Candida* spp. multiply by the production of buds from a blastospore (yeast cell), approximately 1–5.0μm in diameter.

C. albicans produces:

- hyphae—long tubes made up of multiple cell units divided by septa arising from blastospores or as branches of existing hyphae
- pseudohyphae—single elongated cells from blastospore buds with constrictions instead of septa. Each generation remains attached to its parent
- chlamydospores—large refractory bodies, with double-layered cell walls; probably a dormant phase

Mycelium is the entire yeast aggregate (spores, hyphae, and branches). *C. glabrata* does not produce hyphae or pseudohyphae.

Candida spp. contain their own set of virulence factors that may contribute to their ability to cause infection. They include surface molecules that facilitate mucosal adherence, proteases when there is mucositis, and the ability to convert into a hyphal form. *C. albicans* has the greatest ability to adhere and invade the mucosa, enhanced by the production of germ tubes (also useful in species identification), where it may form a reservoir for recurrences.

Epidemiology and transmission

75% of ♀ have at least one episode of genital candidiasis with 40–50% having one or more recurrences. It is much less common for ♂ to present with symptomatic infection. However, in GUM clinics *Candida* spp. colonization of the glans penis has been reported in 16% (unrelated to sexuality or the presence of a prepuce but associated with vaginal carriage in ♀ partners) with ~33% admitting to symptoms.

Candida spp. can be found anywhere on the body but most commonly in the mouth (30–55% of young adults), vagina (8–32% of young ♀, 40% if pregnant), and anorectal canal (40–65%). *C. albicans* accounts for 80–90% of genital yeast isolates and 60–80% of oral carriage although seldom recovered from normal skin (*C. parapsilosis* and *C. gulliermondi* being more prevalent).

Although penovaginal intercourse is a factor in the direct transmission of yeast infection its role is unclear, however it is generally accepted that without predisposing factors, ♂ usually acquire infection sexually. In ♀ it seems that coitus is more likely to act as a trigger by introducing perineal organisms and causing microtrauma breaching mucosal integrity. Hypothetically vaginal intercourse following anal penetration is more likely to introduce infection although there is no data to support this. However there does seem to be an association with recent cunnilingus. This may be by direct transmission, with saliva promoting pathogenesis by moistening and irritating the vulval mucosa and altering the local immunity. Non-specific genital infection and other STIs have been shown to be associated with yeast infection in 39% of ♀ and 29% of ♂.

Frequently asked questions

What is thrush?

It is an infection caused by a yeast, usually *Candida albicans. Candida* spp. commonly lives in small numbers in and around the genitals, especially the vagina. Asymptomatic until candida multiplies and penetrates the skin surface.

Is it sexually transmitted?

Usually not, especially in women. Partners do not need any treatment unless they have symptoms and signs of thrush themselves.

Predisposing factors

Reduction in local mucosal resistance

- Sexual contact causing micro-fissures.
- Inflammation (e.g. eczema related to contact irritants, other dermatoses, tight/non-absorbent clothing though evidence inconclusive).

Diabetes mellitus

Produces a glucose rich environment ideal for the growth of yeasts especially in poorly controlled diabetes. Associated with a 20% ↑ in oral colonization by *Candida* spp.

Hormonal

- Physiological—↑ oestrogen raises the amount of glycogen in the vagina and ↓ cell-mediated immunity and progesterone (also immunosuppressive and stimulates germ tube formation). Therefore, symptomatic candidiasis is uncommon before menarche and after the menopause. In the child-bearing years it is found most commonly:
  - in the luteal phase of the menstrual cycle
  - during pregnancy, especially the 3rd trimester (↑ vaginal glycogen and immunological factors). A large proportion of ♀ who subsequently present with recurrent vulvo-vaginal candidiasis (RVVC), first present with infection during pregnancy.
- Combined oral contraceptives—only associated with high dose oestrogen (50μg) preparations.
- Oestrogen replacement treatment—probable relative ↑.

Impaired immunity

Including HIV, drugs (e.g. corticosteroids, chemotherapeutic agents).

Broad-spectrum antibiotics

↑ vaginal yeast carriage by 10–30%. Although there is an association with candidiasis it is small and the vast majority of ♀ on antibiotic treatment are unaffected.

Other contraceptives

Conflicting evidence of an association with the use of spermicides (cidal effect on lactobacilli), diaphragms, and caps (causing re-infection) and intrauterine devices (IUDs). More likely carriage rather than disease.

Local factors

Lack of consistent evidence relating intimate hygiene practices or menstrual sanitation (use of external towels or pads) with genital candidiasis. Vaginal deodorants, disinfectants, and perfumed products may exacerbate candidiasis by causing dermatitis. No evidence to support re-infection by fomites such as underwear.

Chronic mucocutaneous candidiasis

Characteristically involves skin folds, nails, skin in and around the mouth, and vulva/vagina. If present consider:

- anaemia
- auto-immune conditions, e.g.
  - Addison's disease
  - hypothyroidism
  - hypoparathyroidism
- thymomas.

► These conditions are not associated with simple genital candidiasis.

Clinical features

Women—acute vulvo-vaginitis (90% of presentations)

Symptoms: vulval pruritus, and burning, with external dysuria and dyspareunia being common. Usually start or worsen from mid-menstrual cycle, often improving with menstruation.
Signs: vulval erythema with fissuring is the most common finding. Usually localized to the vulval mucocutaneous margins but can spread to involve the labia majora, perineum, and perigenital skin where satellite lesions (small areas of erythema adjacent to but separate from the main body of inflammation), pathognomonic for candidiasis, may be seen. Vaginal erythema seen in 20% with a thick, white, curdy, adherent discharge in 20%, ↑ to 70% if pregnant, forming plaques on the vagina, cervix, and vulva. Discharge may be purulent or watery.

Women—recurrent vulvo-vaginal candidiasis

Definition: 4 or more episodes of symptomatic candidiasis annually.
Frequency: occurs in ~5% of ♀. Thought to be due to incomplete elimination of infection (usually identical strain), or inadequate treatment with a change in the protective vaginal mucosa cell mediated host defense mechanisms leading to relapses.

Other factors

- *Hypersensitivity*—probably important as shown by associations with perennial allergic rhinitis and a family history of allergies. Compared to ♀ with isolated episodes ♀ with RVVC cannot tolerate small numbers of yeast organisms.
- *Sex*—positive association between the monthly frequency of sexual intercourse and the incidence of RVVC. Asymptomatic penile colonization with *Candida* spp. occurs 4× more commonly in the partners of ♀ with candidiasis.

Clinical features

- *Recurrent candidiasis*—vulval pruritus with burning common but signs (erythema, oedema, fissures, white curdy discharge) are found less commonly than in acute cases.
- *Chronic, persistent candidiasis*—vulval lichenification and local oedema, more commonly found in older, obese diabetics.

Men

In colonized ♂ most common symptom is postcoital itching or burning. Clinically presents as:

- Direct infection with inflammation of glans (balanitis) and/or prepuce (posthitis). More common in the uncircumcised presenting as a glazed erythematous rash, sometimes with white papules/discharge, and if severe, fissuring, oedema, and 2° phimosis.
- Contact hypersensitivity reaction.
- Usually mild to moderate balanoposthitis within 24 hours of contact with vaginal candidiasis. Yeasts are often not detected from the penis.
- ~20% of ♂ contacts of ♀ with RVVC complain of soreness and irritation lasting for 24–48 hours starting shortly after intercourse.
- Rarely as non-gonococcal urethritis.

Diagnosis

Patient's self-assessment is not a reliable method of diagnosing candidiasis and only pruritus and objectively gauged signs are reliable clinical indicators.

Sampling

♀—specimens, using a plastic loop or swab, should be taken from any vaginal discharge and also the lateral vaginal walls. In addition, material can be taken from inflammatory areas on the vulva or surrounding skin.
♂—sampling for microscopy is more difficult and a variety of methods are used including dry or moistened swabs, plastic loops (which may also be moistened with normal saline), skin scrapings and a dry slide (or prepared with double-sided clear adhesive tape) pressed against the penis.

Laboratory culture

Gold standard. Genital specimens usually sent in transport medium (e.g. Amies, Feinberg–Whittington) and cultured on growth medium (e.g. Sabouraud). Culture allows speciation which may be important in the patient's management. Germ tube formation is used in the presumptive identification of *C. albicans* with an accuracy of 95–100%.

As yeasts are commensals, treatment is not required unless clinically indicated.

Direct microscopy

Pseudohyphae and/or spores (*C. glabrata* only produces spores) may be seen in vulvo-vaginal saline suspensions viewed as wet-mount preparations in 40–60% of women with symptomatic candidiasis. If 10–20% potassium hydroxide is used in the wet mount to lyse epithelial and blood cells the sensitivity ↑ by ~10%. Alternatively, vulvo-vaginal material examined by Gram-stain detects infection (Gram-positive spores/pseudohyphae) in ~65% of symptomatic cases (Plate 9).

Other investigations

Latex agglutination test: limited value. Sensitivity ~75%, specificity ~97%.
PCR: not routinely available, doubts about sensitivity and specificity.
Vaginal pH: remains normal at 4.0–4.5. A pH of >5 may suggest bacterial vaginosis (BV). *C. glabrata* grows at a higher pH than *C. albicans* and may be associated with BV.
Urinalysis: for sugar to exclude diabetes (especially ♂ and ♀ with RVVC).

Recurrent vulvo-vaginal candidiasis

Requires clinical examination, culture with speciation as *C. glabrata* (and also *C. krusei*) are more resistant to azoles, and consideration of underlying disease. Penile colonization with candida occurs in ~20% of the uncircumcised partners of ♀ with RVVC, usually with identical strains.

Important to exclude pregnancy, diabetes, and other risk factors e.g. immunodeficiency and repeated antibiotic or corticosteroid use.

Frequently asked questions

Why do I keep getting it?

Treatment of candidiasis may not eliminate it entirely from the vagina and so remaining spores/hyphae may multiply again when the conditions are right, and produce a recurrent attack of thrush. Certain situations make thrush more likely e.g. pregnancy, diabetes, immunosuppression, corticosteroids, and antibiotics. Avoid precipitants and irritants such as bubble baths, perfumed soaps, vaginal douching, and tight fitting synthetic underwear. About 5–10% of cases are due to *C. glabrata*, which may be resistant to azoles but should respond to nystatin pessaries.

Is there anything that I can take to prevent it from coming back?

Recurrent thrush is defined as 4 or more symptomatic episodes in a year. Some people seem to go through phases of recurrences which is probably because of incomplete eradication. A longer course of topical or oral therapy may help. Women with frequent episodes can try prophylactic treatment such as clotrimazole 500mg pessary weekly or oral fluconazole 100mg weekly for up to 6 months. Thrush is associated with recent cunninglingus, therefore avoidance may prevent recurrence.

Does my pill make my thrush worse?

The usual type of contraceptive pill prescribed contains low levels of oestrogen and is not related to ↑ rate of thrush.

Do I need to go on a yeast free diet?

There is no evidence that yeast free diets make any difference to vaginal thrush infections. Studies to eliminate *Candida* spp. from the gut using long-term oral medication have shown that recurrent vaginal thrush is not prevented.

I am pregnant is thrush harmful to my baby?

Thrush is more common in pregnancy. Asymptomatic colonization rates are higher and symptomatic episodes are more common in pregnancy. Thrush can be treated with topical azoles in pregnancy but oral preparations are contraindicated. There is no evidence that colonization with candida in pregnancy affects pregnancy outcome.

Does yoghurt help?

Probably not, but we're not sure. Intravaginal use (by applicator or on a tampon) has been tried with varying degrees of success although it may just sooth irritation. Daily oral ingestion of 8 ounces of active yoghurt has been shown to decrease both candidal colonization and infection although this has not been confirmed in other studies.

Management

Acute vulvo-vaginitis: principles—see Box for drugs

General—bathing in saline or sodium bicarbonate may provide symptomatic relief and if severe, analgesics (e.g. non-steroidal anti-inflammatory drugs) are beneficial.

Little difference in efficacy between the drugs available and their route of administration, though to aid compliance short duration treatments are favoured. Therefore, azole therapies are preferred with a 80–95% clinical and mycological cure rate in acute candidiasis (if non-pregnant). Cure rates for nystatin are slightly lower (70–90%). Oral treatments are contraindicated if pregnant or lactating. If severe, creams may be preferred as they are more soothing than pessaries. They may also produce a more prompt relief of symptoms than oral treatment. Nystatin stains the underwear yellow. Although candidal vulvitis can be treated locally with cream, it is almost always associated with vaginal infection which should also be treated.

► Topical preparations may damage latex in condoms or diaphragms.

If the candidiasis is 2° to dermatitis or there appears to be a hypersensitivity reaction, an antimycotic/hydrocortisone combination should be considered.

Unless symptomatic no action is required for ♂ partners.

Balanoposthitis: principles—see Box for drugs

Mild cases will respond to simple saline lavage. Moderate or severe inflammation usually requires antimycotic treatment commonly prescribed as a cream although similar results are achieved with oral azoles. Consider hydrocortisone containing topical combinations if underlying dermatitis or hypersensitivity.

♀ Sexual partners should be offered screening ± epidemiological treatment.

Drug resistance

~50% of all *C. glabrata* strains have ↓ sensitivity to azoles and there are ↑ levels of resistance with *Saccharomyces cerevisiae* and *C. krusei* (intrinsic resistance to fluconazole). Polyene resistance is rare.

Standard antimycotics for acute genital candidiasis

Available in the UK

Azoles

Intravaginal

- Clotrimazole:
  - pessary—500mg single dose, 200mg for 3 nights, 100mg for 6 nights.
  - cream—10% as a single 5g intravaginal dose.
- Econazole: pessary—150mg single dose or 150mg for 3 nights.
- Miconazole:
  - pessary—100mg for 14 nights (or 200mg for 7 nights).
  - ovule 1.2g single dose.
  - cream—2% 5g dose (in applicator) daily for 10–14 days or twice daily for 7 days.
- Fenticonazole: pessary 200mg for 3 nights (or 600mg single dose).

External

- Clotrimazole cream: 1% and 2%—2–3 times a day.
- Econazole nitrate cream: 1%—twice a day.
- Ketoconazole cream: 2% once or twice a day.
- Miconazole nitrate cream: 2% twice a day.

Oral ► (avoid in pregnancy or breast feeding)

- Fluconazole 150mg as a single dose.
- Itraconazole 200mg twice daily for 1 day.

⚠ Avoid terfenadine as risk of arrhythmias.

Polyenes

Intravaginal

Nystatin:

- pessary—100,000U as single or double dose for 10–14 nights.
- cream—100,000U/4g application for 14 nights.

External

Nystatin cream: 100,000U/g—2–4 times a day.

Topical combinations with hydrocortisone

Canesten HC—clotrimazole 1% + hydrocortisone 1% cream.
Daktacort—miconazole nitrate 2% + hydrocortisone 1% cream.
Econacort—econazole nitrate 1% + hydrocortisone 1% cream.
Nystaform-HC—nystatin 100,000U + hydrocortisone 0.5% cream.

Azoles not available in the UK

Butaconazole: 2% cream—5g daily for 3 days, intravaginal.

- Terconazole:
  - 0.4% cream—5g for 7 days, intravaginal.
  - 0.8% cream—5g for 3 days intravaginal.
  - pessary—80mg pessary for 3 nights.
- Tioconazole:
  - 6.5% ointment—5g single dose, intravaginal.

Management of recurrent vulvo-vaginal candidiasis

Induction Topical treatment for 7–14 days or oral fluconazole 50mg daily (or 150mg every 3rd day for 3 doses). If azole resistance suspected use nystatin.

Maintenance

If regular a pattern is followed, consider maintenance treatment, usually for 6 months initially, e.g.:

- fluconazole: 100mg oral weekly
- itraconazole: 400mg oral monthly
- clotrimazole 500mg pessary weekly
- ketoconazole 100mg daily (risk of hepatotoxicity)
- nystatin pessaries 100,000U can also be considered in resistant cases though there is no data on regimens.

During maintenance 90% remain free from symptomatic recurrences, however, they may occur in 30–40% of ♀ after cessation.

No evidence of ↓ recurrences by:

- Routinely treating asymptomatic ♂ partners. However, limited data suggests treatment benefit if ♂ are colonized (systemic route advocated because of the possibility of oral reservoir of infection).
- Reducing intestinal colonization (e.g. with oral nystatin).
- Zinc supplements (no evidence of association with zinc deficiency).
- Special cleaning of underwear.

Other medications

To consider if persistence encountered (unlicensed preparations):

- Boric acid—600mg vaginally as a gelatin capsule once or twice daily for 10–14 days has shown promising results with mycological cure rates of around 75% for *C. glabrata*. A 300mg dose is suggested if mucositis develops. Contraindicated in pregnancy. Although maintenance has been used (twice a week or for the 5 days during menstruation) data are limited and because of potential toxicity nystatin pessaries are advocated.
- Flucytosine and/or amphotericin in cream or KY jelly for vaginal insertion.
- Gentian violet 1% solution—used widely in the past as a vulval and intravaginal paint but messy, may cause irritation and associated with hepatocellular carcinoma in mice.

Other approaches

- Self-help measures: avoid products that may cause vulval irritation (e.g. vaginal deodorants, perfumed preparations) and wear loose cotton underwear. Avoid douching.
- Desensitization: studies have shown a significant reduction in the frequency of RVVC following immunotherapy with *C. albicans* extract. There is also limited data suggesting that zafirlukast, a leukotriene receptor antagonist may be beneficial.
- Change from combined to progesterone only contraception: limited data.

- Complementary treatment
  - Vaginal or oral lactobacilli are of no value in preventing post-antibiotic candidal vulvo-vaginitis.
  - Yoghurt and milk containing *Lactobacillus acidophilus*—intravaginal use (by applicator or on a tampon) has been tried with varying purported degrees of success. Daily oral ingestion of 8 ounces of yoghurt containing *L. acidophilus* has been shown to ↓ both candidal colonization and infection (not confirmed in other studies).
  - Reduce pH: acetic acid, gel, lactic acid, and vinegar washes (no clear evidence of benefit).
  - Tea tree oil: on a tampon or towel (frequently causes severe allergic reactions).
  - Others: e.g. topical calendula (cream, gel, or pessary), garlic clove wrapped in gauze and inserted into the vagina overnight. Lack of scientific data for benefit.

Candidiasis and HIV infection

- Carriage rates ↑: *C. albicans*—vagina (75–85%), oropharynx (90–95%).
- Although vaginitis due to *Candida* spp. is more common and persistent in ♀ with HIV infection, it is clinically similar to that found in HIV –ve ♀ and can be treated with conventional therapy.
- Recurrent infection is not in itself an indicator of HIV infection.
- In AIDS, ↑ colonization with fluconazole resistant *Candida* spp.

Chapter 17

Tropical genital and sexually acquired infections

Chancroid

Aetiology: *Haemophilus ducreyi*

Small Gram-negative coccobacillus occurring in chains. Culture requires blood enriched medium incubated in an atmosphere of 5–10% carbon dioxide. Most clinical isolates are β-lactamase producers.

Epidemiology and transmission

Highest incidence found in tropical and subtropical countries (especially Africa, S.W. Asia, S. America, Caribbean) with occasional outbreaks in temperate climates. Most common cause of genital ulcer disease (GUD) in developing countries and accounts for 10–30% STIs in Africa.

Sexually transmitted (including oral sex) but also auto-inoculated especially locally by fingers. Infection rate following single exposure from ♂ to ♀ ~60%. Carriage of *H. ducreyi* without symptoms or signs has been reported in prostitutes who may be an important reservoir infection. No evidence of congenital or perinatal transmission.

Associated with: the prepuce (uncircumcised twice as susceptible), prostitution, crack cocaine use (in USA), HIV infection (GUD enhances the transmission of HIV).

Clinical features

Incubation period: 3–7 days (range 1–14 days).

Initial tender red papule which progresses to a pustule forming 1–3 tender ulcers after 2–3 days. Multiple ulcers are common, facilitated by auto-inoculation—'kissing' lesions (Plate 10). Usually 1–2cm in diameter, irregular margins, bleeding on touch, non-indurated ('soft chancre or sore'). May coalesce into giant ulcers. Main features:

- ♂: prepuce (may cause phimosis), coronal sulcus, frenum, anus (homosexuals)
- ♀: vulva, vagina, perianal area, rarely cervix
- extragenital: very unusual (fingers, breasts, conjunctivae)
- inguinal lymphadenopathy: usually unilateral occurring in ~50% as a tender swelling which may develop into a unilocular abscess (bubo) in 25%.

Disseminated infection not reported.

Complications: bacterial superinfection with tissue destruction (phagedenic chancroid); chronic suppurative inguinal sinuses.

Diagnosis

Microscopy: sensitivity 62%, specificity 99%. Smear from cleaned ulcer or bubo by rolling the swab through 180° on the slide and stain with Gram-stain. Typically small Gram-positive rods running in parallel and forming chains, 'shoals of fish' seen (unreliable due to bacterial contamination).

Culture: standard diagnostic tool but only 75% sensitive from ulcer swabs (pus aspirated from intact bubo almost always sterile).

EIA and PCR: still under commercial development.

Management

- Oral ciprofloxacin 500mg twice daily for 3 days (no effect against treponemes therefore will not mask developing syphilis).
- Oral azithromycin 1g single dose.
- IM ceftriaxone 250mg single dose.
- Oral erythromycin 500mg 4 times a day for 7 days.

Fluctuant buboes should be aspirated (by needle).

Partner notification: sexual contacts within 10 days of disease onset should be examined and given epidemiological treatment as for a clinical case.

Other non-sexually transmitted infections (mostly tropical), which may affect the genitalia

- Schistosomiasis (*Schistosoma haematobium*): from swimming in fresh water lakes in Africa (e.g. Lake Malawi). Usual urinary symptoms include dysuria and haematuria. Other features:
  - urethritis, lumpy semen, haematospermia;
  - friable polyps and ulcers of cervix, vagina, and vulva;
  - groin/scrotal cutanea tarda.
- Bancroftian filariasis (E. Africa): spermatic cord inflammation (funiculitis), hydrocele, scrotal, and vulval elephantiasis.
- Onchocerciasis (tropical Africa, Central and S. America): itchy papules and nodules around genitalia similar to scabies.
- Guinea worm infestation (dracunculiasis)—remote parts of Africa, especially Sudan: presents as a blister from which the worm's head protrudes. Usually affects lower limbs but may involve the scrotum.
- Amoebiasis (*Entamoeba histolytica*), especially Africa, Asia, Central, and S. America: perianal, cervical, and penile ulceration especially in homosexuals.
- Leishmaniasis (Middle East, Indian subcontinent): genital ulceration and annular perigenital skin lesions.
- Cutaneous larva migrans (dog hookworm), tropical, and subtropical countries: usually acquired from bare skin contact (e.g. nude sunbathing) with infected tropical beaches. Pruritic erythematous papules or tracts moving several millimetres a day may be seen affecting the glutei and genitalia.
- Myiasis (C. and S. America). Infestation by the larvae of certain fly species, e.g. *Dermatobia hominis* (botfly): may rarely affect healthy external genital tissue, especially the scrotum. Presents as a nodular inflammatory lesion.

Lymphogranuloma venereum (LGV)

Aetiology: L1, L2, L3 serovars of *Chlamydia trachomatis*

Primitive obligatory intracellular bacterium. (See p. 124).

Epidemiology and transmission

Main areas: Africa, India, Caribbean, Central America, S.E. Asia.

Usually sexually transmitted, almost always acquired in tropical and subtropical areas. Highest rates in 20–30 year age group and associated with prostitution, multiple sexual partners, other STIs, and social deprivation.

Since December 2003 outbreaks have been reported from West Europe in homosexual ♂ (mostly white and HIV positive). Associated with sexual networks in large cities especially if involved in 'party' and 'leather' scenes. Sexual practices reported include unprotected anal intercourse, oral contact, fisting, use of sex toys, and use of urine and faeces. Most have anorectal symptoms or proctitis although asymptomatic cases have been found.

Congenital infection does not occur but perinatal infection may be acquired from birth canal.

Clinical features

1° LGV: Incubation period—3–30 days.

Small papule at site of infection progressing to a pustule and asymptomatic ulcer that heals without scarring. 1° lesion reported only by 20–50% of ♂ with 2° LGV. Sites involved include coronal sulcus, prepuce, glans, scrotum, vulva, vagina, cervix (cervicitis). Rarely causes urethritis in ♂. Oral lesions after oral sex have been reported.

2° LGV (inguinal syndrome): Usually 1–6 weeks (up to 6 months) after 1° infection.

In ♂ usual presentation is unilateral lymphadenopathy (~70%). Only 20–30% of ♀ with LGV develop inguinal lymphadenopathy as lesions from the posterior vulva, anus, and vagina drain to perirectal or pelvic nodes. Femoral nodes may also be involved (20%) and the 'groove sign' (enlargement of nodes above and below the inguinal ligament) found in 15–33%. Lymphadenopathy progressing to multilocular abscesses (buboes) occur in ~33% which may rupture producing sinuses. Otherwise, they involute forming firm inguinal masses.

Associated constitutional features include fever, arthritis, aseptic meningitis, hepatitis, perihepatitis, pneumonia, erythema multiforme, and erythema nodosum.

3° LGV (anorectal syndrome): Usually seen in ♀ and homosexual ♂ because of lymphatic drainage from initial infection site. Proctocolitis and lymphorrhoids (hyperplasia of perirectal lymphatic tissue) produce anal discharge with bleeding, rectal pain, tenesmus, fever, and malaise. Chronic infection leads to perirectal fistulae, abscesses, strictures, and scarring. Destructive sclerosing lymphangitis, and oedema of external genitalia (esthiomène—Greek: 'eaten away') may occur with penile and scrotal oedema causing distortion which may produce the 'saxophone penis'.

Complications
Genital lymphoedema (elephantiasis), suppurative fistulae and sinuses, rectal strictures leading to intestinal obstruction, rectal carcinoma.

Diagnosis

- Cell culture: sensitivity ~80% sensitive from ulcer, ~30% bubo pus.
- LGV complement fixation test (response usually in first 4 weeks): 4-fold antibody ↑ or titre ≥1:64 with clinical features considered diagnostic.
- Nucleic acid amplification test. Currently unlicensed and non-validated for anorectal and oropharyngeal specimens although most sensitive method. Positives should be confirmed using another test, which utilizes a different target and genotyped for L1, L2, or L3.

Management

- Oral doxycycline 100mg twice daily for 3 weeks.
- Erythromycin 500mg 4 times a day for 3 weeks.
- Repeat needle aspiration of buboes may be required.

As buboes are multilocular surgical incision of fluctuant glands is contraindicated. Surgery may be required for late manifestations.

Partner notification: sexual contacts within 30 days of disease onset should be assessed and offered treatment as for clinical cases.

Granuloma inguinale (Donovanosis)

Aetiology—*Klebsiella (Calymmatobacterium) granulomatosis*

Human parasite (no animal model). Gram-negative pleomorphic bacterium with a well-defined capsule, 1–1.5μm in length and 0.6μm in width.

Epidemiology and transmission

Main areas: Western New Guinea, S. Africa, Caribbean, southern India, Brazil, S.E. Asia, aboriginal Australia.

Infection routes unclear. Sexual transmission, especially anal intercourse, most likely but accidental inoculation from skin contact and faecal contamination possible.

In support of STI origin

- Most commonly affects sexually active adults aged <30 years.
- Genital infection usual (including cervix as sole site, anus with receptive intercourse).
- Associated with concurrent STIs including HIV.

Against STI origin

- Occurs in young children (allegedly from sitting on lap of infected adult) and the sexually inactive.
- Relatively uncommon in sex workers.
- Rare in partners of those with open lesions.
- An outbreak linked to a healthcare professional.

Clinical features

Incubation period: uncertain (1–360 days), probably ~50 days.

Predilection for moist mucocutaneous and mucous surfaces with external genital involvement in 90%, cervix in 10%, inguinal area (including mons pubis) in 10%, extragenital, usually anal and oral, in 6%.

Starts as a firm pruritic papule or nodule (diameter 5–20mm) that ulcerates. Typically granulomatous, beefy-red, painless, and haemorrhagic (Plate 11). May become necrotic and locally destructive. Less commonly hypertrophic verrucous lesions, resembling warts and dry ulcers followed by scarring.

Lesions gradually spread locally with destruction of genital tissue and a relapsing course. Mean duration ~18 months.

No regional lymphadenopathy (unless there is 2° bacterial infection). Haematogenous spread to bone, liver, and spleen rare.

Complications: include lymphatic genital oedema (elephantiasis) in 15–20%, stenosis (anus, urethra, vagina) and local skin malignancy.

Diagnosis

- Biopsy from lesion stained with Giemsa stain. Intracellular Donovan bodies (bipolar, 'closed safety pin' like organisms) within mononuclear leucocytes.
- Other methods reported include cell culture and PCR but not readily available.

Management

- Oral azithromycin 1g weekly for 4–6 weeks or 500mg daily for 7 days.
- Oral co-trimoxazole 960mg twice daily, doxycycline 100mg twice daily, ciprofloxacin 750mg twice daily (all minimum of 3 weeks or until lesions healed).

Pregnancy: Oral erythromycin 500mg 4 times daily (minimum 3 weeks or until lesions healed) and caesarean section if active cervical lesions (which may complicate delivery).

Partner notification: sexual contacts within 40 days of disease onset should be assessed and offered treatment as for a clinical case.

HIV infection

Associated with:

- chancroid, especially in sub-Saharan Africa;
- outbreaks of anorectal LGV in homosexual ♂ (W. Europe).

Chapter 18

Endemic treponematoses

Introduction

Important differential diagnosis of reactive syphilis serology in those coming from countries where such infections are found. Current available tests cannot distinguish them from venereal syphilis. Identification of scars from old healed lesions may aid diagnosis. However, if there is doubt about the possibility of underlying syphilis or active non-venereal treponematosis, the patient should be fully treated for syphilis.

There are close similarities to syphilis; initial lesions, 2° development, latency, and asymptomatic infection. However, transmission is by close, non-sexual body contact. Found more commonly in remote areas with limited healthcare and associated with poor hygiene. Worldwide prevalence has ↓ since 1952 with global control programmes reinforced in the 1980s.

Yaws

- Causative organism: *Treponema pertenue*.
- Areas found: humid, warm tropical areas of Africa, S. America, the Caribbean, S.E. Asia.
- Transmission: direct contact with infectious lesions, especially in children. No vertical transmission.
- Clinical features:
  - 1° lesion: proliferative papilloma, often ulcerating, at site of infection usually healing after 3–6 months with a scar. Found most commonly on legs.
  - 2° yaws: rashes and mucosal lesions similar to 2° syphilis. Tender plaques on soles. Relapses common in first 5 years but skin lesions heal without scarring. Painful (especially at night) osteoperiostitis with development of sabre tibia.
  - Late yaws: gummatous skin lesions, hyperkeratosis, juxta-articular nodules, nasal and palatal collapse from underlying tissue destruction (gangosa). No cardiovascular and neurological sequelae.

Pinta

- Causative organism: *Treponema carateum*.
- Areas found: warm, semi-arid areas of central and northern S. America.
- Transmission: direct skin contact, especially in children. No vertical transmission.
- Clinical features:
  - 1°: initial papule that may form a plaque, especially affecting limbs, with local lymphadenopathy.
  - 2°: widespread coloured skin rashes and papules with generalized lymphadenopathy, sometimes persisting for years.
  - Late: patchy altered skin pigmentation (hyperpigmentation and leukoderma) with pruritus and skin atrophy. No neurological or cardiovascular involvement.

Endemic syphilis (Bejel)

- Causative organism: *Treponema endemicum*.
- Areas found: hot, dry countries (e.g. Arabian peninsula and Saharan/sub-Saharan Africa).
- Transmission: skin contact, the use of shared eating and drinking utensils, especially in children. No vertical transmission.
- Clinical features:
  - 1°: rarely seen (mucous patches in mouth most common site).
  - 2°: mucocutaneous papules around mouth and genitalia, condylomata lata, painful osteoperiostitis.
  - Late: nasal and palate collapse because of underlying bone and cartilage destruction, skin gummata, periostitis. No neurological or cardiovascular involvement.

Management of endemic treponematoses

IM benzathine penicillin 1.2g as a single dose to patient and contacts, with children <10 years given 600mg, is curative although scars may remain. Alternatives include tetracyclines and erythromycin.

Chapter 19

Proctocolitis and enteric sexually acquired infections

Related to penetrative anorectal intercourse and analingus. Unusual and although found in ♀ most arise in homosexual/bisexual ♂.

No infection demonstrable

- Acute anorectal symptoms related to penoanal intercourse or the insertion of a fist, forearm, or foreign body. May lead to:
  - prolapsed haemorrhoids
  - fissures, ulcers, tears, and rectal perforation
  - retained foreign bodies.
- Chronic symptoms (non-specific proctitis).

Possibly related to recurrent trauma associated with rectal coitus and associated with an 8 fold ↑ in HIV infection.

Infections usually sexually transmitted

- *Neisseria gonorrhoeae* (p. 112)
- *Chlamydia trachomatis* (p. 126)
- *Treponema pallidum* (p. 94)
- Herpes simplex virus (p. 240)
- Tropical STIs—chancroid, lymphogranuloma venereum (recent outbreaks in homosexual men in W. Europe), and granuloma inguinale (see Chapter 17, pp. 215–22).

► Consider empirical treatment for *N. gonorrhoeae* and *C. trachomatis* if suspected clinically.

Infections not usually sexually transmitted

Bacteria

Bacillary dysentery. *Shigella* spp. (usually *sonnei* and *flexneri*).
Usual spread: hand to mouth, fomites, water, and food. Outbreaks reported in homosexual ♂.

Incubation period 2–7 days. Apyrexial, frequent loose stools usually resolving in a week. Occasionally chronic proctocolitis develops. Reactive arthritis may complicate. Prepubertal ♀ may develop vaginitis, especially with *S. flexneri*.

Diagnosed by stool culture. Treated conservatively with bed rest, fluid replacement, and anti-motility drugs if necessary. Unless severe, antibiotics should be avoided to ↓ risk of resistance.

Campylobacter infection. *Campylobacter* spp. (usually *jejuni*).
Usual spread: contaminated water, food, and milk. In homosexual ♂ sporadic case reports and higher rates in those with proctocolitis (compared with asymptomatic controls).

Incubation period up to 10 days. Sudden diarrhoea with abdominal pain, malaise, pyrexia, muscle and joint pains. Usually resolves in 10 days. Reactive arthritis rarely complicates.

Diagnosed by stool culture and serology. No treatment unless severe, then oral erythromycin 500mg twice daily for 5 days.

Helicobacter pylori infection

It has been suggested that *H. pylori* may be transmitted by the ingestion of infected vomit and regurgitated food that may occur during sexual contact, although there is no firm evidence 💣.

Protozoa

Cryptosporidiosis. Cryptosporidium spp. (usually *parvum*)

Usual spread: Usually oral–faecal (in poor social conditions), by water or animal contact. Symptomatic disease more commonly associated with HIV infection, where outbreaks occur. Sporadic cases in immunocompetent homosexual ♂, associated with multiple contacts (especially at sex venues) and insertive anal sex.

Offensive watery diarrhoea with abdominal pain, low-grade pyrexia, anorexia and vomiting, which spontaneously resolve in 1–3 weeks.

Diagnosed by detecting oocysts in faecal samples. No specific treatment, but anti-motility drugs as required.

Giardiasis. *Giardia duodenalis (intestinalis, lamblia)*

Usual spread: water or food contaminated with faecal material. Sexual transmission recognized especially in homosexual ♂ but no ↑ risk with HIV infection.

Incubation period 12–19 days. Sudden onset of foul-smelling diarrhoea, abdominal pain, and distension. Stools float due to steatorrhoea with malabsorption contributing to weight loss. Symptoms resolve in 3 months.

Diagnosed by detecting cysts in stool samples by microscopy or enzyme immunoassay. Jejunal biopsy if clinical suspicion with negative stools.

Treatment: oral metronidazole 2g daily for 3 days, oral mepacrine hydrochloride 100mg 3 times a day for 7 days.

Amoebiasis. *Entamoeba histolytica*

Usual spread: from faecally contaminated water and food (infecting about 10% of the world's population). The non-pathogenic strain, reclassified as *Entamoeba dispar*, is commonly found in faeces of homosexual ♂.

~90% are asymptomatic. Symptoms include bloody diarrhoea, abdominal discomfort, weight loss, and fever with colitis in ~20%. Invasive disease includes hepatic abscess and granulating ulceration around the anus and genitalia but is rare in homosexual ♂.

Diagnosed by detecting trophozoites and cysts on faecal microscopy, stool culture, and serology (for invasive disease). Immediate treatment indicated for invasive disease: oral metronidazole 800mg 3 times a day for 5 days (for trophozoites) followed by oral diloxanide furoate 500mg 4 times a day for 10 days. Hepatic abscesses may require aspiration if large.

Nematodes

Threadworms. *Enterobius vermicularis*
Usual spread: by food or fomites contaminated by ova (especially in children). Associated with analingus in homosexual ♂. Rarely causes vaginal infection in prepubertal girls.

Cause pruritus ani (or vulvo-vaginitis in young girls).

Diagnosed by seeing the adult worm in the anal canal or detecting ova from the perianal skin by microscopy using material collected on transparent adhesive tape.Treatment: oral mebendazole single 100mg dose or oral piperazine, single 4g dose repeated in 14 days. Neither treatment is advised in pregnancy.

Strongyloides stercoralis infection
Reports of detection in faeces of homosexual ♂ STI clinic attenders (probably sexually transmitted).

Chapter 20

Urinary tract infection

Aetiology

Considerable geographical variation in cause but predominant organism is *Escherichia coli* (up to 80%).

Data from UK 12-centre study for community acquired UTI in 1999

Escherichia coli—65.1%	*Pseudomonas* spp.—1.8%
Other coliforms—23.4%	Coagulase-negative staphylococci—1.5%
Proteus and *Morganella* spp.—4.6%	Group B streptococci—0.7%
Enterococci—2.4%	*Staphylococcus aureus*—0.5%

Source: From SP Barrett *et al. J Antimicrob Chemother* 1999, **44**: 359–65. With permission of Oxford University Press.

Bacterial factors

Some strains develop uropathogenic properties including adhesins (e.g. type 1 pili adhesive organelles), serum resistance and cytotoxins (e.g. haemolysins). These are important in overcoming host resistance in uncomplicated urinary tract infections (UTIs) and uropathogenic bacteria have been shown to remain in the bladder epithelium for weeks.

Resistant to the most commonly used antibiotics except for fluoroquinolones. Resistance patterns vary geographically but in the UK 98.9% of community acquired strains are sensitive to fluoroquinolones, 95.7% to co-amoxiclav, 86.8% to nitrofurantoin, 77.4% to cefalexin, 75.6% to trimethoprim, and 51.7% to amoxicillin. Before prescribing, it is important to be aware of local sensitivity patterns.

Women

Host factors with recurrent UTIs (25–35% aged 20–40 years have history of UTI):

- maternal history of UTI
- the use of spermicides alone and with diaphragms (↑ local *E. coli* colonization)
- a shorter distance between urethra and anus (but on average only 0.2cm shorter than controls)
- new sexual partner during the past year
- UTI before the age of 15 years
- sexual activity (coitus >4 times a month)
- non-secretors of blood group antigens and oestrogen deficiency (peri- and postmenopausal ♀)
- diabetes mellitus

Factors **not** implicated in ♀ include:

- voiding habits (e.g. pre- and postcoital micturition)
- lifetime number of sexual partners
- sexually transmitted infections
- personal hygiene (e.g. wiping back to front, tampon use, douching, type of underwear)
- bacterial vaginosis

Acute uncomplicated cystitis

Usually sudden onset of dysuria, ↑ frequency and urgency of micturition and suprapubic or low back pain. Fever, rigor, malaise, loin pain, and vomiting suggest pyelonephritis.

Dysuria alone may indicate urethritis (e.g. by *Chlamydia trachomatis*, *Neisseria gonorrhoeae*, herpes simplex virus) or vulvo-vaginitis (e.g. by *Candida* spp., *Trichomonas vaginalis*).

Chronic urethral syndrome

Recurrent irritative urinary symptoms without pyuria and $>10^2$ bacteria/mL in urine culture.

Associated with previous pelvic and urethral trauma during obstetric or gynaecological procedures (e.g. grand multiparity, delivery without episiotomy, ≥2 abortions).

Men

UTIs: uncommon in ♂ <50 years old but ↑ thereafter as a result of incomplete bladder emptying 2° to prostatism.

In younger ♂, possible underlying urological abnormality but uncomplicated infection (usually cystitis) probably related to uropathogenic strains of *E. coli*. May present as an acute urethritis (purulent urethral discharge and dysuria).

- Risk factors include:
  - calculi and other foreign bodies
  - non-circumcision (enhanced colonization of the glans and subpreputial sac by *E. coli*).
- Others that have been suggested include:
  - anal sex and urethral exposure to coliforms
  - sexual partner with vagina colonized by uropathogens.

Diagnosis

- Clinical features.
- Urine dipstick testing showing leucocytes (leucocyte esterase component has 75–96% sensitivity in detecting infection associated pyuria), nitrites, protein, and often blood.
- Lab. culture (midstream sample of urine) $\geq 10^5$ colony forming units/ml (or less with 10–20 white blood cells/mm^3). UTI can be diagnosed with a count between 10^2–10^5 colony forming units/mL provided that a single organism is isolated and there is pyuria (20% of those diagnosed with UTI).

Management

- Push fluids
- Antibiotics: cefalexin 500mg twice daily, amoxicillin 250–500mg 3 times a day (or two 3g doses 12 hours apart), co-amoxiclav 250mg 3 times a day, nitrofurantoin 50mg 4 times a day, trimethoprim 200mg twice daily, ofloxacin 200–400mg daily (avoid the last two in pregnancy)
  - ♀: simple cystitis—although a 3 day course of antibiotics is widely used, recent data suggest that 5 and 7 day courses are more effective. If acute pyelonephritis—7–10 days.
  - ♂: 7–14 days antibiotics recommended, preferably lipid soluble, low protein bound antibiotics covering prostatic involvement e.g. trimethoprim and fluoroquinolones.
- Urological investigations in ♀ and young ♂ following isolated episode responding to antibiotics are usually unrewarding.

Recurrent UTIs

Prevention. If ≥3 episodes a year:

- self-administered standard treatment (at symptom onset)

- prophylactic low dose antibiotic (e.g. cefalexin 125mg, trimethoprim 100mg, nitrofurantoin 50mg)
    - daily or thrice weekly
    - postcoital if related to intercourse.

Cranberry juice: It has been suggested based on the premise that the hippuric acid contained acts as an antiseptic by reducing bacterial adherence. However, there is no consistent evidence that daily ingestion prevents UTIs and it is unpalatable for many.

Urology referral: (Ultrasound, radiology, cystoscopy) especially in ♂.

Pyuria with no or low bacterial counts

Consider:
Incorrect sampling (disinfectant contamination)
Bacterial infection not growing on standard medium (e.g. *C. trachomatis, N. gonorrhoeae, Mycobacterium tuberculosis*)
Foreign body (also important to consider in recurrent UTI)

- Indigenous
    - Calculi
    - Penetration from G/I tract into bladder (chicken/fish bones, swallowed needles and pins).
- Invasive
    - Parasitic catfish, *Vandellia cirrhosa* (found in the Amazon River) penetrates the urethra of bathers, especially if they urinate in the water (urinophilic organism), and clings to the urethral wall by spines from the gills and jaw.
- Inserted directly (more commonly found in ♂ following sexual activity, especially masturbation) and include:
    - metallic objects (needles, screws, wire)
    - writing implements (pencils, pens, ink cartridges)
    - animals/animal parts (snails, ants, dog penis, decapitated snake)
    - vegetable products (grasses and wood)
    - inserted into bladder via the vagina (usually in relation to masturbation)
    - cucumber, hair pin, wooden shoe tree.

Chapter 21

Anogenital herpes

Introduction

'Herpes' is named from ancient Greek 'to creep or crawl' with the typical spreading skin lesions described by Hippocrates.

Aetiology

Herpes simplex virus (HSV) type 1 and 2—a neurotropic virus, about 200nm in diameter, with a central DNA core covered by an icosahedral capsid and enveloped in a lipid membrane derived from host cell. Two viral types, HSV-1 (usually transmitted by contact with infected oro-labial mucosa) and HSV-2 (usually transmitted by contact with infected genital mucosa sexually or at delivery). HSV is readily inactivated at room temperature and drying therefore fomite and aerosol spread is unusual. Previous oral HSV-1 infection protects against genital HSV-1 but not HSV-2 disease although it reduces severity of 1st episode genital herpes and makes asymptomatic seroconversion more likely.

Terminology

- 1° infection—1st exposure to any type of HSV.
- Initial infection—1st infection by one HSV type. Either 1° (~50%) or non-1° if there has been exposure to other viral type (which may be detected serologically). Generally less severe symptoms if non-1°.
- Latency—dormant HSV in sensory (dorsal root) ganglia of nerves serving affected sites—sacral ganglia (S2–S5) for anogenital herpes (AGH).
- Reactivation—process unclear but precipitating factors include local nerve stimulation (e.g. by trauma, ultraviolet light) and immunosuppression by other infections such as HIV, drugs and malignancy. Persistent stress implicated but association with menstruation unclear.
- Recurrence—occurs when latent virus is reactivated, causing a peripheral lesion to appear.
- Asymptomatic viral shedding—reactivated HSV at nerve periphery without visible lesions. Viral shedding more common with HSV-2 (18–55%) compared with HSV-1 (10–29%). Occurs most commonly in 1st 6 months after infection (during a mean 6% of days) diminishing thereafter and falling by at least 66% after 10 years.

Epidemiology and transmission

HSV-1 antibodies (usually indicating oral infection) ↑ with age up to ~80%, (more common in low socio-economic groups). ↑ prevalence rate at adolescence suggests transmission by sexual contact. HSV-2 antibodies (usually indicating ano-genital infection) appear at puberty and correlate with sexual activity with a lifetime seroprevalence rate of 10–80% ↑ in ♀. <10% of those with HSV-2 antibodies recollect previous symptoms. Over the past 20 years there has been a disproportionate ↑ in HSV-1 as cause of initial AGH especially in young ♀, now with about 60–70% affected, but lower rates are found (35–45%) in ♂.

HSV-2 sexual transmission rate between discordant couples is about 10–15% per year (↑ from ♀ to ♂). Transmission follows direct skin contact rather than from genital fluids.

Frequently asked questions

How have I caught it if my partner does not have symptoms?
It is possible to be infected with HSV without knowing. Two out of three people who contract the virus catch it from someone who is asymptomatic. People who experience recurrent symptoms may also occasionally shed the virus asymptomatically as can those who have never had symptoms. It is also commonly acquired from the lips through oral sex.

Can I catch herpes from a toilet seat?
HSV can only survive for a short time away from the body. The virus may live for a short time on a wet towel and can theoretically be passed on this way. It is not thought possible to catch herpes from a toilet seat.

How often will I get an attack?
Some people have no further episodes after their primary attack, a few get frequent recurrences (i.e. >6 episodes per year). If the infection is due to HSV-2, 90% have a recurrence within the 1st year with the frequency of attacks related to the severity of the initial infection. Frequency of attacks tends to decrease in the 2nd and subsequent years. If the infection is due to HSV-1, 60% will have a recurrence within the 1st year with recurrences unusual beyond the 1st year.

What brings on an attack?
A recurrence occurs when latent virus is reactivated causing a peripheral lesion to appear. It is not clear why but precipitating factors have been recognized. They include: local nerve stimulation such as local trauma or UV light; immunosuppression e.g. HIV, drugs, or malignancies; persistent stress has been implicated. The association with menstruation is unclear.

Will all the attacks be this painful?
The 1st symptomatic attack of herpes is usually the worst attack. Subsequent attacks tend to be shorter and less painful. Patients are advised to use painkillers e.g. codeine phosphate and/or salt baths. Urinating into a bath may be more comfortable particularly for ♀ with painful sores around the urethral orifice.

Clinical features

Initial infection

~70% of new infections acquired from asymptomatic viral shedders. 25% of those presenting with a 1st clinical HSV-2 episode have HSV-2 antibodies indicating previous asymptomatic acquisition (pre-existing genital herpes). Over 60% of newly acquired HSV-2 infections are asymptomatic (↑ in ♂). In those with symptoms, 13% have atypical clinical features.

Incubation period is variable but typically 3–14 days. Clinical features and course of HSV-1 and 2, AGH similar though severity of symptoms (systemic and local) and complications ↑ in ♀.

Constitutional symptoms occur within 1st week in over 50% (fever, headache, malaise, and myalgia). Non-1° infections are less likely to have constitutional or severe symptoms.

Local symptoms include pain, irritation, regional tender lymphadenopathy, and discharge—vaginal and urethral (~33% of ♂ with 1° HSV-2). Typically, vesicles appear over a local area of erythema and may become pustular before breaking down to form multiple tender ulcers with local oedema being common (Plate 12). Persist for 4–15 days before being followed by crusting (if keratinized skin) and re-epithelialization. New lesions (crops) during episode occur in 75%, usually within 1st 10 days. Mean resolution time without treatment 17–20 days (but may take up to 6 weeks) and viral shedding time about 12 days.

In ♀ problems with micturition, including urine retention, more common than in ♂. Cervicitis occurs in 70–90% (with HSV-2). ♂ may develop 2° phimosis.

Anal infection, usually related to anal sexual contact, if symptomatic presents with pain, irritation, discharge, tenesmus, and sacral autonomic dysfunction. External perianal lesions only seen in ~50%.

Extra-anogenital lesions occur around groin, buttocks, lips, fingers (whitlow), eyes (kerato-conjunctivitis), and by infecting eczematous skin (eczema herpeticum).

Complications

- Associated HSV pharyngitis (both HSV-1 and 2). Occurs in ~10% with HSV-2 AGH.
- 2° bacterial and yeast infection.
- Adhesions (especially labial in ♀).
- Aseptic meningitis (symptoms/signs of meningeal involvement found in 36% ♀ and 13% ♂ with 1° HSV-2 AGH).
- Sacral radiculopathy: urine retention, constipation, sacral anaesthesia (in ~1% with HSV-2 AGH).
- Disseminated infection: very rare but more common in the immunosuppressed and pregnant.
- Psychological: including—denial, anger, anxiety, loneliness, fear, poor self-image.

Recurrent infection

Following initial AGH:

- HSV-2: 90% of patients (↑ in ♂) have recurrences in 1st year (median recurrence rate 0.33/month). Frequency of recurrences related to severity of initial infection. Significant reduction in 2nd year and thereafter (though marked individual variability).
- HSV-1: 60% recur clinically in 1st year (median recurrence rate 0.11/month). Recurrences are unusual beyond the 1st year.
- factors increasing risk of symptomatic recurrences include: a severe initial episode, infection with HSV-2, within 3 months of initial episode, immunodeficiency (e.g. HIV infection).

Signs and symptoms confined to affected anogenital site. Prodrome (local skin tingling, sciatic nerve pain) occurs up to 48 hours before appearance of lesions in ~50%. Although symptomatic recurrences are more common in ♂, severity ↑ in ♀. Lesions similar to initial infection but area of skin involvement one-tenth and re-epithelialization occurs in 6–10 days with viral shedding about 4 days. Cervical infection only found in 15–30% of ♀.

Main complication is psychological, especially if recurrences frequent, and include: shame, frustration, depression, and withdrawal from social and sexual interaction.

Rarely erythema multiforme.

Causes of ano-genital ulceration

- Trauma
- Sexually transmitted infections
  - Ano-genital herpes
  - 1° or 2° syphilis
  - Chancroid
  - Lymphogranuloma venereum
  - Granuloma inguinale
- Herpes zoster
- Aphthosis
- Behçet's disease
- Fixed drug eruptions
- Erythema multiforme
- Pyoderma gangrenosum
- Inflammatory bowel disease
- Cicatricial pemphigoid
- Lichen planus
- Lichen sclerosis
- Basal cell carcinoma
- Squamous cell carcinoma
- Melanoma.

Diagnosis

- *Viral cell culture*

Swabs from lesions including vesicle fluid (best source). Sensitivity >90% from fresh lesions. Standard transport medium should be retained at 4°C but systems not requiring refrigeration are commercially available.

- *Real time polymerase chain reaction*

Performed in a closed system (limiting risk of contamination), does not require postamplification manipulation. Swabs from lesions including vesicle fluid. Most sensitive method (detects 11–88% more cases than culture), rapid and highly specific. ↑ cost of consumables, compared with culture, off-set by ↓ labour costs per sample.

- *Immunofluorescent antigen detection*

Smears from lesions. Quick result but ↓ sensitivity.

- *Non-specific serology—complement fixation test (CFT), IgM*

Not type specific. Paired sample needed for CFT (antibody response may take 6 weeks). Of limited value but may be of use in late presentations when material from lesions is not available. In initial AGH positive predictive value of IgM is 100% but its sensitivity is only ~48% due to narrow window of positivity (9–21 days after infection).

- *Type specific serology*

Specific response may take 8–12 weeks to develop. Not widely available. Care with interpretation as HSV-1 and 2 are not site specific. HSV-2 has sensitivity and specificity of 98% and 97%, respectively, which limits value in low prevalence populations.

- Cervical cytology (multinucleate giant cells).

Sensitivity ~60% compared to culture.

Frequently asked questions

Do I need to treat each attack?

Usually only the initial episode of genital herpes is treated with an antiviral preparations, as treatment of subsequent attacks has little influence on the symptoms and their duration. Therefore generally only symptomatic treatment is advised for recurrent attacks e.g. saline baths and simple painkillers. If someone is experiencing symptomatic attacks >6 a year they can consider suppressive treatment (e.g. aciclovir 200mg 4 times a day for 6–12 months).

How do I tell a new partner that I have herpes?

There is a small risk of passing on the infection between symptomatic episodes by asymptomatic shedding, so informing a new partner about having herpes is a difficulty to face up to. Some people find it easier to wait until a relationship has developed and strengthened before disclosing this sensitive information while at the same time being careful to practice safer sex.

Will I give it to a new partner?

The sexual transmission rate between discordant couples is about 10–15% a year. The risk of transmission is reduced by avoiding sex when active lesions are present, but asymptomatic shedding may occur with the subsequent risk of transmission.

Should my partner be seen?

Unless your partner has any symptoms there is little point. However, if your partner wants to discuss the implications of the infection in your relationship then an appointment may be useful. It is also important if there are concerns about other STIs.

Is herpes dangerous in pregnancy?

A 1° attack of herpes in pregnancy may be serious. In the last 6 weeks of pregnancy it is associated with ↑ risk of neonatal herpes infection. The woman should be treated with aciclovir and delivered by caesarean section.

If a ♀ has never had herpes but her partner has then they should use condoms during intercourse throughout the pregnancy. The ♂ partner can be offered suppressive treatment during the duration of the pregnancy to ↓ the risk of a 1° attack of herpes in the ♀ during her pregnancy.

Recurrent attacks of herpes in pregnancy should be treated as though the ♀ were not pregnant. There is now evidence that caesarean section is not necessary for a non-1° attack of herpes in pregnancy even if the attack is in the last 6 weeks of pregnancy.

Management

Initial AGH

- Saline lavage (if severe dysuria, suggest urinating within bath water).
- Analgesia
  - Oral e.g. codeine phosphate 30–60mg 4–6 hourly as required.
  - Topical with caution in view of hypersensitivity risk.
- Rarely hospital admission may be required for urinary retention (for suprapubic catheterization), meningitis, or other severe constitutional symptoms.
- Antiviral management
  - Start within 5 days of onset or while new lesions are appearing.
  - Always use systemic treatment (usually oral).
  - 5 days treatment adequate unless new lesions are still appearing.
  - Duration of symptoms reduced by 50% and viral shedding by ~60%.
  - Antiviral treatment does not seem to influence recurrence rate.
- Antiviral drugs (all 5-day courses)
  - Aciclovir 200mg 5 times a day.
  - Famciclovir 250mg 3 times a day.
  - Valaciclovir 500mg twice daily.

Recurrent AGH

Typically mild and self-limiting. Unless unusually severe antiviral treatment is of limited benefit in reducing duration and viral shedding. General advice and support are often adequate.

Regular recurrences

Episodic treatment

May be considered for infrequent but regular recurrences. Should be commenced as early as possible, ideally at prodrome to reduce duration by a median of 1–2 days. Therefore, provide medication in anticipation of next episode to commence before signs appear. This approach may have a placebo effect as it gives reassurance that medication is available. Treatment regimens are same as for initial herpes except for famciclovir reduced to 125mg twice daily.

Suppressive treatment

Usually considered for >6 recurrences a year. Provide continuous treatment for 6–12 months then discontinue for reassessment. If recurrences resume at a high level, then further suppressive treatment may be required. >90% have a significant reduction in recurrences (mean recurrence rates of 12.8/year pretreatment falling to 1.8 during treatment). ~20% experience a reduction in frequency of recurrences after completion. Limited data on reduced asymptomatic shedding in ♀ and reduced transmission with valaciclovir.

- Aciclovir 200mg 4 times a day or 400mg twice daily.
- Famciclovir 250mg twice daily.
- Valaciclovir 500mg daily.

Aciclovir resistance

Rarely found in immunocompetent patients but reported in ~6% of those with immunosuppression, including HIV infection. Resistant strains can be treated with foscarnet and cidofovir.

Herbal treatment

Extract from the plant *Echinacea purpura* has been advocated in treatment of genital herpes but a double blind trial in recurrent AGH showed no significant benefit when compared with placebo.

Condoms

Laboratory experiments indicate that latex is impervious to HSV-2. Data suggest condoms reduce transmission to ♀ but no evidence of protection to ♂.

Discussion and support

For many patients diagnosis of AGH infection and implications of recurrence can provoke severe emotions often fuelled by misinformation. Time discussing these issues is important in management of AGH and points to consider include:

- accurate information on natural course of infection, recurrences, correction of false ideas.
- relevance of infection to current and potential future relationships.
- usual management and implications of current episode and possible recurrences.
- balanced consideration of potential to transmit infection both with and without symptoms and recognition of prodromes.
- safe sex issues and condom information.
- issues relating to pregnancy.

Pregnancy and neonatal infection

Clinical aspects

Woman: Clinical course of AGH in pregnancy similar to non-pregnant except disseminated infection (visceral) more common with recurrences more frequent and severe.
Pregnancy: Symptomatic 1° HSV-2 genital infection associated with increase in spontaneous abortion (1st trimester), preterm labour, low birth weight (3rd trimester). Complications do not usually arise from recurrent herpes.
Neonate: Incidence of neonatal infection—in UK 1.65/100,000 live births annually from 1986–91; USA 11–29/100,000 with 70–90% due to HSV-2. Maternal antibodies protect neonate so the highest risk of transmitting HSV is when acquisition occurs at or near to labour. Risk of neonatal herpes with 1st episode genital lesions at delivery calculated at ~40%. Rate of neonatal transmission with maternal recurrent herpes is 2–5%.
Clinical features and natural course (without treatment). Signs usually start towards end of the 1st week of life (up to 3 weeks) and include:

- Superficial—skin (vesicular) lesions (often protracted), conjunctivitis, and gingivo-stomatitis—low mortality, but 30% have neurological impairment.
- Encephalitis—50% mortality with most survivors having psychomotor or neurological impairment.
- Disseminated—multi-organ especially CNS, liver, lung, and superficial sites—mortality 80% with most survivors having severe neurological damage.

Diagnosis

- Pregnancy: As above. No value in taking serial swabs in late pregnancy from ♀ with recurrent herpes to detect viral shedding.
- Infant: If infection is suspected, or for babies born to ♀ with initial genital herpes test for HSV—urine, stool, oro-pharyngeal, and conjunctival swabs, skin vesicle fluid.

Management

- Pregnancy (consult local guidelines which may vary).

Prevention: Avoid intercourse during partner's recurrences. Advise about risk of acquiring HSV-1 through cunnilingus.

A strategy to reduce new HSV-2 infection in pregnancy is to identify seronegative pregnant 5 whose partners have recurrent HSV-2 and recommend consistent use of condoms and/or suppressive treatment for the partner. Currently not cost-effective as type-specific HSV-2 antibody testing is insufficiently specific for a low prevalence population.
Treatment: Aciclovir is well tolerated and safe in pregnancy but its use is currently not licensed. Therefore, although it is widely prescribed, this must be discussed with the patient and documented. Suppressive aciclovir has been advocated for recurrences especially during last 4 weeks.
Caesarean section: Routinely advised for all ♀ with initial genital herpes at term, may be considered for those acquiring initial infection in last

6 weeks of pregnancy but not indicated for 1st and 2nd trimester acquisition. Recurrence at term—risks of infection to baby is small, needs to be balanced with operative risks to mother.

- Infant with HSV infection

Intravenous aciclovir 10mg/kg body weight 8-hourly for 10 days.

Herpes and HIV

- Strong association between HSV-2 and HIV infection, increasing transmission of both.
- Viral shedding ↑ with low CD4 counts.
- Some experts advocate 10 days treatment as standard.

Chapter 22

Anogenital warts

Introduction

References to anogenital warts date back to the Roman and Hellenic ages with Celsus observing, in the 1st century AD, that anal warts resulted from sexual intercourse.

Aetiology

Human papilloma virus (HPV) is a genus in the family of papilloma viruses with a double-stranded DNA structure. The virion is 55nm in diameter. The capsid (envelope) comprising 72 capsomeres has an icosahedral symmetry. Hybrid capture II and polymerase chain reaction (PCR) are highly sensitive in detecting HPV.

HPV is classified by the nucleotide sequence of the major capsid gene L1 into >100 types which are identified by a number and are usually site specific (see Table 22.1). Types frequently detected in anogenital squamous cell carcinoma are described as oncogenic ('high risk') and the remainder non-oncogenic ('low risk'). The 'low risk' types HPV 6 and 11 account for ~90% of anogenital warts and 'high risk' HPV is found in >95% of cervical squamous cell carcinoma (type 16 in 50%, 18 in 20%).

Infection begins in the basal stem cells of the epithelium. Active viral replication occurs in the well-differentiated layers near the surface with sudden amplification of virus to 100,000 genomes per cell. Virions are then released from desquamating cells.

Epidemiology and natural history

Genital tract HPV DNA is found in 10–20% of those aged 15–49 years, however, <10% have clinically apparent lesions, i.e. ~1% overall. The peak age of prevalence in ♀ is 20–24 and ♂ 25–34 years. Infection rate is ↑ in smokers (>5-fold).

Median incubation period of exophytic warts is 3 months (range 2 weeks–9 months but can be much longer). In the immunocompetent warts eventually regress with immune response which usually begins after a period of 3–6 months of active growth. Response to E6 antigen leads to clearance but E7 results in persistent or relapsing infection. In ~95% HPV can no longer be detected 2 years after infection.

Transmission

Through contact with apparent or subclinical epithelial lesions and/or genital fluids containing infective virus, usually during sexual intercourse (including non-penetrative contact). Resultant micro-abrasions enable viral inoculation into the basal layers of the epithelium. Occasional reports of anogenital types at other sites (e.g. fingers) and non-anogenital types on anogenital skin suggest digital–genital transmission (including auto-inoculation). This may explain the absence of a history of genital–genital/anal or orogenital/anal sexual contact reported in ~1% of ♀ with anogenital warts (no data available for ♂). The finding of oral, laryngeal, conjunctival, and nasal lesions in those with anogenital warts (~5%), with the same HPV type, suggests orogenital transmission.

Mother to child transmission may occur during vaginal delivery with a 10–70% rate of neonatal infection and has also been reported following caesarean section. In pre-pubertal children digital warts may be transmitted to anogenital regions, up to 20% of which may be due to skin types.

Table 22.1 HPV types in lesions

Lesion	HPV types (more common types in bold)
Skin warts	**1,2,3,10,27,** 4,7,26,28,29,41,49, 57,60,63,65
Anogenital warts	**6,11,** 16,30,40,41,42,43,44,54,55
Squamous intraepithelial lesions*	**6,11,16,18,31,** 30,33,34,35,56,57,58,59,61,62,64,67,68,69,70
Anogenital squamous cell carcinoma	**16,18,31,45,** 33,35,39,51,52,54,56,66,68
Oral warts	**2,6,11,16** (7, 13, 18, and 32 in HIV+ve)
Laryngeal papilloma	**6,11**
Head and neck carcinoma	6,11,16,18,33,57

*Cervical, vaginal, vulval, anal, or penile intra-epithelial neoplasia.

Clinical features

Symptoms

Usually little physical discomfort but disfiguring lesions may lead to psychological distress. Perianal or large growths may cause irritation and soreness. Urethral, anal, and cervical warts may cause bleeding and urethral warts may distort the urinary stream.

Signs (Plate 13)

Warts (usually multiple) appear most commonly at sites likely to be traumatized during sexual intercourse with HPV detectable in apparently normal surrounding skin. Perianal and anal warts (almost always below the pectinate line) may occur in both ♂ and ♀, more commonly but not only with receptive anal sex. May be found on the cervix and in the vagina, anal canal, urethral meatus with rare involvement of urethra and bladder. (Table 22.2)

Lesions are either pedunculated or sessile and sometimes pigmented. They may be:

- condylomata acuminata—soft/non-keratinized, 'cauliflower-like' in appearance, found on mucosae/warm, moist, non-hairy skin.
- keratinized resembling skin warts usually on dry anogenital skin.
- smooth papules on dry skin e.g. penile shaft.

Subclinical infection may be detected as aceto-white patches with 5% acetic acid, better visualized through a colposcope (⚠ Low specificity). Atypical balanoposthitis/vulvitis may be associated with HPV 💣.

Giant condyloma of Buschke and Lowenstein

Usually associated with HPV 6 and 11, resembles a very large wart but invades the dermis and underlying tissue (e.g. corpus cavernosum). Starts as a keratotic papule and grows into a large cauliflower-like lesion. Most commonly located on the glans penis but may occur anywhere on the penis, scrotum, vulva, vagina, rectum, and bladder. It does not metastasize but malignant transformation (verrucous carcinoma) develops in up to 50%. Diagnosed histologically. Liable to recur if not completely excised.

Diagnosis (Table 22.3 for differential diagnosis)

- Usually on clinical appearance.
- Internal examination:
  - speculum for vaginal/cervical warts
  - proctoscopy for anal warts if perianal lesions present
  - urethral meatoscopy (with an otoscope) if meatal warts
- Biopsy under local anaesthetic if in doubt, or lesion atypical or pigmented. This may be aided by the use of a colposcope.
- Routine DNA detection is unnecessary or cost-effective.

Table 22.2 Relative frequency (reported range) of location of genital warts

	% of cases (range)		**% of cases (range)**
Prepuce	65 (49–80)	Posterior aspect of introitus	73 (77–94)
Frenum, corona and glans	46 (22–70)	Labia minora/ majora, clitoris	32
Urethral meatus	34 (24–45)	Cervix	34 (6–64)
Penile shaft	27 (16–55)	Vagina	42 (32–52)
Scrotum	23 (2–25)	Urethra	8
Perianal area	8 (3–15)	Perianal area	18 (13–85)
		Perineum	23

Table 22.3 Differential diagnosis of external anogenital warts

Achrocordon (skin tag)	Molluscum contagiosum
Epidermal/melanocytic naevi	Condylomata lata (secondary syphilis)
Sebaceous glands	Seborrhoeic keratosis
Penile pearly papules	Dermatofibroma
Vulval papillae	Angiokeratoma
Ectopic sebaceous glands (Fordyce spots)	Epidermal cyst
Prominent hair follicles	Lichen planus
Nabothian follicles (cervix)	Psoriasis
	Penile/anal intraepithelial neoplasia
	Giant condyloma of Buschke and Lowenstein
	Squamous cell carcinoma
	Basal cell carcinoma

Pregnancy and infection in the neonate and children

Warts may rapidly enlarge with pronounced vascularity during pregnancy (probably as a result of altered immunocompetence or ↑ oestrogen/progesterone) and regress in the puerperium often with complete resolution. Warts do not usually obstruct vaginal delivery.

Neonatal infection commonly clears within 6 weeks. Persistence is usually subclinical but may lead to recurrent respiratory papillomatosis, anogenital, or extra-genital warts. Recurrent respiratory papillomatosis incidence is 0.25% in children (3 months–5 years of age) born to mothers with warts. Mostly caused by HPV 6 and 11. Usually located on the vocal cords and epiglottis (laryngeal papillomas), rarely the entire larynx, tracheo-bronchial tree or even the lungs.

Perinatal infection is the usual cause of anogenital warts in children up to 3 years of age. However, sexual abuse and non-sexual transmission should be considered in older children.

Management

General principles

The aim of treatment is essentially cosmetic or for symptomatic relief. Treatments have no direct effect against HPV and only limited impact on viral clearance and infectivity. Diagnosis of subclinical infection is of no practical benefit.

Optimal management is enabled by a treatment protocol with clear guidelines on the choice of treatment and arrangements for review. Treatment choice depends on the morphology, number, and distribution of warts and should be made after considering the available options and discussing side-effects, e.g. scarring, with the patient. Serial documentation of the number, size, appearance, and distribution of wart/s in genital maps gives a visual record of treatment response. If the wart area is greater than $4cm^2$ treatment under direct supervision of clinical staff is recommended. No treatment is an option particularly for vaginal/anal warts.

Condom use does not impact on anogenital HPV prevalence but may reduce the incidence of genital warts in ♂ and cervical neoplasia in ♀. Psychological distress may require referral for counselling. The possibility of a long incubation period should be discussed especially if concerns about infidelity.

All treatments have significant failure rates. Soft non-keratinized warts respond well to podophyllotoxin (and podophyllin). Keratinized lesions are better treated with ablative methods e.g. cryotherapy, trichloroacetic acid (TCA), excision, or electrocautery. Imiquimod may be suitable for both types. Preferred initial treatment for small number/low volume warts of either type is ablation.

▶ Risk of scarring and pigment changes should be discussed before treatment.

Frequently asked questions

How have I caught them?
Genital warts are usually sexually transmitted by direct skin to skin contact. It is thought that ~90% of people who are infected with HPV have no visible warts. After infection it takes a mean 3 months for warts to develop but may extend to months or years.

Will they go on their own?
Warts left untreated may disappear on their own (usually within 18 months) but they can also grow and spread becoming unsightly and more difficult to treat.

Will I ever get rid of them?
When warts are treated they should clear but HPV may persist, pending the host's immunological response. Therefore the patient should be warned that they may recur. Recurrences are more likely within 3 months of treatment. HPV usually clears within 24 months although, especially if the patient is immunocompromised, this may be longer.

Am I infectious?
Someone infected with HPV is infectious until it clears. The level of infection is probably greater when warts are present as viral shedding is likely to be greater.

Can I have sex?
It is often recommended that if visible warts are present condoms are used during sex, although there is no clear evidence of benefit. Friction associated with coitus may spread warts. However, it is likely that the regular partner of someone who has warts will also be infected with the wart virus whether they have visible warts or not.

Do they cause cervical cancer?
There are many strains of HPV but those causing genital warts are different from the types associated with cervical cancer. It is recommended that a ♀ attends for routine smear tests which will detect abnormalities associated with the HPV strains that may be related to cervical cancer. ♀ with warts do not need extra smears.

My partner does not have warts; does he/she need to be seen?
Only if there are concerns about possible warts or other STIs.

Specific treatments

- *Podophyllotoxin* (self-applied). The active lignan ingredient of podophyllin resin and an anti-mitotic agent causing local tissue necrosis. Available as 0.5% solution or 0.15% cream. Should be applied twice daily for 3 consecutive days, repeated at weekly intervals for a total of up to 4–5 three-day treatments. Clearance rate 42–88%. Recurrence rate 10–91%. In ♀ 0.15% cream is more effective than 0.5% solution (81% versus 50%).
- *Cryotherapy*. Liquid nitrogen spray (–180°C), swab (–20°C) or probe (–196°C), nitrous oxide probe (–75°C), or carbon dioxide snow (–79°C) may be used to freeze (for ~20 seconds) the wart/s and a margin ('halo') of 1–3mm of surrounding epithelium. The depth of freezing achieved is variable and operator-dependent. Local anaesthetic is usually not needed but may be required depending on pain tolerance and extent of warts. Adequate cryotherapy causes immediate erythema followed in a few hours by blistering due to cytolysis of the epithelial cells. Healing takes 7–10 days with minimal scarring. If the treated area is large severe ulceration may occur causing wound care problems and scarring. Cryotherapy may be repeated at 1–2 week intervals. Clearance rate 63–88% after 1–10 (average 3) weekly treatments. Recurrence rate up to 39%.
- *Trichloracetic acid (TCA)*. Caustic agent causes chemical coagulation leading to necrosis. Applied once a week as a 80–90% solution (unlicensed) ensuring protection of surrounding epithelium with petroleum jelly Treatment induced pain, ulceration, irritation, and scarring limit its use. Clearance rate 50–81%. Recurrence rate 36%.
- *Imiquimod 5% cream* (self-applied). Stimulates innate and acquired immune responses. Applied once a day, 3 times a week for up to 16 weeks. Clearance rate 50–62% with partial clearance (≥50% reduction) in 59–81% of the remainder. Recurrence rate 13–19%. More effective in ♀ than ♂ (64–72% versus 33–42%) and uncircumcised than circumcised ♂ (62% versus 33%). Also used as an adjunct to ablative treatment. Erythema, burning, irritation, and tenderness are common side-effects reflecting effective immune response and do not warrant cessation of treatment unless severe.
- *Podophyllin 15–25%*. A resin extracted from *Podophyllum peltatum* dissolved in alcohol or benzoin. In addition to the active ingredient podophyllotoxin, it contains quercetin and kaempherol which are mutagenic. (Teratogenic and oncogenic effects in animal experiments but no evidence in humans.)

Applied to warts once or twice a week with advice to wash off after 4–6 hours (to limit the inflammatory response). Volume of solution applied in a single treatment session must be ≤0.5mL to avoid risk of systemic toxicity. Less effective than podophyllotoxin (which has largely replaced it) and more likely to cause side-effects. Clearance rate 32–79%. Recurrence rate 11–65%. Its use now is usually in combination with cryotherapy. This gives better results than podophyllin or cryotherapy alone.

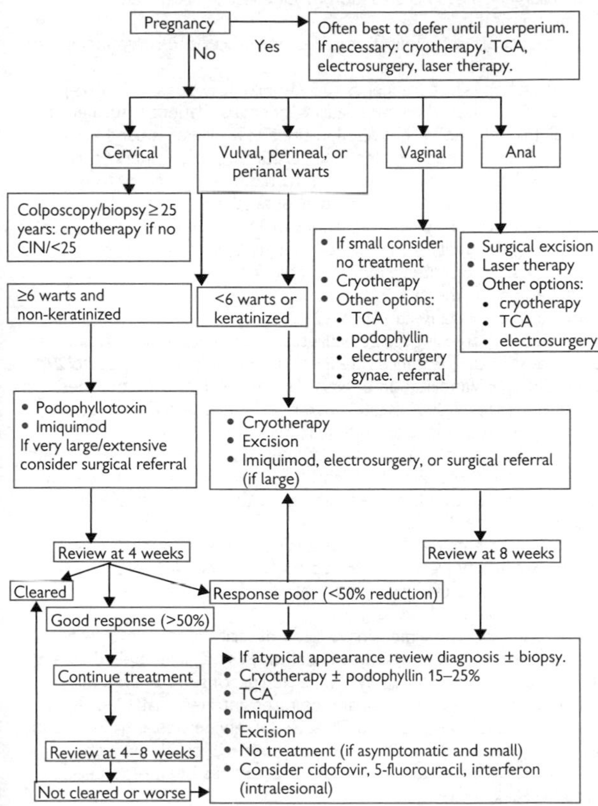

Treatment algorithm for genital warts in ♀

- *Electrosurgery*. Tissue destruction by electrically produced heat. Common methods:
  - electrocautery—application of heat to warts and surrounding tissue under local anaesthesia.
  - hyfrecation—high frequency (0.5–3MHz), low power (1–30W) electricity heats the tissue causing necrosis. Patient return electrode ('diathermy pad') is not needed since low power is used. 2 techniques used are electrofulguration (current sparks across an air gap) and electrodessication (electrode in contact with or penetrating warts). Requires local anaesthesia.
  - surgical diathermy—high frequency (0.5–3MHz), high power (up to 400W) electricity (requiring 'diathermy pad') to produce coagulation or cutting. More suitable for large warts. Requires general anaesthesia.

Clearance rate ~94%. Recurrence ~24%.

- *Excision*. Excision using scalpel, curette, or scissors under local or general anaesthesia. Clearance rate 89–93%. Recurrence rate up to 29%.
- *Laser therapy*. Vaporization of warts under local or general anaesthesia. Clearance rate 27–89%. Recurrence rate 7–45%. Adverse effects include pain, itch, bleeding, and scar formation.
- *Cidofovir 1% cream* (self-applied). Unlicensed for routine use. Applied daily for 5 days, repeated fortnightly (i.e. after 9 treatment-free days) for a total of up to 6 five-day treatments. Clearance rate 27–89%. Recurrence rate 7–45%.
- *5-Flurouracil 5% cream*. Pyrimidine analogue inhibiting RNA/DNA synthesis. Applied twice a week for up to 10 weeks. Not recommended for internal warts (especially urethral). Clearance rate 13–43%. Recurrence rate ~50%.
- *Interferon*. Various regimens have been described using interferon α, β, or γ as intralesional or systemic injection (also as self-applied cream). Its use is, however, limited by a variable response rate, systemic side-effects, and expense. Clearance rates, intralesional 19–62%, systemic 7–51%, and topical 6–90%. Recurrence rates, intralesional up to 33%, systemic up to 23% and topical ~6%. Cyclical low dose injection used as an adjunct to laser therapy has been reported to reduce relapse rate.
- *Isotretinoin*. Conflicting results when used to treat genital warts. A recent study using oral isotretinoin 0.5mg/kg/day showed efficacy in the treatment of recalcitrant cervical warts. However, because of its teratogenicity its use as 1st line therapy for genital warts in ♀ is unacceptable.

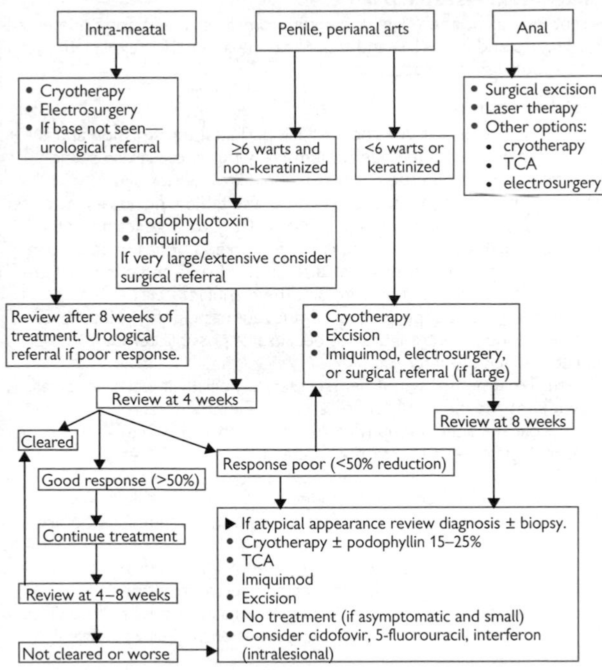

Treatment algorithm for genital warts in ♂

Management—sexual partners

Current sexual partner(s) may benefit from assessment for undetected genital warts and other STI and there may be a need for explanation and advice about disease process.

Special situations

- *Pregnancy*. Treatment does not reduce perinatal transmission and is better deferred until the puerperium. Very rarely caesarean section may be indicated because of obstruction. Cryotherapy, TCA, electrocautery, and laser vaporization are suitable if necessary. Excision may cause severe haemorrhage and diathermy of large lesions intense post-operative pain. Imiquimod is not approved but has been used in exceptional circumstances (after discussion of risks and benefits with the patient and registration with 3M, the manufacturers).
  ⚠ Podophyllin, podophyllotoxin, 5-fluorouracil, cidofovir, interferon, and isotretinoin contra-indicated because of possible teratogenic effects or lack of safety data.
- *Vagina*. Treatment may not be necessary especially if warts are small. Cryotherapy is the usual 1st line therapy. Electrosurgery, trichloroacetic acid, podophyllin (total area treated $<2cm^2$), or gynaecological referral are other options.
- Cervix:
  - Cervical warts—cryotherapy, electrosurgery, or TCA. If ≥25 years of age colposcopy ± biopsy best practice to exclude CIN before treatment
  - Cytology—no changes to routine screening intervals necessary.
- *Urethral meatus*. If base of lesions seen preferred treatment—cryotherapy or electrosurgery. Other options are podophyllotoxin or imiquimod but use with caution. Deeper lesions require surgical ablation under direct vision.
- *Anal canal*. Surgical excision or laser preferred. If small and accessible—cryotherapy, TCA, electrosurgery.
- *Immunosuppressed patients*. Poor treatment response, ↑ relapse, and dysplasia more likely with ↓ cell mediated immunity e.g. following renal transplant or HIV infection. Careful follow up required.

Vaccine

Virus like particle, the capsid without DNA, is immunogenic but non-infectious. Trials have shown that virus like particle vaccines induce a strong antibody response preventing HPV infection during a 4-year observation period. Phase III studies are in progress assessing a tetravalent vaccine against types 6, 11, 16, and 18. If efficacy is proven vaccination before the onset of sexual activity will potentially prevent 70% invasive cervical cancers, 60% high grade CIN, 90% of anogenital warts.

Frequently asked questions

Can I treat them myself?

It is advisable not to treat warts at home with over the counter preparations for warts; these preparations are designed for use on hands or feet and may damage genital skin.

There are special prescription only preparations (podophyllotoxin and imiquimod) for home use although treatments recommended depend on the position, number, and appearance of the warts.

Can I pass them to my children?

The HPV types that usually cause genital infection almost exclusively favour this site so are sexually transmitted. However, occasionally other types, such as those causing warts on the hands, can be spread to the genitals and have been found in children.

I am pregnant, are the warts harmful to my baby?

Warts are common in pregnancy, often grow more quickly and are more difficult to manage as certain treatments cannot be used. They often resolve spontaneously after the pregnancy is over. Although HPV can be transmitted to babies at delivery it is unusual. Treating the warts will not remove the underlying infection.

HPV and HIV

- HPV infection has not been associated with ↑ risk of HIV acquisition.
- Those with HIV infection appear to be at greater risk of acquiring or reactivating HPV.
- Oral warts (due to types 7, 13, 18, and 32) are more common in those with HIV infection.
- Duration and natural history of concurrent HPV infection may be altered leading to ↑ incidence of cervical and anal neoplasia.

Chapter 23

Molluscum contagiosum

Introduction

First described in 1817. Viral origin discovered by Juliusburg in 1905.

Aetiology

Molluscum contagiosum virus (MCV), genus *Molluscipoxvirus*, a poxvirus.
A benign self-limiting skin infection caused by a large DNA virus replicating in cytoplasm of epithelial cells. Two major subtypes MCV-1 (↑ in children) and MCV-2 (↑ in adults and those with HIV infection). Humans the only natural host.

Epidemiology and transmission

Worldwide, more common in warm climates, linked to poor hygiene and overcrowding. Equal sex distribution. Transmitted by direct skin to skin contact. Microscopic abrasions (trauma) and a warm moist environment facilitate transmission. The period of infectivity and viral shedding is thought to be equal to the duration of lesions.

Both sexual and non-sexual spread occurs, the latter more commonly especially in:

- pre-adolescent children (17% in those aged <15 years)
- individuals with impaired cellular immunity
- sports involving skin to skin contact
- those using gyms, swimming pools, and saunas (including fomites e.g. shared towels)

If sexually acquired lesions are usually found around the anogenital area and in:

- sexually active adults aged 20–29 years
- those with a history or presence of other STIs
- those whose partner has molluscum contagiosum (MC).

No documented cases of maternal–fetal transmission.

Clinical features

Incubation period usually 2–12 weeks, up to 6 months.

Smooth, pearly coloured umbilicated lesions growing over several weeks to a diameter of 2–6mm, occasionally larger (Plate 14). In adults, when sexually acquired, found in pubic region, thighs, buttocks, lower abdomen, less commonly external genitalia sparing mucous membranes. Usually up to 10–20 lesions unless immunosuppressed. May appear during pregnancy and generally resolve after delivery. Typically asymptomatic but may cause pruritus (10% develop dermatitis around lesions), leading to auto-inoculation through excoriation. In children lesions characteristically found on face, upper limbs, and trunk but 10–50% have genital lesions.

Spontaneous resolution common within 2–3 months, but recurrences occur in 15–35% over 8–24 months.

Diagnosis

- Characteristic appearance.
- Histology—enlarged epithelial cells with intracytoplasmic molluscum bodies.

Management

As MC frequently resolve without treatment, the benefits of treating lesions must be balanced against the possible risk of post treatment scarring.

Treatment options include:

- curettage, cryotherapy, electrocautery, puncture with sharpened orange stick dipped in 80% phenol
- imiquimod cream 5%
- podophyllotoxin 0.5% (reported but very limited data on efficacy)

Partner notification

Unnecessary. No evidence that treating partner prevents re-infection.

Frequently asked questions

Where have I caught it?

Molluscum contagiosum is a viral infection spread by skin-to-skin contact. If lesions appear around the genitals they have probably been sexually transmitted.

How long has the infection has been there and how long will they stay?

Lesions usually appear after an incubation period of 3 to 12 weeks (although this can be longer) and usually disappear spontaneously within 2–3 months. Clearance depends on the body mounting a suitable immunological response against the causative pox virus.

Does it need treating?

As molluscum resolve spontaneously treatment is offered for cosmetic purposes only. Generally people with genital lesions want them cleared as soon as possible.

Can it be treated?

The usual treatment is by cryotherapy but curettage, diathermy, piercing with an orange stick then applying iodine or phenol have also been used. There is limited data on podophyllotoxin cream and imiquimod cream (currently unlicensed).

Will it recur?

~33% of people will get recurrences over the next 1–2 years.

HIV infection

Mollascum Contagiosum found in 5–18% of those with HIV. Lesions may become wide-spread (commonly affecting the face) and hypertrophic. Use of HAART may lead to resolution of lesions.

Chapter 24

Sexually acquired viral hepatitis

Hepatitis A virus (HAV) infection

Aetiology

A highly infectious RNA picornavirus. Identified in 1972 but condition had been known for a long time as epidemic jaundice, yellow jaundice, or infectious hepatitis.

Epidemiology and transmission

Common in developing countries (poor sanitation) and with close personal contact. Prevalence in USA and Western Europe 10–33%. Transmission usually faeco-oral (contaminated food/water). Associated with urine contamination and contact with infected urine (e.g. europhilia). Most commonly affects children but outbreaks reported in homosexual ♂ (faecal contact), injecting drug users (IDUs), and institutions. Batches of contaminated blood products have been found. Patients are infectious for 2 weeks before and 1 week after the onset of jaundice. After infection immunity is life-long.

Clinical features

Incubation period: usually 2–6 weeks.
Symptoms: most children and upto 50% of all adults are either asymptomatic or have mild non-specific symptoms with no obvious jaundice. An icteric illness with jaundice, anorexia, nausea, and fatigue lasting usually 1–3 weeks (up to 12 weeks) is preceded by prodromal, flu-like symptoms (malaise, myalgia, fatigue, nausea) often with right upper abdominal pain lasting 3–10 days. Pyrexia usually disappears at the beginning of the icteric phase with symptomatic improvement at onset of jaundice.
Signs: jaundice (hepatitic and/or homeostatic) with pale stools and dark urine. Liver tenderness and dehydration may occur.
Complications: fulminant hepatitis in ~0.4% (more common in those with hepatitis C). Up to 15% of symptomatic patients may require hospitalization with 25% having severe hepatitis. HAV associated mortality very low (<0.2%). Chronic infection does not usually occur.
HAV in pregnancy: associated with ↑ rate of premature labour and miscarriage proportional to severity of illness. Vertical transmission rarely reported.

Diagnosis and investigations

- HAV-IgM: positive within 5 days of illness (up to 6 months).
- HAV-IgG: indicates past exposure or response to vaccination.
- Alanine aminotransferase (ALT)/aspartate aminotransferase (AST) and bilirubin can ↑ to 10,000 IU/L and 500μmol/L respectively.
- Alkaline phosphatase (ALP) ↑ modestly but higher with cholestasis.
- Prothrombin time prolongation of >5 seconds suggests decompensation.
- Screen for other hepatotropic infections and STIs if appropriate.

Management

Provision of information and advice (avoid alcohol, stop food handling, and unprotected sexual intercourse until non-infectious). Most cases managed on an outpatient basis. Follow-up only necessary for patients whose ALT or bilirubin does not settle within 4–8 weeks.

HAV infection is a notifiable disease with contacts requiring follow-up by public health authorities including partner notification (PN) for sexual partners. Human normal immunoglobulin (HNIG) or early HAV vaccine may be considered for non-immune close contacts including neonates. Breastfeeding can be continued.

Vaccination

Active vaccination recommended for travellers to endemic countries, and in outbreak situations, chronic liver disease, IDUs and those with human immunodeficiency virus (HIV) infection.

Schedule: 2 doses at 0 and 6–12 months giving 95% protection for 5–10 years. Combination vaccine with hepatitis B follows same schedule as hepatitis B vaccination. HAV vaccine response may be lower in HIV/immunocompromised patients.

Hepatitis B virus (HBV) infection

Aetiology

A Hepadna DNA virus first reported in 1965 (Australia antigen). Six genotypes—A to F.

Epidemiology and transmission

Occurs endemically with high chronic carriage rates (up to 8%) in S.E. Asia, China, Africa, S. and E. Europe, Central and S. America. Low carriage rates in N. America, W. Europe, and Australia (UK < 0.04% but ↑ in IDUs, homosexual ♂, commercial sex workers, and heterosexual HBV contacts).

In homosexual ♂ sexual transmission is associated with multiple partners, unprotected anal sex, oro-anal sex. Mother to child transmission is common, its frequency depending on maternal antigen status (90% if e Ag +ve, 10% if –ve). Other transmission routes include parenteral (IDU, tattoos, blood products, acupuncture). Sporadic infections may occur in healthcare professionals (HCPs) and institutions.

Clinical features

Incubation period: usually 6 weeks to 6 months.
Symptoms: infants and children usually have asymptomatic acute infection. 10–50% of adults are asymptomatic. Symptoms more likely if HIV infected. Prodromal and icteric phases are similar to HAV but may be more severe and prolonged.

Signs

- Acute—similar to HAV.
- Chronic—persistent HB surface antigen (HBsAg). Usually no physical signs. After many years signs of chronic liver disease may emerge including spider naevi, finger clubbing, gynaecomastia, and in end stage disease jaundice, ascites, liver flap, and encephalopathy.

Complications

- Acute infection mortality is <1% due to fulminant hepatitis.
- Chronic infection (defined as >6 months of HBsAg-positivity) develops in 5–10%. More common in HIV infection, chronic renal failure, the immunosuppressed, and >90% of vertically infected children. Immunosuppression can also lead to HBV reactivation. ↑ mortality rate in cirrhosis due to decompensating liver disease and progression to liver cancer. Concurrent infection with hepatitis C virus can lead to more progressive chronic liver disease. Co-infection with hepatitis D (Delta agent), usually IDU associated, may lead to rapid deterioration and its response to treatment is poor.

HBV ↑ rate of miscarriage and premature labour.

Diagnosis

- HBsAg (surface antigen) is positive in acute and chronic infection disappearing in resolved/immune infection. Usually appears within 3 months of infection (rarely up to 6 months).

- HBcAb (core antibody) is a marker of acquired infection and remains positive in resolved infection but is negative in vaccinated patients.
- HBeAg (envelope antigen) is a marker of high viral activity/high infectivity.
- HBV DNA identifies the amount of virus present and correlates with infectivity and hepatic activity.
- HBsAb (surface antibody) is a marker of successful vaccination and its titre determines level of protection. It may be positive in those with resolved/immune hepatitis B.
- Liver function tests may be normal, but often are of variable levels and are usually ↑ during hepatic 'flares'.

Serological, virological, and liver enzyme tests in different stages of viral hepatitis A, B, C

	HAV	HBV	HCV
Acute infection	• HAV IgM +ve • ALT ↑ usually	• Usually HbsAg +ve • Anti HBc IgM +ve • ALT ↑ usually • HBV DNA present	• HCV IgG +/–ve • ALT ↑ often • HCV-RNA +ve (usually)
Chronic infection	Does not usually occur	• HBsAg +ve • HBeAg +/–ve • HBc IgG +ve • ALT ↑ ↓ • HBV-DNA +/–ve	• HCV IgG +ve • ALT ↑ ↓ • HCV-RNA +ve
Recovered infection	• HAV IgG +ve • Normal ALT	• HBs IgG +ve • HBc IgG +ve • ALT normal	• HCV IgG +ve • HCV-RNA –ve • ALT normal
Successful vaccination	HAV IgG +ve	• HBs IgG +ve • HBc IgG –ve	Not available

Management

Information and advice including avoiding unprotected sexual intercourse until non-infectious or partner successfully vaccinated. Stop (or ↓) alcohol consumption. Refer to specialist unit if acute deteriorating liver disease.

Notifiable disease. Partner notification and screening of close family contacts are important with public health involvement for non-sexual contacts. Consider specific HBV immunoglobulin 500 units IM and rapid vaccination of contacts.

Newborn. Vaccination (rapid schedule) and HBV specific immunoglobulin 200 units IM ↓ vertical transmission by 90%. Breastfeeding can continue.

Chronic infection. Specialist referral recommended. High level HBV viraemia predicts progressive liver disease. Some HBeAg negative patients may also progress. Currently three licensed medications:

- lamivudine
- adefovir
- α-interferon.

Newer medications include tenofovir, emtricitabine, entecavir, and pegylated α-interferon. Decision to treat depends on patient's age, severity of liver disease, and co-pathologies. Patients with a high viral load (HBV-DNA > 10^5copies/mL), +ve HBeAg or active liver disease should be considered for:

- either long-term viral suppression with lamivudine 100mg daily (duration not defined but a minimum of 1 year usual).
- or an attempt at inducing HBV seroconversion by using sequential lamivudine/interferon or pegylated interferon monotherapy (unlicensed).

In the UK adefovir is currently limited to lamuvidine resistant virus. Treatment primarily ↓ risk of liver cirrhosis and liver cancer.

► In decompensated liver disease interferon is absolutely contraindicated.

Vaccination

Apart from contacts vaccination should be considered for those at ↑ risk e.g. homosexual ♂, sex workers, association with endemic areas, prisoners, IDUs, those sexually assaulted, occupational/needle-stick risk. Protection of vaccinated patients is assessed by HBsAb level >100mIU/mL is ideal but even with levels >10mIU/mL subsequent HBV infection is very rare. It has been suggested that memory cells provide protection as immunity appears to be maintained even if HBsAb ↓ provided there has been a good initial response.

Schedules

- Ultra-rapid course: of recombinant vaccine schedule: 3 doses and booster at 0, 7, 21/28 days plus 12 month booster.
- Rapid course schedule: 3 doses and booster at 0, 1, 2 months plus 12 month booster.

Note these schedules are not licensed for neonates.

- Standard schedule: 3 doses: 0, 1, 6 months, booster dose if protective antibody level <100mIU/mL.

Protective antibody level in 80–95% after full course of vaccination but lower response rates if aged >40 years or immunocompromised, e.g. HIV infection particularly if CD4 < 200cells/μL (but even <500cells/μL).

Combined hepatitis A and B vaccine overall has a lower response rate but may be useful sometimes. Newer types of vaccines (pre-S formulations, not widely available) or ↑ dosage of HBV vaccine may effect seroconversion.

Active hepatitis A and B vaccines

Hepatitis A vaccine

Havrix monodose®: suspension of formaldehyde-inactivated hepatitis A virus.
Adult dose: 1mL with the deltoid region the preferred site (subcutaneous may be used in those with bleeding disorders).

Hepatitis B vaccine

Engerix B®, HBvaxPRO®: both suspension of HBV surface antigen prepared from yeast cells by recombinant DNA technology.
Adult dose: 1mL with the deltoid region the preferred site (subcutaneous may be used in those with bleeding disorders). Should not be injected into the buttocks (efficacy reduced).

Combined hepatitis A and hepatitis B vaccine

Twinrix®: inactivated HAV and recombinant HBV surface antigen
Adult dose: 1mL with the deltoid region the preferred site (subcutaneous may be used in those with bleeding disorders although immune response may be reduced). Should not be injected into the buttocks (efficacy reduced).

Hepatitis C virus (HCV) infection

Aetiology

RNA virus of the family Flaviviridae discovered in 1989. Six predominant genotypes. In the UK genotype (G) 1 is most common (~50% of cases) followed by G2/G3 (together 40–50%). G1 relatively more common in those infected through blood products and G2/G3 in injecting drug users (IDUs).

Epidemiology and transmission

High prevalence rates found in Egypt (up to 29%), S.E. Asia and E. Europe. UK has a rate of ~0.5% with a higher prevalence in IDUs (20–50% IDUs), people who received a blood transfusion before September 1991 and blood products prior to 1986.

Transmission mainly parenteral through shared needles/syringes/equipment. ~67% are ♂ (more IDUs and haemophiliacs are ♂). Found in up to 1% of GUM patients although <2% of infections are sexually acquired. Outbreaks described in HIV positive homosexual ♂ and there is ↑ prevalence in ♀ sex workers. Vertical transmission occurs in up to 6%.

Clinical features

Incubation period: 4–20 weeks.
Symptoms: acute hepatitis occurs in 20% and is less likely to be followed by chronic infection.
Signs: similar to HAV and HBV.
Complications: acute fulminant hepatitis is rare but can occur in HCV patients with acute HAV infection.
Natural history: >80% become chronically infected with HCV, most unaware. High alcohol intake, co-existing HBV, HIV, and other chronic liver diseases can lead to a more rapid progression to cirrhosis and liver cancer. Progress to cirrhosis in ~20% after 20 years. Thereafter annual rate of developing cancer ~5%. Co-infection with HBV or HIV is associated with ↑ progression. ► ALT may be normal despite severe liver disease.

Diagnosis

- Antibody testing with confirmation by polymerase chain reaction (PCR) test for viral RNA. Antibodies usually appear within 3 (rarely 6) months of infection.
- Genotype testing. Influences duration of treatment and estimates response rate.
- Liver function, clotting tests, and exclusion of other viral hepatotropic infections and liver related diseases are helpful.
- Screening for other blood-borne infections including HIV advised.
- Abdominal ultrasound and α-fetoprotein monitoring recommended.

Screening should be offered to:

- all IDUs (past and present)
- in the UK recipients of—
  - blood (prior to September 1991)
  - blood products pre-1986
  - tissues/organs before 1992

- regular sexual partners of those with HCV infection
- HCP exposure to blood/needlesticks
- those with HIV infection
- people tattooed/skin pierced where poor infection control
- children of mothers with HCV infection.

It may be advised for prisoners/ex-prisoners, those sexually assaulted and homosexual ♂ if outbreak identified.

Management

A notifiable infection with partner notification and public health implications. Provide information and advice (IDU risk of sharing, risks of sexual transmission). Stop (or ↓) alcohol consumption. Consider discussion of insurance issues. If patient amenable to further management refer to specialist.

Acute infection: consider high dose α-interferon (pegylated/non-pegylated) and/or ribavirin.

Chronic infection (persistent HCV-PCR positive): based on genotype and degree of liver disease (biopsy, if indicated). Current guidelines recommend combination treatment:

- ribavirin 800mg–1.2g divided into 2 doses daily by mouth (dependent on genotype, weight, and type of pegylated interferon)
- pegylated interferon once a week by subcutaneous injection:
  - α-2a: 180μg
  - α-2b: 1.5μg/kg body weight.

Duration depends on genotype. People infected with G2, G3 should be treated for 24 weeks. Those with G1, 4, 5, or 6 should be treated for 48 weeks but tested for response at 12 weeks. If there is an undetectable viral load or ↓ in viral load drop (of at least 2-log) then treatment should be continued for full 48 weeks, otherwise stopped.

Combination treatment has multiple side-effects and requires close monitoring of haematology, liver function, thyroid function with psychiatric support if needed. Ribavirin may cause haemolytic anaemia which may require dose reduction or its cessation. Sustained viral response rates vary between 40% and 70% for G1 and G2/3, respectively. Interferon may benefit liver fibrosis independent of viral clearance.

Prevention and prophylaxis: No vaccine available. Currently no treatment for needle-stick injuries recommended. Newly employed HCPs with high risk exposure must declare their HCV status or undergo pre-employment testing.

Chapter 25

Other viral infections

Epstein–Barr virus (EBV)

Aetiology

A DNA herpesvirus consisting of types EBV1 and EBV2. Infects >90% of humans, persisting for life. Probably evolved from a non-human primate virus.

Epidemiology and transmission

Virtually all children infected in developing countries (especially with socio-economic deprivation).

In developed countries most infections are acquired by those aged 15–25 years. Characteristically spread by ingestion of infected saliva from a seropositive carrier during kissing. Although unproven, reports of EBV isolated from a vulval ulcer, semen, and cervical secretions suggest the potential for sexual transmission.

Clinical features

Incubation period 20–50 days. Infection in children usually asymptomatic. In adolescents and young adults >50% present with infectious mononucleosis (glandular fever):

- fever
- lymphadenopathy
- pharyngitis
- >10% develop hepatosplenomegaly and palatal petechiae (Forscheimer spots).

Other less common features include anaemia (haemolytic and aplastic), thrombocytopenia, myocarditis, hepatitis, genital ulcers, Guillain–Barré syndrome, encephalitis, meningitis.

Non-specific diffuse central rashes may be found in up to 50% with an immune complex macular rash in >70% of those taking ampicillin or amoxicillin.

Investigations

- Haematology: leucocytosis of 12–25 x 10^9/L, lymphocytosis of 4.5–5 x 10^9/L with 20% of cells atypical. May also be thrombocytopenia.
- Biochemistry: elevated liver enzymes in up to 100% from week 2–5.
- Antibody testing
  - Monospot test–heterophil antibodies (sensitivity ~80% in adults).
  - EBV antibody tests. IgM to viral capsid antigen IgM (transient) but most reliable test; paired IgG showing > than 4-fold titre rise; IgG to EB nuclear antigen appears in convalescence.

Management

Bed rest, analgesics, antipyretics. Antibiotics (not ampicillin/amoxicillin) if 2° bacterial infection. Steroids if airways obstruction.

Prognosis

Self-limiting though associated with persisting tiredness and possible relapses during the first 6–12 months. Not associated with chronic fatigue syndrome.

Other conditions associated with EBV include

- Burkitt's and Hodgkin's lymphoma
- Nasopharyngeal carcinoma
- Lymphoproliferative disease
- In HIV infection
  - Oral hairy leukoplakia
  - Some non-Hodgkin's lymphomas

Cytomegalovirus (CMV)

The largest known DNA herpesvirus, host-specific, with four human/higher primate subtypes.

Epidemiology and horizontal transmission

Worldwide distribution favouring developing countries and low socio-economic classes. Spread through contact with infected saliva (kissing—↑ infection rates in adolescence), urine, genital fluids (cervical, vaginal seminal), breast milk (via lactation), and blood. Infection with multiple strains reported in sexually active. ↑ rates found in those with history of STIs and seroprevalence proportional to number of lifetime partners. In STI clinics prevalence of CMV antibodies in homosexual ♂ about 1.5 times that of heterosexual ♂.

Epidemiology and vertical/neonatal transmission

Most common vertically transmitted viral infection. Worldwide incidence of fetal CMV acquisition during pregnancy 0.8–4%. In UK ~50% ♀ becoming pregnant are CMV seronegative with ~3% becoming infected during their pregnancy (largely from young children). 30–40% with 1° infection and about 1% with recurrent CMV will infect their fetus (overall congenital infection rates from 0.5–1%).

Transmitted by fetal ingestion of infected intra-amniotic material, haematological transplacental spread, and lactation.

Clinical features—horizontal transmission

Generally causes asymptomatic infection unless immunosuppressed.
Only 10% of 1° infections cause an infectious mononucleosis type illness consisting of fever, myalgia, cervical lymphadenopathy, and less commonly pneumonitis and hepatitis.

Illness self-limiting, though life-long viral persistence often with extended periods of asymptomatic viral shedding (e.g. during pregnancy).

Clinical features—vertical transmission

Severity of neonatal symptoms/signs less if mother seropositive (neutralizing antibodies). Range from none (in about 80%) to the classical congenital syndrome—hepatosplenomegaly (with jaundice), thrombocytopenia (with purpura), which are self-limiting. Less common but permanent CNS features include microcephaly, chorioretinitis, progressive senso-neuronal deafness.

Diagnosis

- Immunocompetent adults—serology; 4-fold ↑ in IgG CMV antibodies from paired blood samples taken 10–14 days apart or IgM from single specimen (persists up to 20 weeks).
- Fetal infection: CMV detection from amniotic fluid by PCR after 21 weeks gestation.
- Congenital/neonatal infection: CMV culture or PCR from urine and pharynx.

Management

Symptomatic treatment (as for EBV infection).
For CMV associated with HIV infection see p. 436.

Human T-cell lymphotropic virus (HTLV)-1

Single-stranded RNA retrovirus.

Epidemiology and transmission

Endemic in Japan, and parts of the Caribbean, S. America, and sub-Saharan Africa. Main transmission routes are breastfeeding and sexual intercourse but also from blood products and the sharing of injecting drug equipment.

Diagnosis

Serology: enzyme immunoassay or gelatin particle agglutination.

Clinical features

Most infected remain healthy carriers but up to 5% develop adult T-cell leukaemia/lymphoma and ~2–3% myelopathy.

Adult T-cell leukaemia/lymphoma

Leukaemic involvement in 80% with wide-ranging skin lesions in ~40%. Other manifestations include hepatosplenomegaly, lymphadenopathy, hypercalcaemia, and sometimes immunosuppression.

Myelopathy (tropical spastic parapheresis)

Demyelination of long motor neurons of spinal cord producing lower extremity weakness, spasticity, urinary incontinence, and erectile dysfunction.

Management

Trial data shows some success in treating adult T-cell leukaemia/lymphoma with HAART +/– interferon. Without treatment median survival is <1 year.

Human herpes virus-8 (HHV-8)

Herpes virus with five major variants, A–E. B and C predominate in Europe and USA.

Transmission

Sexual, including mouth to mouth contact as HHV-8 is found in saliva. Implicated in close family contact in endemic areas (Africa), especially when associated with poor hygiene. In developed countries ↑ rates among homosexual ♂. Transmission does not appear to be related to pregnancy or breastfeeding.

Clinical features

HHV-8 associated with >95% of cases of Kaposi's sarcoma with immunosuppression an important co-factor. See p. 498.

Chapter 26

Scabies (*Sarcoptes scabiei var hominis*)

Introduction

Discovered in 1687 by Bonomo, arthropod class Arachnida, subclass Acari, family Sarcoptidae.

Aetiology

A parasitic mite with no natural enemies. The ♀ penetrates the stratum corneum constructing short burrows where it lays 1–3 eggs daily during its lifespan of 4–6 weeks. Eggs are oval and 0.1–0.15mm in length. Six-legged larvae hatch in 3–4 days then moult to form an eight-legged nymph. After a further moult the adult develops. The total time to maturity is 10 days with females becoming gravid within 14 days.

The adult is tortoise-like in shape with 8 legs (Fig. 26.1). The two sets of anterior legs end in stalked pulvilli (suckers) which allow the mite to grip the host's skin aiding its movement. Spines and bristles cover the body. Mites are blind with no eyes. The adult female measures 0.4 x $0.3mm^2$ although the male is smaller and dies after mating. It has no spiracles, trachea, or body armour and obtains its oxygen through its surface. Mites can move rapidly on warm skin at ~2.5cm/minute. Burrows are created at variable rates (0.5–5.0mm per day) and lined with scar tissue to prevent them collapsing, thus allowing the mite to breathe and larva to escape. Mites feed on the lymph and lysed tissue. Survival of the mite away from its host is contentious but is unlikely to be >48–72 hours and is probably much less 💣.

Classification

Classical scabies

Found in immunocompetent people with an average of 5–10 mites.

Norwegian scabies (crusted scabies)

Found in the immunocompromised and elderly, may be related to failure of sensitization to mite antigen. Highly contagious, with honeycombed cavities in the skin containing many thousands of mites. Extensive crusted lesions with thick hyperkeratotic scales ('bread crumb') develop over the elbows, palms, knees, and soles of the feet.

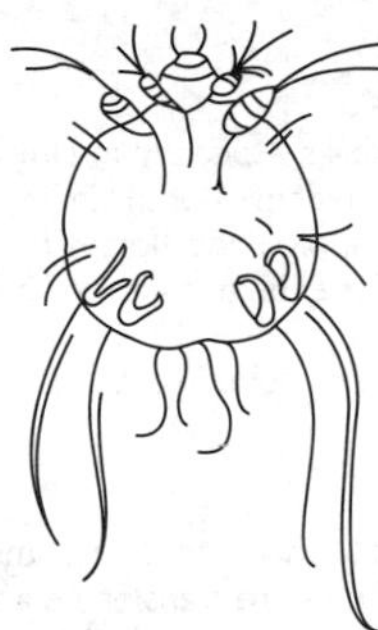

Fig. 26.1 Sarcoptes scabiei

Frequently asked questions

Is it always sexually transmitted?

No. The majority of cases are not sexually transmitted. It commonly occurs in people living closely together and is spread by prolonged skin contact, including holding hands.

Do I just need to treat my body from the neck down?

No. Although this still may be suggested we advise that all skin surfaces are treated, taking care around mucous membranes. Even the scalp should be treated if you are bald. Relapses occur because of failure to treat all sites that may be infected.

Does anyone else require treatment?

Treatment is advised for current sexual partners and intimate household contacts.

I finished the treatment 2 weeks ago but still have some itching. Do I need to repeat it again?

No. Not if you have used it properly and not been re-infected. Symptoms often take 4–5 weeks to resolve as they are due to a hypersensitivity reaction stimulated by mite products. It usually takes this time for them to be expelled from the skin and for the reaction to settle. If relief is required topical crotamiton or antihistamines should help.

Epidemiology

Appears as sporadic outbreaks especially in families, schools, dormitories, institutions, and nurseries. Epidemics occur in 15–30 year cycles. Mammals such as domestic cats, dogs, pigs, and horses may be infected with other sarcoptidae (mange) which may be transferred to humans resulting in irritation without infestation.

Associated with previous or concurrent STIs.

Transmission

Holding hands is the most likely route of transmission. Prolonged skin to skin contact is necessary. Mites are transferred after about 10–20 minutes of close contact and can penetrate the epidermis within 30 minutes. Not vectors of other infections.

Clinical features

In 1° infection patients may be asymptomatic for the first 4–6 weeks. Intense irritation only occurs after immunological reactivity develops (less common in Norwegian scabies). In re-infestation signs and symptoms become evident in 24–48 hours due to previous sensitization.

- Symmetrical, polymorphic, lesions appear, most commonly on hands (especially finger webs), wrists, axillae, genitals, buttocks, and extensor aspect of elbows (Fig. 26.2). They are usually eczematous and associated with burrows (fine, short, serpiginous grey/black channels 5–10mm in length often with a small associated papule or vesicle).
- Indurated nodules (nodular scabies) are commonly found affecting the scrotum, penis, and groin. Mites usually cannot be recovered from these lesions.
- Urticarial papular rash, without mites, may be found in the axillae, upper abdomen, loins, and inner thighs.

Excoriation may lead to 2° bacterial infection.

Diagnosis

Clinical appearance

Burrows may be identified by:

- staining the suspected site with a washable felt tip marker. After removal by washing, the ink will be found to have delineated the burrow
- applying topical tetracycline to the skin and washing off the excess. Burrows retain tetracycline which will fluoresce under Wood's light.

Material for microscopy can be obtained by:

- Extraction of mites (or eggs) from their burrows with a needle
- Scraping the skin using a scalpel blade, following the local application of liquid paraffin.

Mites may be recovered from the wrists (63%), extensor aspect of elbows (11%), feet and ankles (9%), genitals (9%), buttocks (4%), and axillae (2%).

Other possible methods of diagnosis include videodermatoscopy, epiluminescence microscopy, or skin biopsy.

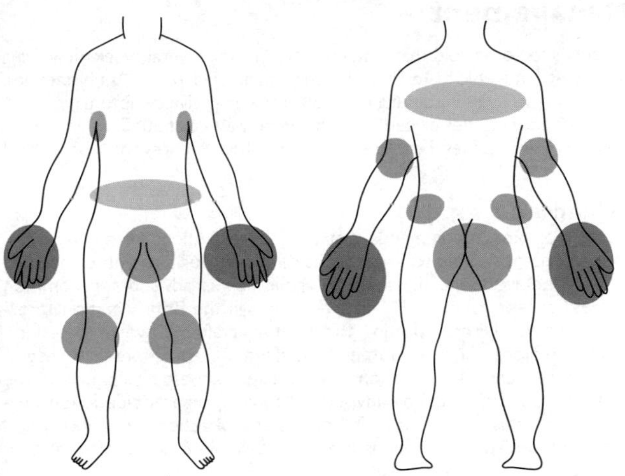

Fig. 26.2 Distribution of scabies

Management

Patients should be told that irritation may last for several weeks following treatment (antigenic material in the dermis and epidermis). Antihistamines, crotamiton 10% cream or calamine 15% lotion may give symptomatic relief. Contaminated clothes or bed linen should be washed at 50°C.

Norwegian scabies best treated in isolation to prevent nosocomial spread.

Treatment

Current opinion recommends that topical preparations be applied head to toe (except for the scalp unless bald) and left for a period of not less than 12 hours. Generally a single application is advised for common scabies (except for benzyl benzoate) although the British National Formulary now advises repeating the treatment after 1 week (based on expert opinion). Aqueous rather than alcohol preparations are recommended because of ↑ irritation of excoriated skin especially around the genitalia. Patients should be advised not to apply an acaricide following a hot bath as this may remove it from its site of action by ↑ absorption into the bloodstream. If hands are washed within 8 hours of treatment a repeat application is required.

Common scabies

- Permethrin 5% cream.
- Malathion 0.5% aqueous lotion.
- Benzyl benzoate—leave for 24 hours (2–3 applications on consecutive days).

Norwegian scabies

- Topical—repeat applications required for all products
- Ivermectin (named patient basis)—200µg/kg (single dose) in addition if no response to topical agents alone.

Pregnancy/breast feeding

Permethrin is the treatment of choice.

Partner notification

Sexual and household contacts should be treated.

Chapter 27

Pediculosis

Introduction

Pthiriasis (pediculosis) is an ancient disease. Nits (eggs of lice) have been discovered on the pubic hair of a 2000-year-old Chilean mummy, and also in fossilized form dating back to ~10,000 years.

Aetiology

Belonging to the sub-order of Anoplura (sucking lice), the families of Pediculidae (body lice) and Pthiridae (pubic lice) are wingless insects unable to fly or jump. *Pthirus pubis* (the crab louse) (Fig. 27.1) is classified as a species of the genus Pthirus. *Pediculus humanus capitis* (head lice) and *Pediculus humanus humanus* and *corporis* (body lice) are morphologically similar and easily distinguished from pubic lice (smaller and squatter). Life cycle of pubic lice ~15–25 days occurring in 3 stages.

The nit

- White oval egg <0.8mm attached to the hair base by a chitinous envelope.
- Encased by a proteinaceous sheath except for the operculum, allowing ventilation.
- Appears to move up the hair and away from the skin as hair grows.

The nymph

- Resembles a pubic louse but is smaller.
- Hatches in 7 days by releasing itself from the egg with air expelled from its anus.
- Migrates back to the hair base to suck blood and mature.

The adult

- ~1–2mm in length, dark grey to brown in colour. The ♂ is smaller and has a more pointed tail.
- Three distinct pairs of legs each with claw-like appendages whose grasp is designed to match the diameter of pubic or axillary hair in contrast to the finer scalp hair. Can move ~10cm in a day.
- Sensory antennae detect human smell and tactile hairs on its body determine surface type. Eyes faceted, almost blind but photophobic.
- Buries sharp mouthpiece stylets inside a pubic hair follicle to obtain a constant blood supply. Ingests several times its own weight in blood during each feed. May feed at the same place for days.
- Single pair of spiracles allow gaseous exchange and prevent dehydration.
- ♀ will lay two to three eggs during a 24-hour period and 15–50 eggs over a lifetime.

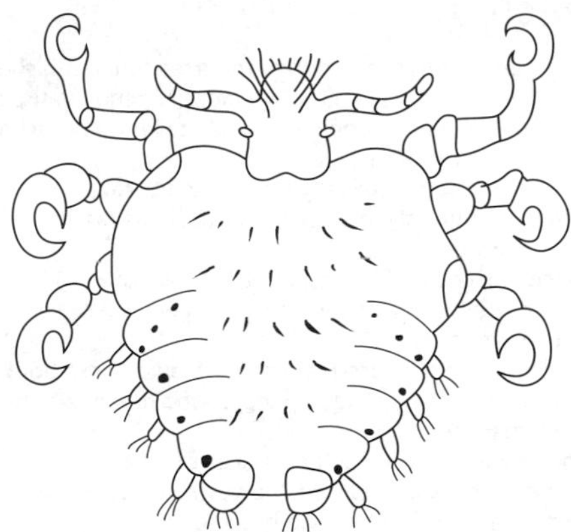

Fig. 27.1 Pthirus pubis

Frequently asked questions

How have I got them?

The crab louse is transmitted by close body contact hence during sexual contact. More rarely infestation can be spread through contact with an infested person's bed linen, towel, or clothes.

Do I need to treat all of my body hair?

Yes, a lotion should be applied to all of the body hair including a beard and moustache if necessary.

Will shaving get rid of the lice?

Lice are treated with carbaryl, malathion, or permethrin preparations. All of the body hairs need to be treated, not just the pubic hair. Therefore shaving is not recommended as treatment.

Do I need to wash all of my bedding?

Yes, it is recommended that all clothes and bed linen should be machine washed on a hot water cycle.

Does my partner need treatment?

Yes. Current sexual partners need treatment. Avoid close body contact until partner and partner(s) completed treatment. Contact tracing of all partners in the previous 3 months is recommended.

Pthirus or Phthirus?

Spelling varies with both Pthirus and Phthirus widely used. Although derived from the Greek *phtheir* (louse), the former is used more widely.

Epidemiology

- Essentially a human parasite although reported to infest higher apes.
- Does not occur in epidemics although more common in the cooler months of the year (unlike body and head lice which occur more often in the warmer months).
- Considered to be usually sexually transmitted because:
  - found most commonly in sexually active adults (aged 16–25 years), especially homosexual ♂.
  - associated with other STIs, especially chlamydia.
- Related to crowded living conditions, poor personal hygiene, and low socio-economic status.
- Infestation of the scalp is rare (about 1% of louse infestation) but occurs more often in red-headed people, who have fewer hairs per unit area than others.
- Rarely reported in the scalp and eyelashes of children, in whom sexual abuse may need to be considered. However, acquisition from nipple hairs during breast feeding has also been reported.
- Not known to be vectors of human disease (unlike body and head lice which may carry organisms responsible for epidemic or louse borne typhus, trench fever, and louse borne relapsing fever).

Transmission

- Usually by skin to skin contact with up to 95% of sexual contacts of an active carrier developing an infestation.
- Occasionally by clothing, bedding, or towels.
- It is unlikely that lice can survive for more than 24–48 hours if removed from host.

Clinical features

~76% complain of intense irritation in the genital area due to hypersensitivity with ~40% of patients experiencing erythema. In the hirsute infestation may spread to the thighs, perineum, trunk, abdomen, or axillary hair. Eyebrows and eyelashes (pthiriasis palpebrarum) may also be infested with the possibility of 2° conjunctivitis.

Blue macules (maculae caeruleae) caused by an enzyme secreted from the salivary glands of the lice may be visible at feeding sites. 0.2 to 0.3cm in diameter, with an irregular outline, painless, do not disappear on pressure, and appear to be in the deeper tissues. Apparent some hours after the louse has fed, lasting several days. 'Black spots' on underwear or in the genital area, usually indicate insect faecal matter or blood spots.

Diagnosis

Identify lice, eggs, or maculae caeruleae with the naked eye. Low power microscopy of the louse may show movement, sucking pumps in the head and a blood filled oesophagus.

Management

Offer full screening for STIs and advise avoidance of close body contact until patient and partner(s) complete treatment. Clothes and bed linen should be washed at 50°C or dry-cleaned.

Due to the delicate nature of the genital skin aqueous rather than alcohol based preparations are recommended with lotions more effective than shampoos. All body hair should be treated (not just groins and axillae) and left for 12 hours (or overnight). A second application after 7 days is advisable to kill lice emerging from any surviving nits. Dead nits may continue to adhere to hairs for several weeks following treatment and can be removed with a fine tooth comb.

Suggested treatments

- malathion 0.5%
- carbaryl 1% (unlicensed for pubic lice)
- permethrin 1% (recommended in pregnancy or during lactation)
- phenothrin 0.2%

Eyelashes

- permethrin 1% lotion ensuring patient keeps eyes closed throughout the procedure and for the following 10 minutes.
- aqueous malathion (unlicensed for eyelashes).
- pilocarpine hydrochloride 4% (Pilogel).
- physostigmine.
- application of yellow soft paraffin or vaseline killing the lice by occluding their spiracles.
- removal of lice with forceps.

Partner notification

Sexual partners within the previous 3 months should be advised to seek screening and treatment. The latter may also be required for those sharing the same bedding.

Chapter 28

Anogenital dermatoses

Variations and anomalies

Maculo-papular

- Haemangioma: red macule up to 3–5 mm in diameter on glans penis, less commonly vulval mucosa.
- Pigmentary changes
  - Vitiligo: depigmentation (may also affect hair). Association with autoimmunity, especially thyroiditis.
  - Melanocytic naevi (moles): genital lesions (keratinised skin) found in ~15% of the population.
  - Mucosal melanosis (genital lentiginosis): more commonly in ♀.

Papular

- ***Achrocordon (skin tags).*** Common around the groin and thighs especially in those aged >50 years.
- ***Angiokeratomas.*** Purple/dark red papules on labia majora, scrotum, and penile shaft. ↑ in those aged >50 years. Benign hyperkeratosis with dilated capillaries. Rarely associated with Anderson–Fabry disease.
- ***Dermatofibroma (fibrous histiocytoma).*** Firm indolent dermal nodule usually <5mm diameter. Benign reactive fibroblast proliferation that may resemble a wart.
- ***Ectopic sebaceous glands (Fordyce spots).*** Tiny yellow grouped papules. Occasionally form larger nodules. Usually found on the mucosal surface of the prepuce and upper/inner labia minora.
- ***Epidermal cysts.*** White or creamy coloured nodules commonly found over scrotum and labia majora. Hair follicles blocked with keratin and filled with sebaceous matter. If required remove surgically.
- ***Epidermal naevi.*** Epidermal outgrowths present at birth (50%) or developing during childhood.
- ***Nabothian follicles.*** Bluish or yellow coloured translucent lumps on cervix. Retention cysts from cervical 'glands'.
- ***Pearly penile papules (hirsutes papillaris penis).*** White dome-shaped papules found at the corona and adjacent to the frenum. Sometimes confused with warts. Reported in 20–50% ♂, usually <1mm in size, may extend to 3mm. Consist of connective tissue core with central thinned epidermis. Removal generally not recommended but clearance possible with cryosurgery and carbon dioxide laser ablation.
- ***Prominent hair follicles.*** Found on penile shaft, scrotum, labia majora.
- ***Seborrhoeic keratosis/wart.*** Domed, heavily pigmented papule usually ~ 1cm in diameter. Eccrine poroma (benign neoplasm that shows differentiation towards glandular ductal cells). Commonly found on mons pubis, penile shaft, labia majora usually in those aged >50 years. If removal required cryosurgery (repeated) or curettage normally effective.
- ***Vulval papillae.*** Fleshy, filiform papules commonly found within the labia minora, and often confused with warts. Typically soft, symmetrical, linear, and pink with separate bases.

Degenerative

Ovarian failure, usually 2° to the menopause, leads to urogenital atrophy, symptomatic in >50%. Symptoms include vulvo-vaginal dryness with discomfort, irritation, and dyspaerunia. Often associated with other systemic symptoms which may influence management. Treat with oestrogen-based hormone replacement therapy which can be administered by various routes (oral, transdermal, subcutaneous, vaginal, and intranasal). Urogenital symptoms may take a year to respond.

Infective conditions

Tinea cruris

Dermatophytic fungal infection commonly due to *Tinea rubrum*, *T. mentagrophytes*, *Epidermophyton floccosum*. Found in those sharing communal facilities (e.g. towels) and auto-inoculation from tinea pedis. More common in ♂. Pruritic plaques in the groin, spreading out to the thigh, with well-defined erythematous scaly edge and central clearing.
Diagnosis: appearance, scraping from margins for microscopy (de-keratinize with potassium hydroxide) or culture.
Management: topical imidazoles (2–8 weeks), oral griseofulvin (0.5g daily for 2–6 weeks).

Erythrasma

Chronic infection of crural folds (especially axilla and groin) caused by *Corynebacterium minutissimum*. Associated with hyperhydrosis, diabetes mellitus, and living in crowded conditions. Dull red or brownish uniform scaly patch with little or no pruritus.
Diagnosis: coral-pink fluorescence with Wood's light. Scale culture.
Management: sodium fusidate ointment 2%, erythromycin gel 2% twice daily for 2 weeks.

Hidradenitis suppurativa

Chronic inflammatory disorder of apocrine glands in the presence of local bacterial infection. Associated with acne, obesity, androgens (in ♀), familial predisposition. Painful nodules which may progress to abscesses, sinuses, fistulae, and scarring. Found in axillae, groin, buttocks, perianal skin.
Diagnosis: clinical appearance.
Management: weight reduction, chlorhexidine disinfectants, long-term tetracyclines, local steroids (for isolated lesions), anti-androgenic high oestrogen oral contraception (♀), and surgery for severe disease.

Inflammatory conditions

Irritant and contact dermatitis (see Box opposite)

- Irritant—direct response to noxious agent, e.g. chemicals, certain soaps, disinfectants, products containing bleach.
- Allergic—idiosyncratic hypersensitivity reaction, e.g. spermicides, semen, or its contents (e.g. antibiotics), local anaesthetics, latex, deodorants, fragrances, lubricants and body lotions containing propylene glycol or glycerin, *Candida* spp., anti-mycotic creams and other topical medications (including local anaesthetic preparations).

Erythema, excoriation, pruritus. Thin, mucosal skin more prone to react to contact agents. May become chronic (lichen simplex chronicus) with excoriation producing lichenification and erythema or hyperpigmentation).
Diagnosis: history, appearance, exclude infection. For contact dermatitis patch testing can be considered although results are often difficult to interpret. Radioallergosorbent and skin prick tests can be performed for suspected Type I immediate hypersensitivity.
Management: advice on avoiding irritants. If moderate to severe—topical steroids, low, or if chronic, medium potency.

Genital hypersensitivity

Sexually related

- Seminal fluid or its contents (e.g. antibiotics)—often associated with systemic symptoms.
- Spermicides and lubricants (may cause irritant or contact dermatitis).
- Latex or products used in condom manufacturing (e.g. carbamates). Polyurethane seems to be safe.
- Topical skin preparations or chemicals (e.g. on fingers). May cause irritant or contact dermatitis).

Not sexually related

- Topical medications (e.g. steroid preparations, anaesthetics, imidazoles)
- Perfumes and cosmetic preparations
  - Female hygiene sprays or wipes
  - Bubble baths, scented soaps, hair shampoos
- Sanitary pads and towels (may be chemically treated)
- *Candida* spp.
- Urine (irritant dermatitis).

Seborrhoeic dermatitis

Scaly inflammation of hairy sebaceous skin. Familial tendency. More common with HIV infection. Presents as dry erythema with serous transudation (mons pubis, labia majora, scrotum, and penile shaft); discoid lesions with 2° infection and crusting; shiny, well-defined erythema with tenderness (labia minora, subpreputial sac, and glans penis).
Diagnosis: appearance and erythematous lesions covered with greasy yellowish scales at other typical sites (scalp, eyebrows, naso-labial folds, sternum, axillae, umbilicus, natal cleft). Histology.
Management: low potency topical steroids and antimicrobials including ketoconazole (if infected).

Fixed drug eruption

Reaction at the same site in an individual to repeated use of a systemic agent. Over 500 drugs implicated including tetracyclines, barbiturates, phenolphthalein (laxative chocolate), sulfonamides, paracetamol. Preferentially affects genitals (especially glans penis). Sudden onset of erythematous macule or bulla with irritation or pain.
Diagnosis: history and appearance.
Management: stop drug. Spontaneously resolves but may leave hyperpigmentation.

Erythema multiforme (EM) and Stevens–Johnson syndrome (S–JS)

Acute skin reaction of unknown aetiology but precipitated by infection (e.g. Herpes simplex virus, *Mycoplasma pneumoniae*, *Histoplasma capsulatum*), drugs (e.g. sulfonamides, phenytoin, penicillin), autoimmune diseases (e.g. polyarteritis nodosa), sarcoidosis, malignancy. ↑ frequency of S–JS with HIV infection. Non-pruritic maculo-papular circular lesions with a deep red centre (may form bullae) and erythema producing target or iris lesions, typically found around the hands and feet. The severe bullous form (S–JS) includes orogenital bullae with ulceration, urethritis, conjunctivitis and keratitis, pyrexia, and multi-system disease.
Diagnosis: clinical features.
Management: EM resolves without scarring in 2–3 weeks. Systemic steroids may be required for severe S–JS.

Psoriasis

Affects ~1% of population, 30% familial incidence, ↑ severity with HIV infection. Anogenital/perigenital lesions common which may be:

- papular—well demarcated erythematous, scaly, plaques, or sheets. Usually found on skin around genitalia, labia majora, scrotum, penile shaft and occasionally glans penis.
- inversed—macular, erythematous, non-scaly moist patches arising in perigenital flexures, perianal, labia minora, sub-preputial sac, and glans penis.

Diagnosis: appearance, lesions in classic sites (knees, elbows, scalp, nails with pitting) and histology.
Management: reassure not infection. Low potency topical steroids, 2% coal tar solution.

Lichen planus and lichen nitidus

Inflammatory condition, unknown aetiology. Polygonal, violaceous papules (2–10mm) or annular lesions which may be covered by white streaks (Wickham's striae). Usually found around flexor aspect of wrists but genital involvement common and may cause erosions on mucous epithelium. A network of small white threads or papules over the buccal mucosa is characteristic. Lichen nitidus, a probable variant, presents as small flesh coloured papules (genitals/lower abdomen), similar to molluscum contagiosum, without the 'umbilicus'.
Diagnosis: appearance, classic sites, and histology.
Management: reassure not infection (self-limiting). Low potency topical steroids.

Plasma cell balanitis (of Zoon)

Simple condition of unknown aetiology usually in middle aged/older uncircumcised ♂. Moist shiny area of speckled erythema on glans or mucosal aspect of prepuce.
Diagnosis: histology—heavy plasma cell infiltration.
Management: topical hydrocortisone. Persistent cases respond well to circumcision.
Plasma cell vulvitis, with similar features, occasionally found in ♀.

Lichen sclerosis (LS). Also called balanitis xerotica obliterans (in ♂)

Condition of unknown aetiology. Familial predisposition with onset in up to 50% before puberty. Associated with autoimmune conditions and trauma (Koebner phenomenon). Anogenital skin involvement common. May be asymptomatic or cause pruritus, discomfort or painful intercourse, micturition and defecation if associated with scarring.

Although there may be signs of acute inflammation typical finding is ivory-white polygonal lesions which become confluent and are associated with atrophy, telangiectasia, purpura, erosions, lichenification, and sclerosis. ♂ may develop 2° phimosis and meatal strictures and ♀ labial adhesions with fusion and anal fissuring or stenosis and a loss of clitoral architecture. LS may simulate signs of sexual abuse in prepubertal girls, though it has been alleged that abuse may be related to its aetiology through trauma. Also may cause phimosis in prepubertal boys.

► Penile carcinoma rarely reported with LS but up to 5% ♀ with LS develop squamous cell carcinoma (SCC) of the vulva.
Diagnosis: histology.
Management: if active high dose topical fluorinated steroids for 3 months with careful review and annual assessment for 5 years. Lubricants may help with intercourse. Potassium permanganate soaks are useful for moist inflamed lesions, especially in ♀. Surgical intervention may be required for urethral stenosis and circumcision for phimosis.

Ulcerative conditions

Aphthosis

Common condition of unknown aetiology. Recurrent oral ulcers, rarely genital (especially vulva and scrotum). Associated with trauma and chronic cyclic neutropenia. Shallow painful ulcers about 1–10mm in diameter.
Diagnosis: clinical features. Exclude HSV infection and Behçet's disease.
Management: topical steroids (if severe).

Behçet's Disease

Multisystem disease of unknown aetiology but more commonly found in the E. Mediterranean, Middle East, and Far East. Associated with certain human leucocyte antigen types, especially B51.
Diagnosis: based on defined clinical features.
Recurrent oral ulceration (as aphthosis) >3 times/year and 2 of the following:

- recurrent genital ulcers (as aphthosis)—found in 80%.
- eye lesions (anterior/posterior uveitis, cells in vitreous on slit-lamp examination, retinal vasculitis).
- skin lesions (erythema nodosum, pseudofolliculitis, or papulo-pustular lesions, acneiform nodules in post-adolescence).
- positive pathergy test (papule/pustule developing at site of hypodermic needle puncture, read at 24–48 hours).

Neurological (meningoencephalitis, nerve palsies, brain-stem, and spinal cord lesions) and gastrointestinal (diarrhoea, abdominal pain) features may appear.
Management: local topical steroids. Severe disease—systemic steroids, azathioprine, cyclophosphamide, colchicine, chlorambucil, thalidomide.

Pyoderma gangrenosum

Associated with inflammatory bowel disease, seropositive and seronegative arthritis. Initial pustule progressing to a painful necrotic ulcer occasionally affecting the vulva, penis, or scrotum.
Diagnosis: appearance and associated pathology. Histology.
Management: treat underlying condition. Systemic steroids, dapsone.

Pemphigus vulgaris

Commonest type of pemphigus. Autoimmune condition. Age group usually affected 50–60 years.

Cutaneous lesions appear as flaccid bullae which burst to form painful ulcers. The mucosae, especially the mouth, are ultimately involved in all cases. Genital ulcers are slow to heal but only occasionally scar. Finger pressure on skin may cause epidermis to separate due to its poor attach ment (Nikolsky's sign) and when applied to the edge of a bulla spreads it to adjacent clinically unaffected skin (Asboe–Hansen sign).
Diagnosis: histology, direct or indirect immunofluorescence to show intercellular deposits of IgG and complement.
Management: local or systemic steroids, antibiotics, immunosuppressants (dapsone, azathioprine, cyclophosphamide).

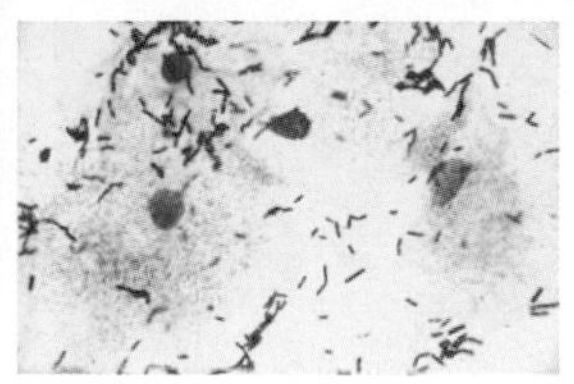

Plate 1 Gram-smear lactobacilli

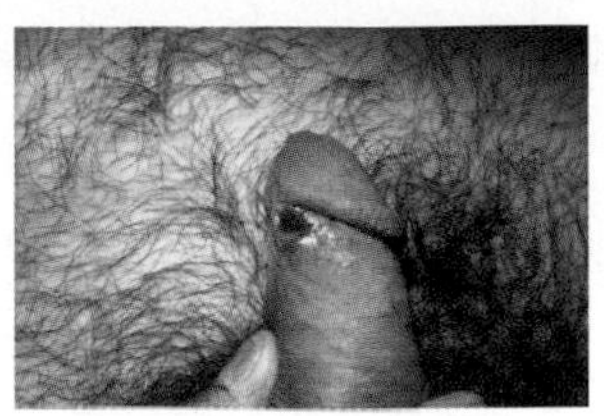

Plate 2 Classic primary chancre

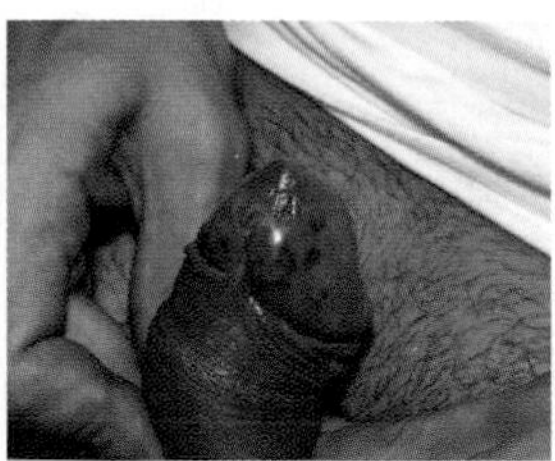

Plate 3 'Contemporary' chancre

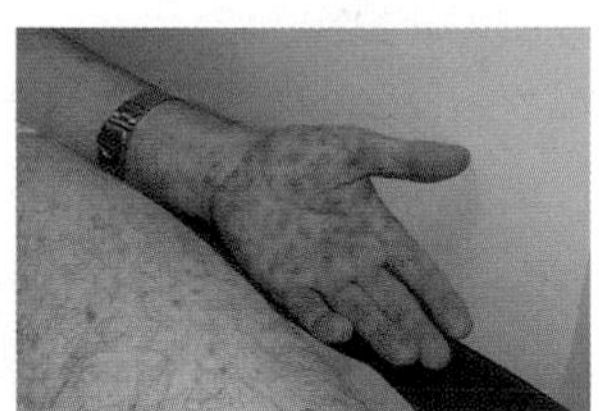

Plate 4 Secondary syphilis

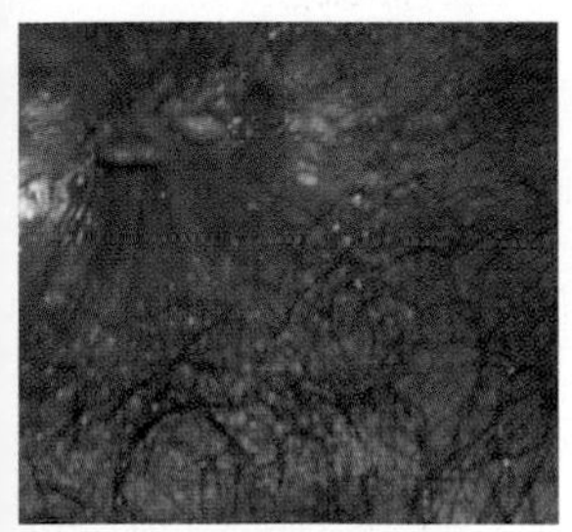

Plate 5 Condolymata lata

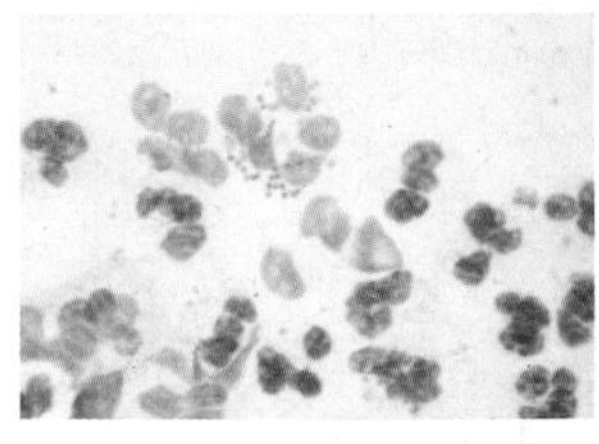

Plate 6 Gram-smear gonorrhoea

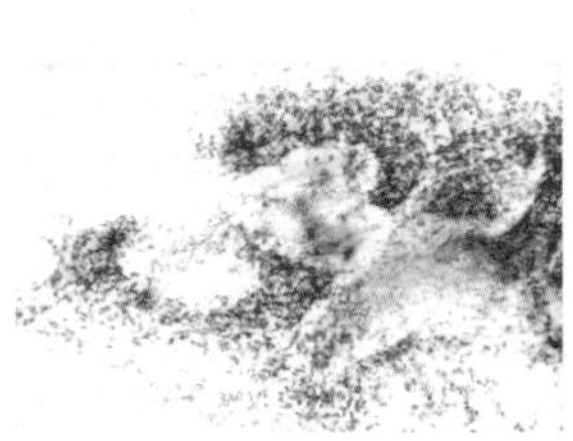

Plate 7 Gram-smear BV

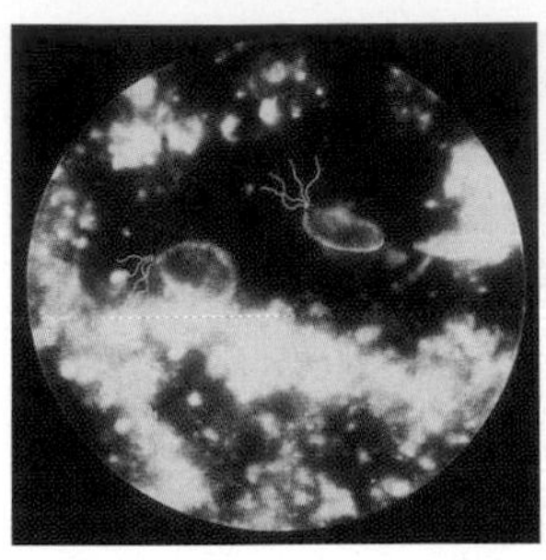

Plate 8 Dark-ground trichomonas vaginalis

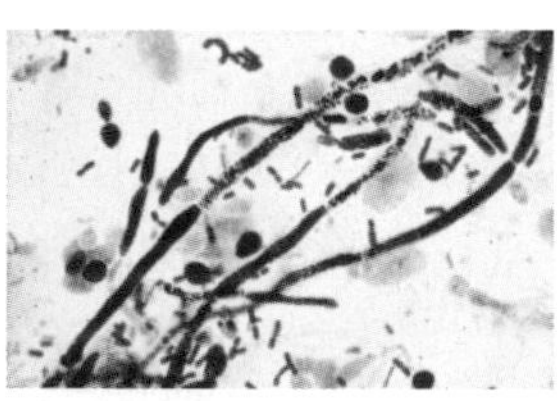

Plate 9 Gram-smear candidiasis

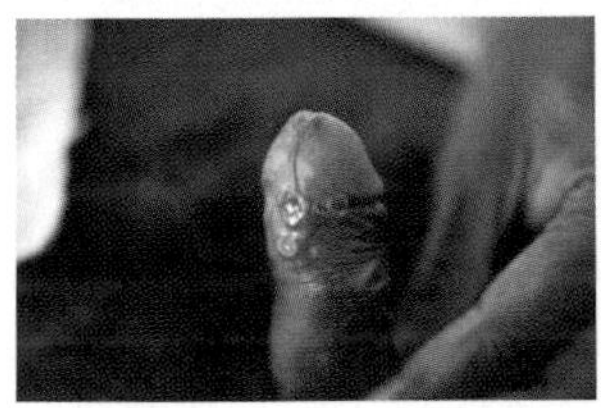

Plate 10 Chancroid

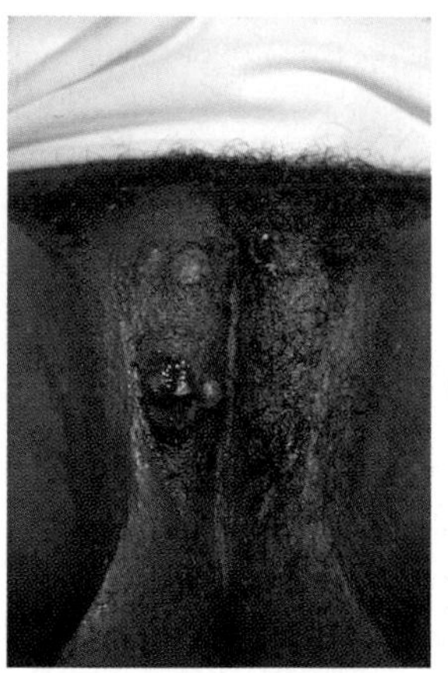

Plate 11 Granuloma inguinale

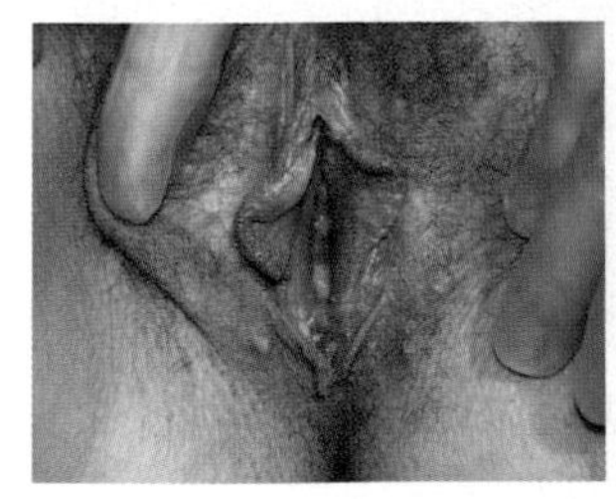

Plate 12 Vulval herpes

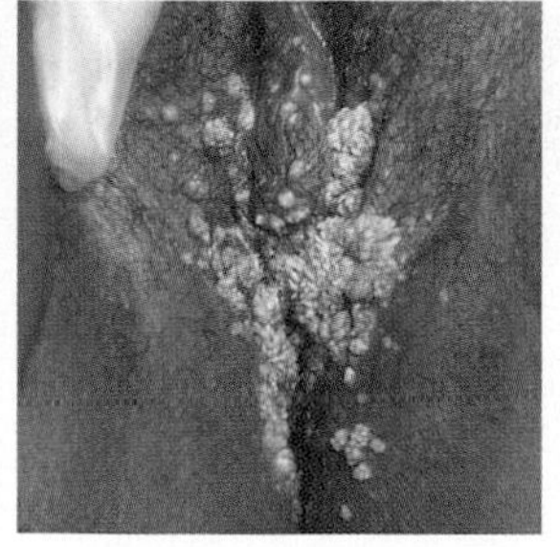

Plate 13 Anogenital warts

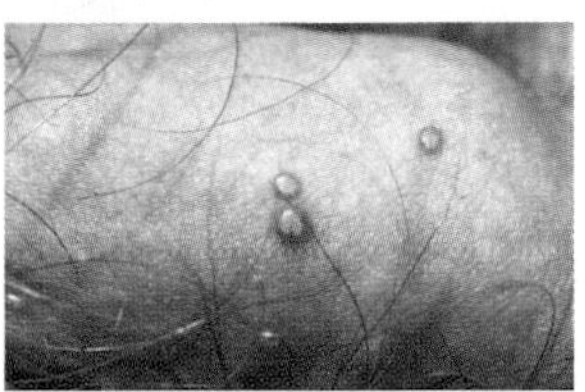

Plate 14 Molluscum contagiosum

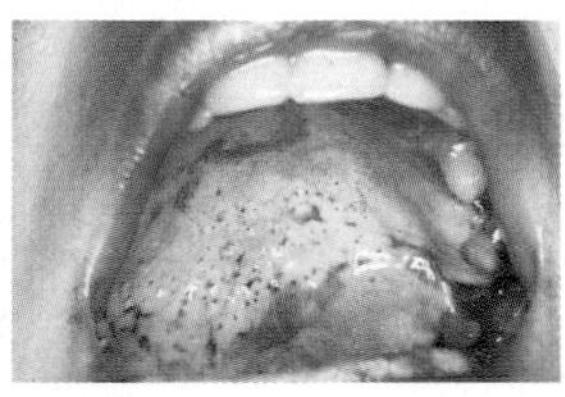

Plate 15 Oral candidiasis and HIV

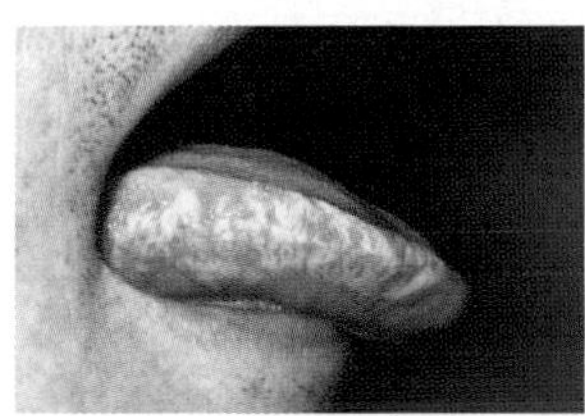

Plate 16 HIV—oral hairy leukoplakia

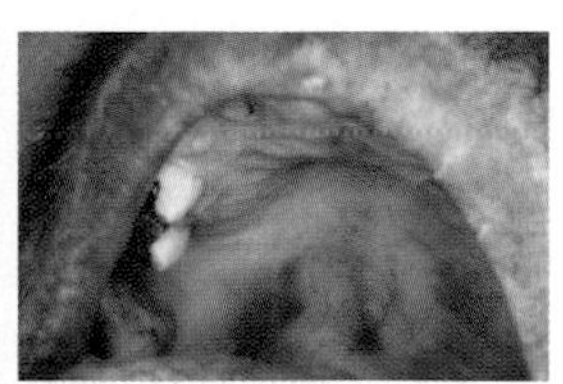

Plate 17 Oral Kaposi's sarcoma

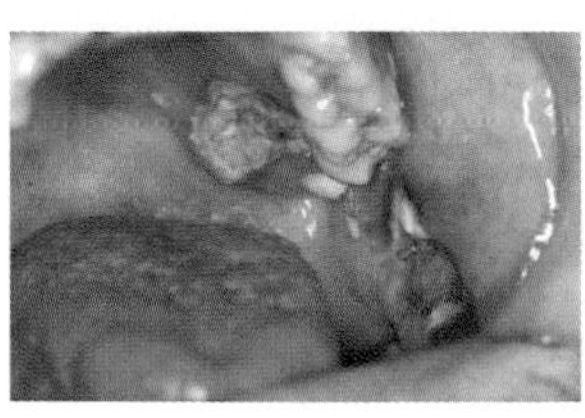

Plate 18 Oral lymphoma and HIV

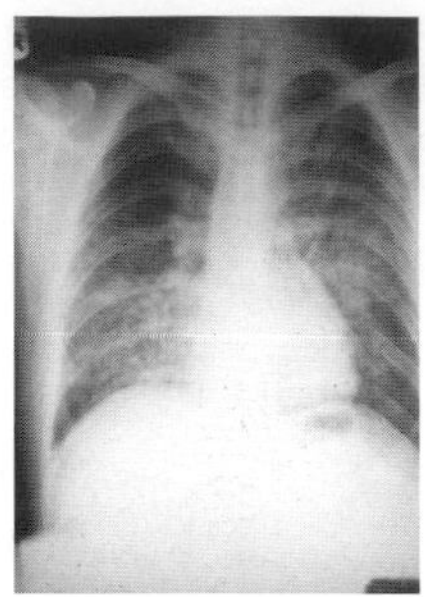

Plate 19 Chest x-ray—PCP

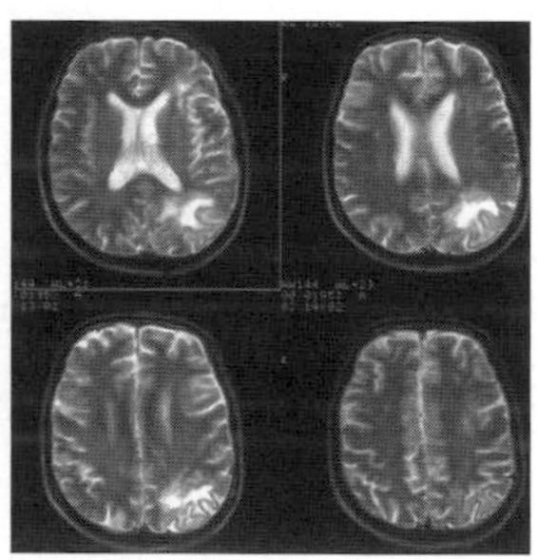

Plate 20 Brain scan—progressive multifocal leukoencephalopathy

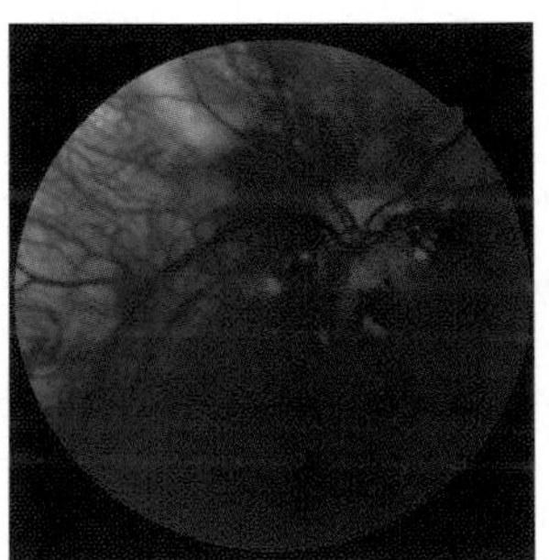

Plate 21 CMV retinitis

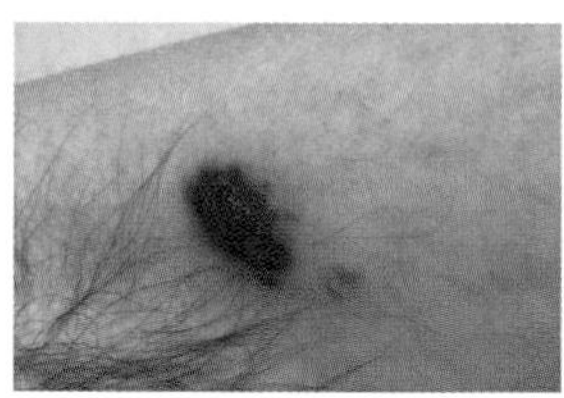

Plate 22 Cutaneous Kaposi's sarcoma

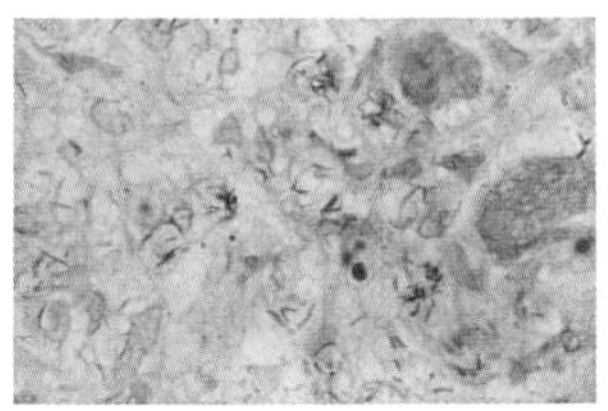

Plate 23 Mycobacteria in lymph node biopsy Ziehl-Neelsen stain

Cicatricial pemphigoid

Autoimmune condition usually affecting older people. Involves skin and mucosa, which may be the only site. Eye involvement (kerato-conjunctivitis with scarring) common. Tense blisters which ulcerate with secondary scarring and adhesions of genital and oral mucosa.

Diagnosis: as pemphigus vulgaris.

Management: as pemphigus vulgaris.

Premalignant conditions

Extramammary Paget's disease

Most commonly found around anus and genitals, especially labia majora, typically presenting as infiltrative plaques. Anal involvement almost always associated with underlying carcinoma, possibly of sweat glands.
Diagnosis: histology
Management: excision.

Vulval, penile, and anal intraepithelial neoplasia (VIN, PIN, AIN)

These pathological descriptive names encompass and replace other terms used to describe dysplasia and squamous cell carcinoma *in situ* (CIS) including Bowen's disease and erythroplasia of Queyrat. Intraepithelial neoplasia (IN) is commonly associated with LS, high-risk HPV infection, ↑ risk of neoplasia elsewhere (e.g. cervical IN) and is also found more frequently in those immunosuppressed (e.g. with HIV infection). Graded by the level of epidermal involvement:

- IN1 (mild dysplasia)—lowest 1/3rd involved
- IN2 (moderate dysplasia)—involves lower 2/3rds
- IN3 (severe dysplasia/CIS)— >2/3rds involved

Diagnosis therefore made on histology.

- VIN
  - Bowenoid VIN (classic type)—more common form of VIN. Usually ♀ aged 30–40 years, 70% current or past cigarette smokers, 50–90% association with HPV, especially type 16. Clinical appearance varies but often presents as white plaques or nodular lesions, which may be pigmented, with multifocal involvement in 40%. 'Bowenoid papulosis' has been used to describe multiple small papules or condylomatous lesions with IN histology. Less likely to develop into SCC than CIS.
  - Simplex VIN (differentiated)—2–10% of VIN. Most common in post-menopausal ♀, 25% current or past cigarette smokers. Small grey/white roughened lesions which may be multifocal. Strong link with HPV negative vulval carcinoma.
- PIN

Associated with HPV (especially type 16), smoking and possibly agricultural chemicals. High grade lesions found most commonly in the 6th decade. Usually presents as multiple lesions ('bowenoid papulosis') which may be:

- flat (grey/red, well demarcated with increased vascularity)
- small plaques of leukoplakia (hyperkeratinised)
- papular and pigmented

In addition, usually in older, uncircumcised ♂ there may be mucosal erythroplastic lesions (shiny, friable, red, moist lesions on glans penis or mucosal surface of prepuce), also known as erythroplasia of Queyrat.

- AIN

Found most commonly in homosexual and bisexual ♂, especially those with HIV infection, and in ♀ with a history of anal sex. HPV 16 associated with anal SCC.

Management of external anogenital IN

There is little evidence based data on the management of this group of conditions. Current practice depends on the grading and extent of the pathology influenced by clinical factors such as appearance and symptoms.

- IN1 and IN2 have a low rate of progression and may resolve spontaneously. It is common practice to keep such cases under supervision (though may be discharged if no cytological progression after 3 consecutive 6 monthly visits). If HIV +ve review should be maintained indefinitely.
- IN3 carries a 5–10% risk of subsequent SCC therefore treatment is usually advised. These include:

Excision biopsy (if complete).
Cryotherapy.
Electrosurgery.
Laser evaporation.
Topical imiquimod 5%.
Topical 5-fluorouracil 5%.
Surgical excision (usual treatment for AIN).
Review after treatment required as ~30% recur within 5 years.

Malignant conditions

Rarely seen in the GUM clinic but require urgent referral elsewhere.

- SCC: associated with intraepithelial neoplasia, lichen sclerosis and high-risk HPV infection (see above).
- Melanoma; very rare on penis but genital lesions account for 3% of melanomas in ♀.
- Basal cell carcinoma rare on surfaces not commonly exposed to the sun, however, genital lesions have been reported especially scrotal.

Conditions exacerbated by or found more frequently with HIV infection

- Seborrhoeic dermatitis
- Psoriasis
- Stevens–Johnson syndrome
- Anogenital intraepithelial neoplasia

Chapter 29

Cervical neoplasia

Introduction

The vagina and ectocervix are lined by stratified squamous and the endocervix with columnar epithelium. The position of the squamo-columnar junction (SCJ) varies throughout life. Hormonal changes of puberty and pregnancy (or the use of hormonal contraception) lead to eversion of the endocervical columnar epithelium moving the SCJ distally. This is counterbalanced by squamous metaplasia (the normal process of reversion to squamous epithelium). The area between the original and receding SCJ is known as transformation zone (TZ), which is susceptible to malignant change when exposed to oncogenic stimuli, especially high-risk human papilloma virus (HPV).

Atypia: cells in the epithelium show nuclear or cytoplasmic abnormalities not considered to be malignant or premalignant. Koilocytotic atypia or koiloctytosis refers to the presence of cells with a perinuclear halo associated with HPV infection.

Cervical intraepithelial neoplasia (CIN): squamous cell premalignant lesion also known as dysplasia. Identified by architectural and cytological changes in the epithelium with the underlying basement membrane intact (essential feature). There are 3 grades of CIN based on the level of epithelial involvement:

- CIN1—lowest 1/3rd (mild dysplasia)
- CIN2—lower 2/3rd (moderate dysplasia)
- CIN3—> 2/3rds (severe dysplasia or carcinoma *in situ*).

Cervical glandular intraepithelial neoplasia (CGIN): columnar cell premalignant lesions. Less common than CIN. Identified by nuclear, nucleolar, and gland structure abnormalities. Low-grade (LCGIN) is also known as endocervical gland dysplasia (EGD) and high-grade (HCGIN) as adenocarcinoma *in situ* (AIS).

Invasive cervical carcinoma (ICC): penetration of the basement membrane by malignant epithelial cells. 85–90% are squamous cell carcinoma (SCC) and the remainder adeno/adenosquamous.

Epidemiology

Cervical carcinoma is the 2nd most common malignancy in ♀ worldwide, ~80% of cases arising in developing countries (rates 25–45/100,000). Variations between and within countries occur due to differing HPV infection rates, other aetiological factors and uptake of screening (2% of all ♀ cancers in UK). Most frequently diagnosed in those aged 40–50 years. The reciprocal association between vaginal/anal and cervical SCC demonstrates the multifocal nature of high-risk HPV infection.

Natural history

Untreated, 25–60% of CIN3 will progress to ICC over 20 years, and ~20% of CIN1 and ~30% of CIN2 to higher grade lesions. 25–50% of CIN1 may regress to normal, especially, in younger ♀. Persistence of high-risk HPV infection is associated with progression to CIN2–3, 10–40% in 2 years.

Cervical cytology—comparison of classifications by British Society for Cervical Cytology (BSCC) and Bethesda system (2001)

BSCC	**Bethesda system (2001)**
Borderline nuclear changes	Atypical squamous cells of uncertain significance (ASCUS)
Borderline nuclear changes with koiloctytosis Mild dyskaryosis	Low-grade squamous intraepithelial lesion
Moderate dyskaryosis Severe dyskaryosis	High-grade squamous intraepithelial lesion
Suspected invasive carcinoma	Squamous cell carcinoma
Borderline nuclear changes, endocervical	Atypical glandular cells (endocervical/endometrial/glandular)
Suspected glandular neoplasia (in Scotland 'adenocarcinoma' if invasive adenocarcinoma suggested, otherwise 'glandular neoplasia')	Atypical glandular cells (endocervical/ glandular) favour neoplastic
	Endocervical adenocarcinoma *in situ*
	Adenocarcinoma (endocervical, endometrial, extrauterine, other)

Risk factors

- Infection
  - Human Papilloma Virus (HPV): high-risk HPV in >99% of SCC (usually 16 (50%) and 18 (20%), also 31, 35, 39, 45, 51, 52, 56 and 58). The relative risk of SCC is ↑ ≥15x. However, the probability of an individual with high-risk HPV developing SCC is <2% with other factors important for malignant transformation. In adeno/adenosquamous carcinoma HPV 18 (50%), 16 (30%).
  - Other genital infections: cervicitis is considered to be a reason for the association between *Chlamydia trachomatis* and CIN3/SCC (2-fold ↑). Conflicting evidence implicating herpes simplex virus type 2, *Neisseria gonorrhoeae* and *Trichomonas vaginalis.*
- Sexual activity: age of coitarche is linked to ↑ risk of SCC e.g. relative risk 2.5 if <18 years compared with >21. Risk ↑ by multiple sexual partners e.g. ↑ 14-fold if >5 lifetime partners.
- Parity: incidence of SCC ↑ with parity independent of other risks. Young age at 1st pregnancy also appears to be a risk marker.
- Male factor: ↑ incidence of CIN and ICC in partners of ♂ with high-risk HPV infection or a history of multiple sexual contacts.
- Smoking: appears to ↑ risk of CIN and SCC.
- Oral contraception: long-term use (>5 years) is associated with ↑ risk of ICC/CIN (3× if >5 and 4× if >10 years).
- Immunosuppression: ↑ risk with immunodeficiency e.g. HIV infection, Hodgkin's disease, treatment causing immunosuppression.

Condoms offer some protection especially in delaying CIN progression.

Clinical features

- CIN is typically asymptomatic but important to exclude in those with postcoital bleeding (PCB) or intermenstrual bleeding (IMB).
- ICC diagnosed in up to 4% of ♀ with PCB and 1.5% with postmenopausal bleeding. If symptomatic, it is usually more advanced so signs are generally evident (pronounced cervical contact bleeding, hard, irregular and enlarged or ulcerated cervix, profuse offensive vaginal discharge) but subtle signs of early stages may be missed. In advanced ICC:
  - Bimanual and rectal examination may demonstrate a fixed uterus and parametrial/posterior pelvic induration.
  - General examination may show hepatosplenomegaly or inguinal/supraclavicular lymph node enlargement.

Screening

- Cervical cytology—Papanicolaou smear

Introduced in the 1940s to screen for premalignant exfoliated cervical cells. Adequate sampling of TZ is achieved by visualizing the full circumference of the cervix. If incomplete, it can lead to false negative results (2–25%). 'Unsatisfactory' results are due to insufficient epithelial cells or presence of blood or pus cells (~10% with slide preparations, <2% using liquid based cytology).

Exfoliated cells display nuclear and cytoplasmic characteristics that correspond to the underlying pathology. Dyskaryosis is the nuclear abnormality of exfoliated cells, graded as mild, moderate, and severe. This indicates the minimum degree of CIN likely to be present as 1, 2, and 3, respectively. Cells suggesting possible invasive carcinoma show coarse chromatin clumps and extensive keratinization with bizarre forms. False negative results may be found in established ICC due to cell necrosis. Closer correlation between cytological and histological findings occurs with higher degrees of abnormality.

► Cytology laboratories will advise on the correct management and follow-up of abnormal cytology.

- High-risk HPV DNA detection

Role in 1° screening unproven although more sensitive than cytology in predicting CIN2/3. Low specificity, especially in those <30 years, due to the high prevalence of transient HPV infection.

Cervical cytology guidance

Using a computerized call-recall system, ♀ who are registered with a general practitioner are invited for screening, 3 yearly if 25–49 and 5 yearly if 50–64. (♀ aged 65+, only if not screened since age 50 or have had a recent abnormality).

It is important not to commence routine screening below the age of 25 because much of the low-grade abnormality due to high HPV prevalence resolves spontaneously and the rate of cervical carcinoma is extremely low with cytology screening not having any impact. Screening is best provided in primary care but if taken in GUM, arrangements should be made for a copy of the result to go to the patient's general practitioner.

Cervical cytology technique

- Take cervical smear before cleaning the cervix and taking endocervical swabs for *N. gonorrhoeae* and *C. trachomatis.*
- Note the macroscopic appearance of the cervix. Defer cytology if in menses or marked cervicitis.
- Sweep 360° around the cervix being sure to sample the transitional zone.
  - Liquid based cytology. The end of sampling brush is rinsed or broken off into the preservative medium.
  - Alcohol fixed smear. Aylesbury spatula (if the SCJ is within the endocervical canal a spatula/endocervical brush combination is recommended).

Diagnosis

CIN

Colposcopy is an essential investigation of cervical premalignancy. Using up to 40x magnification and acetic acid ± iodine, it enables visual grading of CIN and highlights optimal sites for biopsy.

- Cytological indications for colposcopy
  - Suspected invasive carcinoma or glandular neoplasia. Urgent ⚠
  - Moderate/severe dyskaryosis or borderline endocervical changes
  - Mild dyskaryosis/borderline nuclear changes—indicated if any repeat cytology at 6, 12, or 24 months is abnormal (if mild dykaryosis initial colposcopy rather than repeat cytology may be advised).
  - Unsatisfactory/inadequate samples—indicated if 3 consecutive unsatisfactory smears (3 monthly intervals)
  - Any dyskaryosis with a history of CIN
- Clinical indications for colposcopy/gynaecological assessment
  - Symptoms raising suspicion of carcinoma after excluding infection e.g. postcoital/intermenstrual bleeding in ♀ >40 years, postmenopausal bleeding.

ICC

- Biopsy, loop or needle excision depending on appearance.
- For staging
  - Bimanual vaginal and rectal examination under anaesthesia (EUA) with proctoscopy and sigmoidoscopy if rectal spread suspected.
  - Chest and skeletal radiographs, intravenous urogram and barium enema.
- Routine general haematological assessment and other investigations to exclude or gauge metastases e.g. magnetic resonance imaging with a transvaginal coil, lymph node dissection.

Management

CIN

CIN should be managed by accredited colposcopists following clear policies and protocols with multidisciplinary links being essential. ♀ with CIN should receive clear information and have access to appropriate counselling. Treatment options:

- Ablation: by cryotherapy (only for small size CIN1) or laser vaporization (unless suspected invasion, glandular disease, SCJ not visualized or previous treatment for CIN).
- Excision: has largely replaced ablation because of better results, greater applicability, more rapid treatment with less bleeding and lower cost of equipment.
- Cone biopsy: preferred method for AIS.

Histology report should indicate if any excision is complete. If not repeat is required. Cytological follow-up is recommended with repeat colposcopy for abnormal results (at 6 and 12 months followed by annual repeat for 10 years after treatment of CIN2/3 and 2 years after CIN1).

Carcinoma

Histological diagnosis and clinical staging are the basis of treatment decision ranging from cone biopsy to surgery, radiotherapy, and chemotherapy in various combinations. Age, fertility requirements, and general fitness are individual factors influencing management. 5 year survival rates vary from ~100% (≤3mm micro-invasion) to 5–15% (extension beyond pelvis).

Pregnancy

Routine cervical cytology should be postponed until after delivery but repeat following a previous abnormality may be taken in mid-trimester. Incidence of ICC is low and pregnancy does not have an adverse impact. Management of CIN (biopsy and treatment) can be deferred till the postpartum period but colposcopic suggestion of ICC requires urgent biopsy. Treatment of ICC will entail termination or preterm delivery.

Prevention

- Screening prevents ~5000 cases a year in the UK by reducing the lifetime risk of SCC from 1.7% to 0.7%.
- Vaccines against types 6, 11, 16, and 18 are under assessment in phase IV studies. If efficacy is confirmed, vaccination given before the onset of sexual activity and exposure to HPV, may potentially prevent ~70% invasive cervical cancers and ~60% high-grade CIN.

HIV and cervical carcinoma

- ↑ high-risk HPV infection and persistence.
- ↑ in incidence (>4-fold) of CIN2/3.
- Annual cervical cytology recommended.
- Colposcopy and biopsy recommended for borderline changes, mild dyskaryosis.
- ↑ recurrence of CIN after treatment (which should be by excision).
- Cervical carcinoma is an AIDS defining condition.

Chapter 30

Vulval pain syndromes

Introduction

There are various classifications of vulval pain syndrome although these may merely indicate different spectra of a common disorder. Considerable overlap exists with regards to aetiology and clinical features. Recognition and appreciation of a defined clinical entity is important and reassuring to the patient.

Vulval dysaesthesia or (essential) vulvodynia

Aetiology

Conflicting data on association with relationship conflict, depression, or anxiety. Usually Caucasian, aged 40 years (peri/post-menopausal) and beyond. Often long history of multiple inappropriate topical skin applications.

Clinical features

Chronic constant neuralgic type vulval discomfort characterized usually by burning, stinging, irritation, rawness, not especially localized. Symptoms may be hyperaesthetic (exaggerated) or described as allodynia (when sensation different to that applied). Commonly associated with low back pain and urinary symptoms. Libido diminished but dyspaerunia is unusual. Symptoms worsen while sitting and towards the end of the day. No signs.

Management

- Tricyclic antidepressants: amitriptyline 10mg/day gradually increasing to 75–100mg, for 3–6 months (at least 25% improve).
- Anticonvulsants: gabapentin 300mg daily building up to 4 times daily for up to 3 months. Data limited but >80% response reported.
- Carbamazepine has also been advocated.

Prognosis

Usually improves with time but may remit over months and years.

Vulval vestibulitis (vestibulodynia)

Aetiology

No substantiated cause but factors proposed include recurrent candidiasis, human papilloma virus infection or treatment for it (e.g. cryosurgery), irritant dermatitis, hormonal factors (e.g. early menarche/use of oral contraceptives), pelvic floor muscle disorder, vestibular neural hyperplasia, genetic, excess urinary calcium oxalate, psychological stress, sexual abuse, or trauma. Typically affects nulliparous Caucasians aged 20–40 years.

Clinical features

1° if occurs from coitarche, or 2° following a period of pain-free intercourse. Associated with intolerance of tampon insertion because of local pain. Symptoms confined to a specific area of the vaginal vestibule (usually 3–9 o'clock) with pain on touch or attempted vaginal entry (superficial dyspaerunia).

Signs limited to the area of extreme vestibular tenderness on pressure (cotton-swab test) associated with varying degree of erythema.

Management

- Avoid local irritants.
- Topical agents (generally ineffective in most cases)—low concentration hydrocortisone cream/ointment, anaesthetics (e.g. lignocaine gel) although it may cause skin sensitivity, antimycotics, lubricants, short duration high potency steroids.
- Reduce urinary oxalate concentration—low oxalate diet and calcium citrate without vitamin D.
- Others—oral antifungal drugs, intralesional alpha-interferon, intramuscular beta-interferon.
- Surgery—should be avoided wherever possible (as often self-limiting) but ranges from vestibuloplasty to total vestibulectomy.

Prognosis

Partial relief of symptoms occurs in 40–50% cases (regardless of approach) and 50% improve spontaneously within 1 year of diagnosis.

Chapter 31

Streptococcal and staphylococcal infections

Group A—*Streptococcus pyogenes*

- Unusual cause of acute purulent vaginitis, generally related to obstetric or other trauma. May lead to necrotizing fasciitis.
- Recognized cause of acute vaginitis in prepubertal girls.
- May rarely cause balanitis (e.g. pyoderma following fellatio).

Management

For simple infections pending antibiotic sensitivities:
Phenoxymethylpenicillin (penicillin V) 500mg 4 times a day for 7–10 days.

Group B β-haemolytic streptococci (GBS)—*Streptococcus agalactiae*

Found in 12–37% in ♀ attending GUM clinics. Usually not pathogenic (except in pregnancy) but associated with bacterial vaginosis.

Pregnancy

Carriage rate is 6–28%. Intra-amniotic infection and postpartum endometritis if heavily colonized. ~35% of babies of carriers become colonized with ~1% developing invasive neonatal infection. GBS is the most frequent cause of any severe infection in infants aged <7 days. Septicaemia, meningitis, pulmonary infection, and shock may follow in up to 50% of infected infants with a mortality of 6% if full term and 18% if preterm.

Risk factors for neonatal infection are:

- labour <37 weeks
- prolonged rupture of membranes (PROM) >18 hours
- intrapartum pyrexia
- GBS bacteriuria in current pregnancy
- previous infant with GBS.

In the UK, women identified with these risk factors are offered intrapartum antibiotics to prevent neonatal infection. Recommended regimen is IV benzyl penicillin 3g (5 MU) at onset of labour then 1.5g (2.5 MU) 4 hourly until delivery. Clindamycin 900mg should be given IV 8 hourly to those allergic to penicillin.

Practice varies worldwide e.g. US guidelines recommend that all women are screened (vaginal/rectal swabs) at 35–37 weeks for GBS and prophylactic intrapartum antibiotics offered to those testing positive (or not tested). Risk-factor based approach is estimated to ↓ early onset of the GBS disease of the neonate by 50–69% while prophylaxis based on routine swabs may ↓ it by 86%.

Men

Urethral colonization in 38–46% of ♂ attending GUM clinics.

GBS may cause balanitis, usually mild rarely progressing to cellulitis. Group G β-haemolytic streptococci also occasionally implicated in balanitis.

Staphylococcus aureus

Vaginal carriage rate ~10%

- Folliculitis
- Local genital or perigenital infection especially in traumatized skin (e.g. excoriation with scabies).
- Toxic shock syndrome. Due to an exotoxin produced by phage group 1 *Staph. aureus* colonizing the vagina. Arises usually midway through menstruation and associated with super-absorbent tampons (now discontinued), infrequent tampon changing or rarely the use of the contraceptive diaphragm. Typically sudden onset of: sore throat, pyrexia, headache, myalgia, vomiting, diarrhoea, abdominal pain, and vaginal irritation. Followed by a generalized rash, inflammation of oral and vaginal mucosae, vasoconstriction, hypotension, and shock. Skin desquamation and necrosis are common sequelae. Tampons should be changed regularly and diaphragms should not be left *in situ* for longer than the contraceptive needs dictate.

Management

Simple infections pending antibiotic sensitivities—flucloxacillin 250–500mg 4 times a day for 5 days.

Toxic shock syndrome—supportive treatment (for shock), removal of retained tampon or diaphragm, treat with high dose antibiotics.

Current recommendations by the Royal College of Obstetricians and Gynaecologists (UK) for prevention of neonatal GBS

- Intrapartum prophylaxis should be offered to those ♀ with risk factors.
- Intrapartum prophylaxis is not indicated if GBS carriage was detected in a previous pregnancy.
- Routine screening for antenatal GBS carriage is not recommended.
- Intrapartum antibiotic prophylaxis should be considered if GBS is incidentally detected in a vaginal/rectal swab. However, treatment before labour is not recommended (recolonization likely).

Chapter 32

Genital anomalies

Men

Epispadias: absence of upper wall of urethra. Frequency ~1 in 30,000. Urethra opens onto the dorsum of the glans penis or penile shaft as an epithelial-lined groove.

Hypospadias: termination of urethra ventral and posterior to its normal opening. Frequency 1 in 160–1800. Orifice found anywhere from the usual site (with backward extension) to the perineum. Often associated with other local anomalies (e.g. redundant prepuce, absent frenum, meatal stenosis).

Lymphocele: non-tender, cord-like, firm swelling in coronal sulcus. Probably related to sexual trauma (prolonged or frequent intercourse). May be associated with preputial oedema. Self-limiting (usually within days, up to 3 weeks), just requires reassurance.

Paraphimosis: strangulation of the glans penis by retracted prepuce. Usually results from partially phimotic prepuce which has been retracted and cannot be reduced. However, may follow trauma with swelling of the glans (e.g. from vigorous sexual activity) with a retracted normal calibre prepuce. Requires urgent intervention either by manual reduction (using anaesthetic cream and ice to reduce oedema) or surgical intervention to prevent 2° infection and gangrene.

Peyronie's disease: fibrous infiltration of the penile intracavernous septum. Leads to plaque formation causing curvature and angulation of the erect penis. Cause unknown but associated with trauma, diabetes mellitus, and Dupuytren's contracture. Medical treatments with proven control matched benefit include intralesional collagenease, verapamil, interferon, and oral acetyl/propionyl-L-carnitine, colchicine. There is no data to support the use of vitamin E, para-aminobenzoate, intralesional corticosteroids, or laser therapy. If severe, the plaque can be removed surgically (but reduction in penile length).

Phimosis: tight constriction of the prepuce preventing retraction over the glans penis. Aetiology includes:

- congenital (physiological in 1st year of life).
- acute: 2° to underlying infection e.g. syphilis (subpreputial chancre), genital herpes, candidiasis.
- chronic and progressive: 2° to repeated trauma (physical, chemical, repeated infections), skin disorders e.g. lichen sclerosis, local malignancy.

Surgical referral for circumcision may be required.

Priapism: pathologically prolonged erection without libido. May be associated with blood disorders (e.g. sickle-cell disease, leukaemia), drugs used to manage erectile dysfunction and rarely infection (e.g. gonorrhoea). ► Failure to achieve detumescence using ice packs requires urgent urological referral.

Spermatoceles and epididymal cysts: commonly detected as incidental findings or raised by concerned patient, especially in those aged >40 years. Usually <1cm in diameter and filled with spermatozoa (spermatoceles) or serum (epididymal cysts), therefore transilluminate well. They arise from the epididymis (not testis) and generally reassurance can be given. If large or painful, they can be aspirated by needle but surgical removal is not advised as there is a risk of sterility. For intrascrotal lumps or swellings where malignancy is considered ultrasonography is recommended.

Urethral channels (accessory): open dorsal or ventral to urethra and usually blind-ending, rudimentary tracts although may terminate in bladder or posterior urethra. Accessory periurethral ducts are commonly found in ♂ opening into or around the meatus and are blind tracts extending from 2–10mm.

Varicocele: dilatation and tortuosity of the veins of the scrotal pampiniform plexus (along the spermatic cord). 10–17% of young ♂ affected with spontaneous regression common. Swollen veins within the scrotum are bluish and feel like a 'bag of worms'. Most commonly diagnosed because of sterility in ♂ but ~67% ♂ with varicoceles are fertile. Generally no treatment is required although further assessment and surgical intervention should be considered if clinically apparent and has concerns about infertility.

Women

Bartholin gland cyst and abscess: cysts arise following obstruction of the drainage duct whereas abscesses are caused by local pathogens, most commonly *Neisseria gonorrhoeae* (up to 80% of abscesses) but also *Chlamydia trachomatis*, staphylococci, streptococci, and Gram-negative enteric bacteria. Found most commonly in ♀ aged 20–29 years with abscesses occurring about 3× as commonly as cysts. Most small abscesses respond well to appropriate antibiotics although needle aspiration may be required. Chronic or recurrent cysts may require duct catheterization or marsupialization. In ♀ >40 years cyst edges should be examined histologically to exclude carcinoma. Recurrences may occur in up to 20%.

Cervical polyp: often an incidental finding during routine examination but may present with postcoital or intermenstrual bleeding. Red fleshy cervical projections, ~1–2cm in length, containing both squamous and columnar cell epithelium. Found more commonly in multiparous ♀, >20 years and may be associated with chronic local inflammation. 1.7% are malignant and 27% are associated with an endometrial polyp. Usually removed by gently twisting its base (which should be sent for histology to exclude malignancy). Excision with basal electrocautery or laser vaporization may be required for larger lesions.

Developmental anomalies: seen uncommonly in ♀ at GUM clinics. Epispadias is rare and usually severe, diagnosed in childhood.
Abnormalities in vaginal development, unless minor are likely to present at a younger age, including puberty if the menstrual flow is impeded (e.g. atresia or septal obstruction). It is estimated that vaginal malformations arise in between 1/4000 and 1/10,000 ♀ births. Septa may be seen which are vertical (transverse) or lateral (longitudinal).
Vertical defects: may be found anywhere along the length of the vagina and are usually present in the teens with cryptomenorrhoea, cyclical abdominal pain, and haematocolpos. Partial vertical septa may be seen as an incidental finding but can obscure the cervix and may cause dyspaerunia.
Lateral fusion disorders: more common and often asymptomatic. The septum may create two vaginal passages (one usually larger) leading to a didelphic uterus with twin uterine cavities and cervices opening to each vagina. Important to sample both cervices when screening.

Female genital mutilation (FGM) or circumcision: illegal in the UK. It is estimated that 74,000 1st-generation immigrant ♀ have undergone FGM especially in those from Africa, north of the equator excluding Arabic speaking countries other than Egypt. Although associated with some Muslim communities it is not exclusively linked with Islam.

There are three forms of FGM.

- 'Clitoridectomy'—partial or complete removal of the clitoris.
- 'Excision'—removal of both the clitoris and labia minora.
- 'Infibulation' (pharaonic circumcision)—as above with stitching of raw labial surfaces to produce a small hole to allow urine and menses to escape. Found in ~15% of circumcised ♀.

Chapter 33

Infection reduction, emergency contraception, and contraception in HIV infection

Infection reduction

The only absolute form of 'safe sex' is mutual monogamy with an uninfected partner. Non-penetrative sex (e.g. mutual masturbation, body rubbing) is often defined as 'safe sex' although infection can be spread by manual contact, especially with infected body fluids. Any form of penetrative sex ↑ the risk of infection although the use of barriers (especially condoms) ↓ the transmission of most STIs.

Condoms (use dates back to 1550 BC in Egypt)

Intact condoms are impermeable to particles the size of STI pathogens including the smallest virus, hepatitis B. Condoms should be applied before any genital contact commences and not removed until all genital contact has ended. Care should be taken to ensure that ejaculate does not leak from the condom and that it is disposed of safely. Condoms ↓ (but do not eliminate) the risk of STIs only if used consistently for every act of sex. Condom use provides efficient protection in conditions with low infectivity rates such as HIV, but is less effective against highly infectious STIs such as gonorrhoea (see Box). The degree of protection is difficult to assess due to difficulties in interpreting self-reported data regarding frequency/consistency of condom use and levels of breakage or slippage.

- ♂ ***condoms***: usually latex and may be lubricated with a spermicidal preparation, commonly nonoxynol-9 or a simple lubricant, often promoted for those with skin sensitivities (e.g. Sensilube, Aquagel, or KY jelly). Oil-based products, such as body oils, creams, lotions sun tan creams, or petroleum jelly, pessaries, and suppositories will adversely affect the integrity of latex condoms. Reported rates of slippage or breakage have been estimated at 0.5–3.7% with 13% failing to apply condoms before initial penetration. Failure to withdraw the detumescent penis promptly after ejaculation can result in leakage of semen.
- ♀ ***condoms***: made of pre-lubricated polyurethane and can be used with oil- or water-based lubricants. The sheath has two flexible rings one of which fits high into the vagina and the other covering the introitus. The probability of vaginal exposure to semen using a ♀ condom has been estimated at 3% (♂ condom ~12%). Data on disease protection is limited but in theory they should be more effective than ♂ condoms as a larger surface area of skin is protected.

Risk of pregnancy

Protection against pregnancy with correct and consistent use of the ♂ or ♀ condom is estimated at 85–98%.

Other barriers to infection

Spermicides

Chemical compounds in the form of jellies, creams, foams, films, or pessaries that are inserted into the vagina prior to intercourse. The main chemicals used in spermicides are nonoxynol-9, octoxynol-9, menfegol, and benzalkonium chloride. Nonoxynol-9, the most commonly used, has little activity against *Neisseria gonorrhoeae*, *Trichomonas vaginalis*, herpes simplex virus, HIV, and *Treponema pallidum*. It has also been found to cause disruption to the epithelial lining of the vagina and rectum, potentially ↑ the risk of acquiring infection. Therefore, it should not be used by those who are at high risk of contracting HIV or other STIs. Studies on the effects of spermicides on *Chlamydia trachomatis* are conflicting.

Diaphragm/cap (such devices date back to 1850 BC)

A thin latex rubber dome shaped device that fits over the cervix. When used in conjunction with spermicidal preparations, it has been found to provide >50% reduction against gonorrhoea and trichomoniasis. No evidence of protection against HIV infection.

Dental dams

A small sheet of material (latex or non-latex) which acts as a barrier between the vagina or anus and the mouth. May be used in conjunction with a water-based lubricant to ↑ stimulation. Dental dams must be held in place during use, however, some include adhesive strips. A harness (dammit) that holds the dental dam in place may be used. There is little data available on their effectiveness in preventing STIs. Dental dams should not be used as a method of contraception.

Estimated minimum level of protection against infection provided by consistent condom use

- HIV 85%
- *C. trachomatis* 40%
- *T. vaginalis* 60%
- *N. gonorrhoeae* 49%

HSV infection in ♀ may be reduced but no evidence ♂.

Conflicting data on HPV infection, but may ↓ incidence in ♂ and delay progression of CIN in ♀.

Emergency (postcoital) contraception

Two methods recommended:

- Oral progesterone-only emergency contraception (POEC) as levonorgestrel 1.5mg.
- Insertion of a copper intrauterine device (IUD).

Risk of pregnancy following one act of unprotected sexual intercourse (UPSI) at any time in the menstrual cycle is estimated at 2–4%. Failure rates of POEC range from 1–3% and for a copper IUD <1%.

Levonorgestrel (Levonelle)

- Single dose of 1.5mg levonorgestrel provided within 12 hours and no later than 72 hours following UPSI or potential contraceptive failure.
- If vomiting within 3 hours provide a further 1.5mg levonorgestrel.
- POEC is not licensed for use more than once in a menstrual cycle, but may be used if clinically indicated.

Caution

- If taking liver enzyme inducing medication (e.g. antiretrovirals) give 1.5mg levonorgestrel followed by 0.75mg 12 hours later. IUD may be a better option.
- Interaction with warfarin can alter international normalized ratio (INR) therefore IUD is recommended.
- No absolute contraindications, but caution with porphyria or severe liver disease.
- Theoretical risk of ectopic pregnancy—if pregnancy occurs following levonorgestrel this should be excluded.
- Patient should return for pregnancy test if period >7 days late. Levonorgestrel can cause menstrual delay >7 days in 10%.

Copper IUD

- Can be inserted up to 5 days (120 hours) after the first episode of UPSI at any time in the menstrual cycle or up to 5 days after the expected date of ovulation in a regular cycle.
- An IUD containing >300mm^2 copper should be used if possible.
- For ♀ at high risk of infection undergoing emergency IUD insertion, epidemiological antibiotic treatment should be advised, ideally preceded by testing. Azithromycin 1g stat or doxycycline 100mg twice daily for 7 days are suitable regimens. Further sexual intercourse should be avoided until screening test results are available and partner(s) treated (if necessary).

General advice

- ♀ should be instructed to return for a pregnancy test if their expected menstruation is >7 days late or lighter than usual.
- POEC does not provide contraceptive cover for the remainder of the cycle and effective contraception or abstinence must be advised.
- An IUD can be removed any time after the next menstruation if no unprotected sexual intercourse occurs since menses or if hormonal contraception is started within the 1st 5 days of the next cycle.
- Information and counselling should be provided on future contraceptive needs.

HIV positive women

Why is the discussion of contraception important?

- Vast majority of ♀ infected with HIV are of reproductive age.
- Effect of some antiretrovirals on fetus may be severe (e.g. efavirenz resulting in anencephaly in animal studies). Long-term effects are unknown, with concerns over carcinogenesis and mitochondrial disease.
- Drug interactions with hormonal contraception, antiretrovirals, and certain antibiotics (see Box).
- Evidence that hormonal contraception may ↑ cervical HIV shedding.
- Possible HIV transmission to the ♂ partner in an unplanned pregnancy.
- Methods inducing amenorrhoea e.g. depot medroxyprogesterone acetate may ↓ HIV transmission risk.

Male condom

Can be recommended for use by all HIV positive ♀ and ♂, preferably in combination with another contraceptive method if contraception is essential. If ♂ condom is unacceptable ♀ condom should be considered.

Male/female sterilization

Both are safe in HIV infection as operative risks are no greater than in those who are HIV negative. However, should complications occur they could be more serious in those with advanced HIV disease, so other methods may be more acceptable. Caution should also be exercised in newly diagnosed patients who may be coming to terms with their condition and could change their views with regard to future pregnancies. A longer term reversible method may be preferable.

Combined oral contraceptive (COC)

There are no HIV-specific contraindications in those who are well and not on any treatment. However, in those taking antiretroviral or anti biotics treatment numerous interactions may occur (see Box). Therefore, if a ♀ is stable on an antiretroviral regimen it may be preferable to consider an alternative contraceptive method.

Progestogen-only pill/subdermal implant

As with the COC, there are no specific contraindications, but care needs to be taken to avoid drug interactions.

Depot medroxyprogesterone acetate (DMPA)

Due to a theoretical risk that the contraceptive efficacy of DMPA may be reduced towards the end of the 12 week period, it has been recommended that the injection interval be shortened to 10 weeks, or 8 weeks when potent enzyme inducers are used (e.g. rifampicin).

Intrauterine devices (IUD)

- Copper IUDs—highly effective and cost-effective. No drug interactions. Risks of complications and pelvic infection following IUD insertion are similar to HIV negative ♀.

- Levonorgestrel intrauterine system (LNG-IUS)—low failure rate (0.1–0.2/100 ♀ years) and ↓ rate of ectopic pregnancy and pelvic inflammatory disease than copper IUDs. After 1 year, 94–97% ↓ in menstrual flow with amenorrhoea in 10–15%.

Sexual transmission of HIV may be ↑ by genital inflammation and penile microtrauma by IUD threads. ↑ menstrual flow, associated with copper IUDs also ↑ viral shedding. This does not apply to LNG-IUS and with its ↓ failure rate it is a good option for HIV positive ♀.

Interactions and hormonal contraception

Antibiotics and COC

- Rifampicin and rifabutin: powerful enzyme inducers. COC not advised and alternative contraceptive measures required for 4–8 weeks following their discontinuation.
- Certain broad-spectrum antibiotics (e.g. penicillin, tetracycline, erythromycin): COC efficacy ↓ by altering large bowel flora. Additional contraception required while taking antibiotics and for 7 days thereafter (continue next pill packet without a break if necessary). If antibiotic treatment >3 weeks, no additional precautions required as bowel flora becomes antibiotic resistant.

Antibiotics and progestogen-only contraception (POC)

- Rifampicin and rifabutin: powerful enzyme inducers, reducing efficacy of POC. For:
  - DMPA—reduce treatment interval to 8 weeks.
  - implant—not recommended.
  - oral—not recommended. Alternative contraception required for 4–8 weeks following their cessation.
- Broad-spectrum antibiotics: not affected.

Antiretroviral drugs

- May ↑ or ↓ hormonal levels.
- All nucleoside reverse transcriptase inhibitors, indinavir, and saquinavir can be used safely.
- Efavirenz not compatible with COC.
- Amprenavir, lopinavir, nelfinavir, ritonavir, and nevirapine not compatible with any hormonal contraception.

Chapter 34

Psychological aspects and sexual dysfunction

Psychological aspects

Personality types

In those attending clinics for STIs:

- extroversion—associated with ↑ sexual partners, varied sexual behaviour, and ↑ STIs.
- psychoticism—related to ↑ sexual curiosity, promiscuity, and hostility.
- neuroticism—associated with ↓ sexual satisfaction but ↑ sexual guilt, inhibition, and exaggerated concerns about STIs.

Clinic patients

20–40% of new patients attending clinics for STIs have been classified as 'psychiatric cases' based on general health questionnaire scores showing high levels of anxiety. It is important to recognize and manage this during the consultation to help address the presenting problem as well as improve subsequent attendance. New diagnoses of HIV infection, anogenital herpes, and syphilis generate the greatest anxiety and are also the most common STIs associated with phobias.

The greatest psychological reaction usually arises from a diagnosis of HIV infection. It does not necessarily relate to the stage of the disease and may exhibit a 'bereavement'-type reaction—disbelief, denial, anxiety, and depression. There may also be suicidal tendencies. In addition, such feelings may be complicated by guilt, resentment, and stigmatization. Regular support is important ensuring that information is given at and over a time best suited to the individual. Referral for specialist advice/ reatment may also be required.

Certain procedures, e.g. colposcopy for abnormal cervical cytology, are associated with very high levels of anxiety. Stress and depression are common features of chronic conditions e.g. HIV infection, vulval vestibulitis, chronic pelvic pain, prostatitis, and persistent anogenital warts. They are also reported with conditions that may recur e.g. anogenital herpes, warts, and vaginal candidiasis. Patient needs sufficient time to express his/her anxiety and a careful explanation of the condition (with written information) is important. Therapeutic intervention (e.g. antiretroviral treatment for HIV and suppressive treatment for frequent recurrences of herpes) ↓ psychological morbidity.

Neuroses associated with STIs

Over-reaction and hypochondriasis

Examples include:

- inappropriate reaction to the condition diagnosed
- undue vigorous penile squeezing to produce a urethral discharge
- obsessional attention to genital marks and irregularities.

May be a symptom of some other underlying problem (e.g. rumours about a sexual partner). Managed by exploring the patient's anxieties and correcting misinformation.

Phobias

Often triggered by stress and media publicity. Now largely related to HIV infection though previously common for syphilis (e.g. patient fails to believe and accept the results of negative tests). Often prompted by underlying guilt or a sexual concern which should be addressed when formulating management strategies.

Factitious illness and Munchausen's syndrome

In GUM often related to HIV infection with imagined positive test result. Reasons and motivation are often unclear but may be used to gain sympathy, hospital care, or social benefits. Psychiatric referral is often required.

Psychosexual involvement

In managing sexual dysfunction the cooperation and support of both partners is essential. Emotional issues which may underlie or complicate the presenting problem are explored and addressed through counselling. Simple counselling, provided to an individual or couple, is often brief and:
- Provides basic information and corrects false ideas.
- Makes suggestions—e.g. positions during intercourse.
- Provides permission and reassures—often linked with a new suggestion (e.g. the use of vibrators and other sex aids).
- Facilitates communication between partners in particular to develop self-assertiveness and self-protection.

This may lead to behavioural psychotherapy to individuals, couples, or sometimes groups. The framework consists of:
- The setting of behavioural tasks (i.e. 'homework').
- An analysis of the patient's or couple's success, identifying obstacles or difficulties.
- The provision of help, support, and advice to address the obstacles and problems.
- A review of the new situation with new tasks set or revised.

Common sexual dysfunction problems in women

Classified by the American Foundation of Urological Disease as disorders of: hypoactive sexual desire, sexual arousal, orgasm, and sexual pain.

Low sexual desire/arousal (sexual anhedonia) and orgasmic dysfunction

Heterogeneous condition

Causal factors include:
- Partner conflict and disharmony.
- Ignorance.
- Psychological causes: e.g. anxiety, depression, body dysmorphism.
- Physical causes: local (e.g. endometriosis, cystitis), systemic (e.g. diabetes mellitus, multiple sclerosis), drugs (e.g. oral contraceptives, hypotensives, tranquillisers), surgery affecting body image (e.g. hysterectomy, mastectomy).
- Postmenopause: ~15% significant decline in arousal.

Management
- Definition and management of any underlying problem. In postmenopausal ♀ hormone replacement treatment with androgenic activity e.g. tibolone or androgen supplementation is sometimes effective.
- Sensate focus (of benefit despite level of inhibition)—a 3-stage programme in which the couple progresses stepwise from non-genital pleasuring through genital pleasuring to non-demanding coitus under the control of the ♀.
- Insufficient data on drugs but apomorphine may benefit some with arousal and hypoactive sexual disorders. Phosphodiesterase-5 inhibitors appear to be disappointing.

Vaginismus and sexual pain

A learned response, often due to dyspaerunia, leading to an involuntary contraction of the perineal muscles making sexual intercourse difficult or impossible. Other causes include a fear of pregnancy, loss of control, association of intercourse with violence or sexual abuse.

Tampons usually avoided with external towels used for menstruation. Involuntary perineal spasms may occur while preparing for/conducting a pelvic examination which is often evaded.

Management—in stages

- Exclude or manage physical causes and psychological factors.
- Encourage ♀ to become comfortable touching her genitalia and inserting a finger into the vagina.
- Consider the self-use of lubricated graded dilators.
- Advise Kegel's exercise—perineal contraction (against inserted finger(s) or dilators) followed by relaxation, to help muscle control.
- Suggest partner involvement—gentle introduction of a finger into the vagina slowly escalating to dilators.
- When comfortable proceed to penetrative sexual intercourse with the ♀ adopting a position (e.g. superior) to maintain control.

Dyspareunia

- Psychological (e.g. vaginismus).
- Obstruction (e.g. developmental anomalies, genital mutilation).
- Inadequate lubrication (e.g. insufficient foreplay, postmenopausal).
- Trauma (e.g. laceration/tears at introitus following sexual contact or childbirth).
- Vulvo-vaginal infection (e.g. herpes, candidiasis, trichomoniasis, Bartholinitis).
- Local inflammatory (e.g. atopic/contact vulvitis, lichen sclerosis, vulval vestibulitis).
- Pelvic disorders (e.g. cystitis, pelvic inflammatory disease, endometriosis, retroflexed uterus with ovarian prolapse, colitis/proctitis).
- Iatrogenic (e.g. episiotomy, vulval/vaginal/pelvic surgery, radiation therapy).

Common sexual dysfunction problems in men

Erectile dysfunction (ED)

Common, affecting over 50% aged 40–70 years (although only 10% fail to achieve nocturnal erections). 60% organic, 15% psychogenic, 25% mixed.

Main causes

- Lifestyle factors: obesity, smoking (×1.5), alcohol, recreational drugs.
- Trauma and iatrogenic: e.g. prolonged bicycle riding, prostatic/pelvic surgery, pelvic fracture, and local radiation treatment.
- Drugs: e.g. antidepressants (most), antipsychotics (many), hypotensives (most), androgen inhibitors (e.g. finasteride for benign prostatic hypertrophy).
- Vascular: responsible for nearly 50% of cases in those aged >50 years e.g. ischaemic heart disease (IHD), hypertension, peripheral vascular disease. Coexisting IHD (up to 40%) manifests a mean of ~38 months after ED (penile arteries 1–2mm, coronary 3–4mm).
- Endocrine:
  - diabetes mellitus (~50% have ED), neurogenic and vascular factors
  - hyper/hypothyroidism
  - hypogonadism, both physiological and pathological
  - hyperprolactinaemia.
- Neurological:
  - multiple sclerosis
  - Parkinson's disease.
- Psychogenic (depression, anxiety): ↑ sympathetic tone. Performance anxiety may become self-perpetuating.

Basic assessment

- History: for risk factors; libido, shaving (need and frequency).
- Examination: genital abnormalities including hypogonadism, facial/body hair, neurological (S2–S4 dermatomes), blood pressure/peripheral pulses.
- Investigations: exclude diabetes (urinalysis/blood glucose), consider serum testosterone, prolactin + other endocrine tests (thyroid, pituitary function). Ultrasonography and angiography rarely required.

Management—first line

- Psychosexual therapy (alone or in combination).
- Phosphodiesterase-5 inhibitors.

Success rates (erection suitable for intercourse) up to 75% (but high placebo rates 22–38%). Contraindicated in patients taking nitrates (both therapeutic and recreational) and those with hypotension, unstable angina, recent cerebrovascular accident or myocardial infarction.

  - Sildenafil: recommended dose 50mg (range 25–100mg) 1 hour pre-intercourse. Advise 1 dose in 24 hours (100mg maximum) 29% ↓ in plasma concentration with food. Half life—4–5 hours.
  - Vardenafil: recommended dose 10mg (range 2.5–20mg) 25–60 minutes pre-intercourse. Advise 1 dose in 24 hours (20mg maximum). 20% ↓ in plasma concentration with food. Half life—4.8–6 hours.
  - Tadalafil: recommended dose 10mg (range 10–20mg) 30 minutes–12 hours pre-intercourse. Maximum dose over 24 hours—20mg. No ↓ in plasma concentration with food. Half life—17.5–21 hours.

Management—alternatives

- *Central dopamine agonist*

Apomorphine: recommended dose 2mg (up to 3mg) sublingually 20 minutes before intercourse, minimum of 8 hours between doses. Success rate ~50% (32% with placebo). Contraindications include hypotension, severe unstable angina, severe heart failure, or recent myocardial infarction. With the exception of Parkinson's disease ♂ with neurological disease do not respond.

- *Synthetic prostaglandin E1 agent (e.g. alprostadil)*

Available as intraurethral pellets, (usual starting dose 250μg up to 1mg) or as intracavernosal injection (usual dose ranges from 5–20μg). Up to 90% response rate with injection and 40–60% with pellets.

- *Testosterone*

Intramuscular or transdermal. Should only be considered when ED is related to hypogonadism, otherwise no evidence of benefit. Hepatotoxic.

- *Pelvic floor exercises with biofeedback (including perineal muscle electrical stimulation)*

Only if ED related to venous leakage or occlusion (success rate ~50%).

- *Mechanical aids*
  - Vacuum devices: sucks venous blood into the penis causing an erection maintained by a firm constricting band. Lacks spontaneity, may cause bruising and produces a venous (cold/blue) erection.
  - Implants: e.g. inflatable devices, malleable rods.

International index of erectile function-5 (IIEF-5) scoring system

Over the past 6 months	Score				
	1	2	3	4	5
Confidence in getting and keeping an erection	Very low	Low	Moderate	High	Very high
Erections on sexual stimulation hard enough for penetration	Never/ almost never	<50% of the time	~50% of the time	>50% of the time	Always/ almost always
Maintaining erection after penetration	Never/ almost never	<50% of the time	~50% of the time	>50% of the time	Always/ almost always
Maintaining erection to completion of intercourse	Extremely difficult	Very difficult	Difficult	Slightly difficult	Not difficult
Satisfactory intercourse	Never/ almost never	<50% of the time	~50% of the time	>50% of the time	Always/ almost always

IIEF-5 score ≤21 correlates with ED (98% sensitive and 88% specific).

Premature ejaculation

Most common sexual dysfunction in ♂ under 40 years, reported in ~40%. Difficult to define as dependent on sexual partner and may indicate delayed ♀ orgasm. Generally considered to be a psychological problem, rarely reported with chronic prostatitis.

- Primary

Patient has always ejaculated prematurely. Often considered to be a conditioned response from teenage masturbatory practices but may reflect deep sexual anxiety from childhood traumatic experiences including sexual assault and/or familial conflict. Current research suggests genetic susceptibility and ↓ central serotonin/5-hydroxy tryptamine (5-HT) mediated neurotransmission are also important factors.

- Secondary

Previous ejaculatory control. Probably largely related to performance anxiety.

Management

- Stop/start: manual stimulation (initially) by partner or patient until ejaculation is imminent then cease for 30 seconds before resuming. The sequence is repeated until ejaculation is required.
- Squeeze technique: similar approach but firm pressure is applied across the penis at the frenum aborting imminent ejaculation.

Over time these methods progress to vulval contact then vaginal penetration (♀ superior) stopping for 30 seconds or withdrawing and squeezing as ejaculation approaches.

Success rate 65–90% with active participation of partner.

- Ejaculation 1–2 hours before coitus: young ♂—longer latent period for coital ejaculation. (Older ♂ may have problems attaining erection even after 2 hours.)
- Reduce sensation
  - local anaesthetic gel/ointment e.g. lidocaine (providing no allergy)
  - use of less sensitive condoms.
- Drug treatment

  Selective serotonin re-uptake inhibitors (SSRIs) and clomipramine delay ejaculation by their effect on central 5-HT receptors. SSRIs take at least 3 weeks to produce the effect but lomipramine is effective after a single dose. Regimens shown to be effective:
  - Daily—clomipramine 10–40mg or SSRI (paroxetine 20–40mg, sertraline 50–100mg, or fluexitine 20mg).
  - 'On-demand'—clomipramine 10–50mg 5–6 hours before coitus.

HIV infection

- May be associated with reduced testosterone levels leading to a ↓ in libido and ED.
- Bereavement reaction with new HIV positive result.
- Extreme anxiety and phobia generated by HIV.

HIV/AIDS

Chapter 35

HIV: Introduction and epidemiology

History

In 1981 an epidemic of a previously unknown acquired immune deficiency syndrome (AIDS) was described in the USA. A lentivirus (subfamily of retroviruses) was subsequently identified. Lentus (in Latin = slow) denotes the long latent phase between infection and the development of symptoms. Retroviruses use the enzyme reverse transcriptase (RT) to generate proviral DNA from RNA (reverse of the usual direction of genetic transcription). The term human immunodeficiency virus (HIV) was accepted in 1986. In the same year a related virus (HIV-2), endemic in W. Africa, and sharing common features including the induction of immune deficiency, was identified.

Origin of HIV

There are structural and genomic organizational similarities between HIV and simian immune deficiency virus (SIV). Despite similarity between HIV-1 and 2, there is little sequence homology with HIV-2 more closely related to SIV than to HIV-1. Phylogenetically, HIV-1 and HIV-2 cluster with chimpanzee (Pan Troglodytes) and sooty mangabey simian retroviruses, respectively. SIVcpz is almost identical to HIV-1. It appears likely that the virus at some point crossed species from chimpanzees to man.

Evidence that the virus existed for some time before its effects became clinically apparent in 1981 is supported by the following:

- HIV detected in a blood sample taken in 1959 from an adult male living in the former Zaire.
- HIV found in tissue samples from an African American teenager who died in St Louis, USA in 1969.
- HIV found in tissue samples from a Norwegian sailor who died around 1976.

Prevalence

Worldwide

38 million people, 2.1 million of them children, were living with HIV/AIDS by the end of 2003 (two-thirds in sub-Saharan Africa). An estimated 4.8 million new infections occurred in 2003.

The number of people living with HIV is ↑ because of the continuing epidemic and the availability of life prolonging drugs. Infection rates are likely to ↑ in countries with poverty, inadequate healthcare, and limited resources for prevention. The socio-economic impact is greater in developing countries.

UK (Fig. 35.1)

Cumulative total of 60,000 reported cases of HIV in the UK by the end of 2003 with an estimated 50,000 living with HIV of whom one-third are unaware of their infection.

Over the past 10 years the migration of HIV infected people from high prevalence areas of the world has contributed significantly to heterosexually acquired infections. New infections have accelerated among homosexual/bisexual ♂ since 1999, but only one-third of ♂ diagnosed with HIV infection during 2003 were homosexual/bisexual.

Heterosexually acquired infections have been ↑ since the early years of the epidemic and now outnumber those acquired through sex between ♂.

Injecting drug use plays a small role in the UK epidemic. The age at diagnosis of this group has risen suggesting that new diagnoses are being made on a population mostly infected in the mid-1980s.

Screening blood donations and heat treatment of blood products to inactivate HIV was introduced in the UK in 1985. Since then there have been no recorded transmissions of HIV through contaminated clotting factors given to haemophilia patients. However, there have been five cases where HIV infection could have been acquired through blood transfusion. Current estimated blood transfusion risk in the UK <1 in a million units.

HIV seroprevalence rates in adults aged 15–49 years (based on UNAIDS data, 2003)

Heterosexuals (%)	Homosexual men (%)
• UK: 0.1	• London: 15
• Rest of Europe: <0.1–1.4	• Rest of UK: 2–3
• N. America: 0.3–0.6	Injecting drug users (%)
• S. America and Caribbean: <0.1–5.6	• London: 4.7
• S., E., S.E. Asia and Pacific: <0.1–2.6	• Rest of UK: 0.2
• Australia and New Zealand: <0.1	
• N. Africa and Middle East: <0.1–2.6	
• Sub-Saharan Africa: 0.1–38.8	

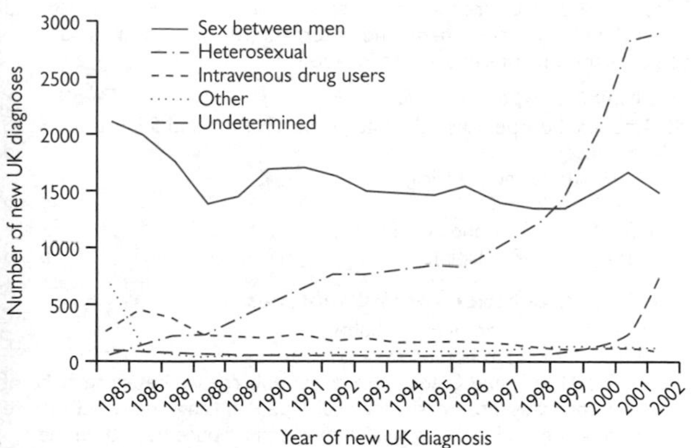

Fig. 35.1 UK HIV prevalence by risk factor. *Source*: From the Health Protection Agency. www.hpa.org.uk/

The viruses and their epidemiology

HIV-1 and HIV-2

Differ in several aspects:

- HIV-1: a rapidly mutating virus eventually producing divergent quasi-species. More virulent and rapidly progressive than HIV-2.
- HIV-2: predominantly found in W. Africa but has been recently reported in India and S. America. ↓ viral loads (VLs) independent of the duration of infection. Rate of vertical transmission ↓ than HIV-1.

HIV-1 and 2 are classified into groups according to their genetic diversity.

HIV-1

- Group M (main group): further divided into subtypes or clades with at least 11 genetically distinct subtypes, A1, A2, B, C, D, (E now considered a circulating recombinant form, CRF01_AE), F1, F2, G, H, J, and K (I now considered a circulating recombinant form). Some variants are termed U category i.e. uncertain or unclassifiable, which may represent new subtypes, or recombinant forms. At least 15 circulating recombinant forms have been described so far and are likely to increase as is their proportion in the pandemic.
- Group O (outlier group).
- Group N (new group).

HIV-2

Divided into group (rather than subtype) A to G.

Geographic distribution of HIV groups and subtypes

Group M is the most common group worldwide. Majority of its subtypes are found in Africa, while certain subtypes predominate in other regions.

Groups N and O are rare and remain confined to W. and Central Africa. Population movement and international travel will erode the geographic boundaries of subtype location.

Predominant subtype distribution

- B: America, Europe, Australia, and Japan. Thailand and S.E. Asia (IV drug users).
- A and D: sub-Saharan Africa.
- C: S. Africa and India.
- E (CRF01_AE): Thailand and S.E. Asia.
- F: Brazil (also in Romania).

Biological implications of HIV subtypes

- Mode of transmission of HIV-1 subtypes:
  - B mainly found in homosexual ♂.
  - E (CRF01_AE) and C are more commonly seen in heterosexuals. They replicate more easily than subtype B in Langerhans' cells (normally found in the vagina, cervix, and prepuce but not in the rectum).
- Infectivity: subtype E (CRF01_AE) is transmitted more easily than subtype B.

- Response to therapy:
  - Implications of subtype diversity need continuous assessment as they may influence the response to treatment.
  - HIV-2 is intrinsically resistant to non-nucleoside reverse transcriptase inhibitors.
- Vaccine production: unclear whether a vaccine provides subtype cross-protection. Genetic variations may be important and necessitate periodic vaccine modification (as with influenza vaccine).
- Diagnosis and screening strategies: diagnostic tests must reliably detect the various strains, subtypes, and circulating recombinant forms. Modifications of tests can be made to ensure that all those with HIV infection are detected. This is also important for ensuring safety of the blood supply.

Phenotypic classification

HIV can also be classified on its ability to form a syncytium with CD4 cells in vitro. This ability is not directly related to the genotypic characteristic of the virus. Therefore, within each HIV subtype there are isolates that are syncytium-inducing (SI) and non-syncytium-inducing (NSI). Most 1° HIV strains are NSI while SI strains tend to appear with disease progression. This switch is dependant on cellular tropism for macrophages or T-cells and on the chemokine co-receptor used to gain entry into the CD4 cell. Most NSI strains use CCR5 and most SI strains CXCR4 co-receptors.

Risk factors and routes of transmission (see Table 35.1)

HIV is exclusively transmitted through body fluids. Routes of transmission include:

- Sexual intercourse: between ♂ and ♀, ♂ and ♂, and rarely ♀ and ♀. Although sex between ♂ characterized the initial HIV epidemic seen in the USA, W. Europe, and Australasia, elsewhere it was typically found to be spread heterosexually. The relative risk of infection depends on the local prevalence and also type of sexual practice.
- Sharing infected needles and syringes among drug users.
- Transfusion of blood and blood products: now very rare in countries where blood is screened for HIV. Transmission may still occur in the developing world through re-use of contaminated surgical equipment and needles.
- Vertically from an infected mother to baby: antepartum, intrapartum, and postpartum (breastfeeding).
- Occupational exposure: to healthcare professional (HCP). Only one documented case of an HCP transmitting HIV to patients.

Table 35.1 HIV transmission risk following single exposure with HIV infection*

Sexual intercourse	
Anal: receptive	0.1–3%
Anal: insertive	0.06%
Vaginal: receptive	0.1–0.2%
Vaginal: insertive	0.03–0.09%
Oral (fellatio): receptive	Up to 0.04%
Oral: cunnilingus and insertive fellatio	No data but estimated to be at least half receptive rate.
Sharing injecting equipment	0.7%
Single unit of blood	90–100%
Occupational	
Needle-stick injury	0.3%
Mucous membrane contact	0.1%

* Influenced by: plasma and genital VLs; breaks in mucosal surfaces e.g. trauma, genital ulcer disease.

Frequently asked questions

What is HIV?

HIV (human immunodeficiency virus) is a virus which damages the body's immune system. HIV destroys a type of white blood cell called the CD4 cell. This cell spearheads/leads the body's defence against infection. When a person's CD4 count becomes low he/she is more susceptible to certain infections.

What is AIDS?

AIDS (acquired immune deficiency syndrome) is the final stage of HIV infection. When the CD4 cells drop to a very low level, (usually <200cells/μL) the ability to resist certain infections is seriously impaired. Certain opportunistic conditions (AIDS-defining illnesses) can develop e.g. *Pneumocystis jiroveci* (*carinii*) pneumonia (PCP), Kaposi's sarcoma.

How is HIV transmitted?

- Having unprotected sex with an infected person.
- Sharing a needle/equipment to take drugs.
- Receiving a blood transfusion from an infected person (unlikely in UK where blood has been tested for HIV since 1985).
- Transmission from a positive mother to her baby during pregnancy, delivery, and by breastfeeding.

Can it be passed on by kissing?

There is no evidence of transmission by kissing and viral levels in saliva are very low. Body fluids which contain high levels of HIV correlating with infection are: blood, seminal fluid, vaginal/menstrual fluid, and breast milk.

Can it be passed on by oral sex?

Yes, especially with receptive fellatio.

Does HIV have symptoms?

Some people get flu like symptoms 4–8 weeks after infection. They usually settle within a 1–2 weeks. A person can have HIV for many years before developing symptoms (and may never do so).

What is the window period?

The delay between infection and a positive HIV antibody test. Although most infected people test positive within 2–6 weeks it can take up to 3 months for enough antibodies to be produced to give a positive HIV antibody test. During this time the person is often very infectious with a high viral load.

Chapter 36

Pathogenesis of HIV infection

HIV structure

HIV-1 and 2 are structurally similar (icosahedral) with the following components (see Fig. 36.1).

Envelope: a lipid bilayer formed from host cell lipids and viral proteins. Embedded in the envelope is a complex protein env containing the viral surface glycoprotein, gp120 and a transmembrane glycoprotein, gp41. Both are derived from a precursor, gp160.

Matrix: encapsulated by the envelope, made up of viral protein p17.

Core: it comprises

- RNA dimer. Two identical copies of single-stranded RNA linked together, each containing ~9500 nucleotides. Associated with a nucleocapsid (p9) and its precursor protein (p6).
- Capsid protein p24 encapsulates the ribonucleoprotein core which contains three enzymes; reverse transcriptase (p51), integrase (p32), and protease (p11).

Genetic organization of HIV

- Genetic information is stored as RNA.
- Gene maps for HIV-1 and HIV-2 are similar except that HIV-2 has *vpu* instead of *vpx*.
- Both sides of the HIV provirus are flanked by a repeated sequence known as the long terminal repeat.

HIV genes and their major functions

Major structural proteins	*gag*	Encodes for capsid, matrix, and nucleocapsid
	pol	Encodes for viral enzymes
	env	Encodes for envelope glycoproteins
Regulatory proteins	*tat*	Regulates HIV transcription
	rev	Induces transition from early to late genes
Accessory proteins	*vpu*	Enhances virus particle release
	vpr	Facilitates import of prointegration complex and cell growth arrest
	vif	Maintains replication of HIV in lymphocytes and macrophages
	nef	Down-regulates CD4 receptors and stimulates HIV infectivity

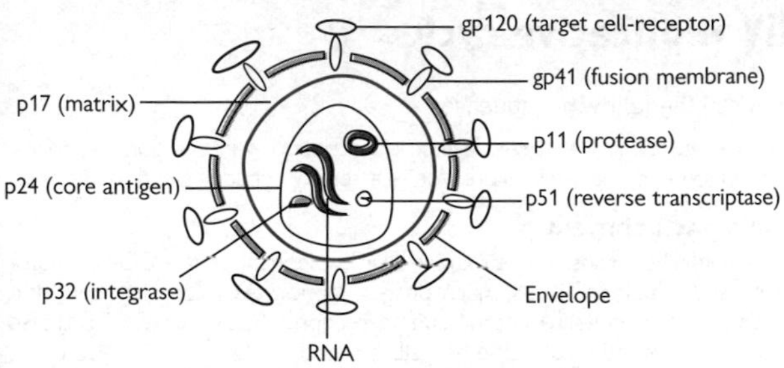

Fig. 36.1 HIV structure. gp and p refer to glycoprotein and protein respectively and the numeric values ($\times 10^3$) indicate molecular weight.

HIV replicative cycle

Occurs in the following sequence:

Binding → fusion and entry → reverse transcription → integration → proviral transcription → cytoplasmic expression → assembly → budding and maturation.

Binding/attachment

Glycoprotein120 binds to the extracellular component of the CD4 receptor (expressed in helper T-cells, macrophages, monocytes, microglial, dendritic, and Langerhans' cells). A chemokine co-receptor (CCR5 or CXCR4) also required for infection of helper T-cells or macrophages.

Fusion

Binding of gp120, CD4, and co-receptors produces a conformational change in gp41 leading to virion and cell membrane fusion and release of the viral core into the cell.

Reverse transcription

Viral reverse transcription complex includes viral RNA, transfer RNA ($tRNA^{Lys}$), viral reverse transcriptase, integrase, matrix and nucleocapsid proteins, viral protein R (*vpr*), and various host proteins. Reverse transcription yields HIV pre-integration complex, composed of double-stranded viral cDNA, integrase, matrix, *vpr*, reverse transcriptase, and the high mobility group DNA-binding cellular protein HMGI (Y). Pre-integration complex travels towards the nucleus using microtubules. Reverse transcription is error-prone producing a mistake every cycle generating multiple mutations instrumental in both the development of drug resistance and escape from immune surveillance.

Integration

Integrase mediates the integration of the viral DNA into the host cell chromosome. It also removes terminal nucleotides from the proviral DNA correcting the ragged ends generated by the terminal activity of reverse transcriptase.

Proviral transcription

Host factors regulate transcription of provirus. Transcription generates different multiple spliced HIV-specific transcripts, which are transported rapidly into the cytoplasm and encode *nef, tat, and rev.* Singly spliced or unspliced viral transcripts remain in the nucleus and encode the structural, enzymatic, and accessory proteins that are needed for the assembly of fully infectious virions.

rev-independent and rev-dependent cytoplasmic expression

During early HIV synthesis only multiple spliced mRNA transcripts are available for translation. Later on unspliced and singly spliced mNRAs diffuse into the cytoplasm where translation to structural protein synthesis starts.

Virion assembly

HIV particles generated assemble at the host cell surface.

Virion budding and maturation

- *env* proteins are synthesized in the endoplasmic reticulum and transported to the cell surface.
- *gag* and *gag–pol* proteins are cleaved by viral proteases during budding to produce mature products.

Mature virions are released ready to infect new cells and begin the replication cycle once again. The entire process is extremely active, with 10^{8-10} viral particles produced each day.

HIV and its receptors

- CD4 antigen is the principal receptor, mainly expressed on the surface of helper T lymphocytes. It is also expressed but to a lesser degree in CD4 dendritic cells including Langerhans' cells and CD4 monocytes, macrophages, and microglial cells.
- Co-receptors—several chemokine receptors have been described but CCR5 and CXCR4 are the most important co-receptors for HIV attachment *in vivo*. CCR5 is the co-receptor for non-syncytium-inducing (NSI) and CXCR4 for syncytium-inducing (SI) strains.
- gp120: contains hypervariable regions (V1–V5) that vary from one HIV isolate to another. V3 loop is not involved in CD4 binding but important for HIV tropism for macrophages or T-lymphoid cell lines. It is also the target for neutralizing antibodies that block HIV 1 infectivity.

Factors influencing HIV disease progression

Host factors

- Age: ↑ age is associated with ↑ progression.
- Co-infection: may affect immune system resulting in ↑ progression (e.g. tuberculosis and hepatitis C). Cytomegalovirus associated with ↑ progression in haemophiliacs.
- Gender: ♀ appear to have higher viral loads at any CD4 level and may progress more rapidly.
- Psychosocial factors: depression, impaired intellectual functioning, drug use, social deprivation may be associated with ↑ progression.
- Genetic susceptibility:
  - Up to 20% of individuals of northern European descent have a deletion in the CCR5 gene resulting in a mutant (CCR5Δ32). Homozygous individuals (1–2% of the Caucasian population) are almost resistant to HIV infection and heterozygotes slow progressors. CCR2 (a minor co-receptor) deletion (CCR-V641) is widespread in all ethnic groups and results in slower progression to AIDS.
  - Certain HLA types associated with ↓ or ↑ progression.
- Nutrition: poor premorbid state associated with ↑ progression.
- Pharmacological variability: individual drug metabolism and elimination modifies response to therapy.

Viral factors

Changes in the phenotype and genotype of the virus enable it to 'escape' control by the immune system. In late HIV infection switching from CCR5 to CXCR4 (i.e. from NSI to SI) leads to infection of both active and resting immune cells resulting in ↑ disease progression. Mutations may alter viral 'fitness' influencing pathogenicity. Gene mutation involving *nef*, is associated with ↓ progression and some drug resistant mutations (e.g. M184V which induces lamivudine resistance) may ↓ viral fitness.

Drug susceptibility depends largely on HIV genotypic and phenotypic characteristics with genotype mutations rendering some drugs ineffective. Other factors such as efflux pumps may also be involved.

Chapter 37

Staging, classification, and natural history of HIV disease

Clinical staging

Early in the epidemic, before HIV was discovered, diagnosis of AIDS was largely based on finding *Pneumocystis jiroveci* (previously *carinii*) pneumonia (PCP) or Kaposi's sarcoma. HIV antibody testing led to patients being identified as having asymptomatic infection, AIDS-related complex or AIDS. The Centers for Disease Control and Prevention (CDC) devised a classification system, revised in 1993, based on clinical features, AIDS defining illnesses and CD4 counts (see Table 37.1). The CD4 count is a useful predictor for the development of opportunistic infections (OIs) and malignancies but it should be recognized that this may be influenced by other factors such as inter-current infection.

This system was originally designed as a categorization tool for public health purposes and not intended for staging.

Table 37.1 Revised classification of HIV disease (CDC, January 1993)*

CD4 (count/μL)	A	B	C
>500	A1	B1	C1
200–500	A2	B2	C2
<200	A3	B3	C3

* Those in categories A3, B3, C1, C2, C3 have AIDS under the 1993 surveillance case definition.

Category A

- Asymptomatic HIV infection
- Persistent generalized lymphadenopathy
- Acute retroviral syndrome

Category B

- Bacillary angiomatosis
- Candidiasis
  - Oral
  - Recurrent vaginal
- Cervical dysplasia
- Constitutional symptoms
- Oral hairy leukoplakia
- Herpes zoster
- Idiopathic thrombocytopenic purpura
- Listeriosis
- Pelvic inflammatory disease
- Peripheral neuropathy

Category C (AIDS defining conditions)

- CD4 count <200cells/mm^3
- Candidiasis
  - Pulmonary
  - Oesophageal
- Cerebral toxoplasmosis
- Cervical cancer
- Coccidioidomycosis
- Cryptosporidiosis
- Cytomegalovirus
- Herpes simplex
  - Chronic (>1 month)
  - Oesophageal
- HIV encephalopathy
- Histoplasmosis
- Isosporiasis
- Lymphoma
- *Mycobacterium avium* complex
- *Mycobacterium tuberculosis*
- *Pneumocystis jiroveci*
- Pneumonia (recurrent)
- Progressive multifocal leukoencephalopathy
- Salmonellosis
- Wasting syndrome due to HIV

Natural history of untreated HIV infection (Fig. 37.1)

Characterized by progressive loss of immune function allowing the development of some virulent bacterial infections, certain opportunistic infections, and malignancies that define AIDS. Progression rate varies depending on interactions between host, viral, and environmental factors. The average time between HIV acquisition and AIDS is ~10 years if untreated.

Course can be divided into 5 continuous stages: 1° infection, early, middle, advanced, and late-stage disease. There is significant individual variation between patients in the same clinical stage.

- 1° HIV infection: Disseminates widely in the body at seroconversion, usually with a very high VL and a rapid, spontaneously but not fully reversible CD4 cell ↓.
- Early stage: CD4 count >500cells/μL. After 1° stage viraemia ↓ (rarely becoming undetectable). Usually asymptomatic apart from generalized lymphadenopathy and certain skin disorders (e.g. seborrhoeic dermatitis, aphthous ulcers, eosinophilic dermatitis, and psoriasis) which may deteriorate or appear for the first time.
- Middle stage: CD4 count 200–500cells/μL. Mostly asymptomatic/mildly symptomatic. Skin disorders of early stage may worsen. Recurrent herpes simplex infection, varicella zoster, diarrhoea, weight loss, and intermittent fever may develop. Lung infections caused by community acquired organisms such as *Streptococcus pneumoniae*, *Haemophilus influenzae*, and *Mycobacterium tuberculosis* become more common.
- Advanced stage: CD4 count 50–200cells/μL. ↑ VL with classical manifestations of AIDS, especially PCP, Kaposi's sarcoma, lymphomas, and *Mycobacterium avium* complex (MAC) infection.
- Late stage: CD4 count <50cells/μL. Very high levels of viraemia. Further development of conditions associated with severe immune deficiency e.g. CMV retinitis, disseminated MAC. Neurological manifestations ↑ due to 1° brain lymphoma, multifocal leukoencephalopathy, and dementia. HIV wasting disease is commonly seen at this stage.

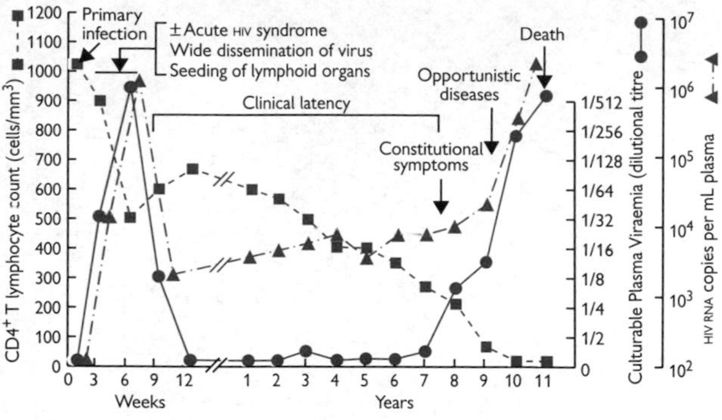

Fig. 37.1 Schematic representation of progression of HIV infection with time. *Source*: Reproduced with permission of Prof. Giussepe Pantaleo from: www.cloettastiftung.ch

Chapter 38

HIV: diagnosis and assessment

HIV pre-test discussion

HIV infection is usually diagnosed by detecting antibodies in a serum sample. However, in suspected 1° infections or 2–4 weeks after a specific high-risk incident (e.g. needle-stick injury) plasma should be tested for HIV p24 antigen and RNA by a nucleic acid amplification technique (e.g. PCR). Testing should always be done with informed consent and assurance about the confidential nature of the process. Points to cover include:

- Risk assessment: e.g. sex practices, travel, drug use, occupation, blood/blood products prior to 1985 (in the UK).
  Very high risk:
  - unprotected sexual contact with an HIV infected partner
  - receipt of infected blood products
  - sharing injecting equipment with HIV infected person.

If risk within 72 hours consider post-exposure prophylaxis (see p. 532)

  High risk:
  - ♂ to ♂ unprotected anal sex (especially receptive)
  - sex or sharing injecting equipment with people from countries with a high HIV prevalence.
- Assess patient knowledge: ensure that the individual understands the nature and transmission of HIV. Advise on risk reduction.
- The standard antibody test—serum (saliva and finger prick tests available if venepuncture impossible):
  - detects antibodies to HIV 1 and 2, does not diagnose AIDS.
  - seroconversion often within 4–6 weeks but may take up to 12 weeks, 'window period', therefore repeat testing may be required. Repeat saliva testing advised 14 weeks after risk. It is therefore important to determine the date of the last risk.
  - positive standard screening tests need to be validated by different method(s) which may incur delays. Rarely indeterminate results are obtained requiring repeat sampling.
- Implications of testing
  - Early diagnosis allows monitoring with pre-symptomatic HAART if appropriate and development of strategies to avoid transmission including post exposure prophylaxis
  - In pregnancy: allows informed choices about the management of pregnancy, especially the use of antiretroviral treatment (both mother and infant), and avoidance of breastfeeding to ↓ vertical transmission. Arrangements for early monitoring of the infant's health
  - If negative, elimination of needless anxiety

But if positive:

  - psychological impact of result
  - social and work implications (e.g. surgeon). May affect travel to, or work in certain countries
  - life insurance restrictions/weightings. A positive result (or awaiting a test result) must be declared on application forms

- Arrangements for giving results
  - How/when the result will be provided (especially in high-risk situations)
  - If positive who will he/she tell, how will the individual cope, what support is available.
- Document that information has been provided on
  - positive, negative, and indeterminate results
  - how, when, and where results will be given and whether written confirmation is required
  - follow up and the possible need for repeat testing to confirm positive results or cover the window period.
- Obtain and document informed consent.

Suggested HIV pre-test check-list

Risk assessment	Yes	No	Further inform.
Prior HIV test			When:
Blood transfusion/products			When: Where:
Injecting drug user (shared equipment)			Last time:
Sex with people from countries with a high HIV prevalence			Last time:
Homosexual/bisexual man or sex with homosexual/bisexual man			Last time:
Contact with HIV			Last time:
No risk			
Low/medium risk			
High risk			
Information provided			
Benefits of early identification and treatment explained			
Implication of positive result (especially if high risk)			
3-month window explained			
Insurance explained			
Result giving explained			
Consent to test obtained			
HIV test taken			
Repeat test required			When:

Post-test counselling

The content and timing of the discussion will depend upon the patient's reaction to a positive or negative result.

The aims of post-test counselling are to:

- address the immediate concerns and provide support for those who are positive and also negative (especially the very anxious)
- provide information on the prevention of HIV transmission
- ensure patient is aware of need for confirmatory/repeat testing if appropriate.

If HIV positive:

- address immediate reactions and assess need for psychological intervention.
- provide further basic information about the natural history of HIV, reinforcing the difference between HIV and AIDS and efficacy of treatment.
- construct a management plan which meets the needs of the patient.
- give details of support services.
- offer follow-up appointments and ongoing support which may include addressing issues concerned with employment, travel, legal matters, and support for carers and partners.
- provide information on what further investigations will be required.

Seronegative HIV infection

Negative HIV antibody test with HIV infection (after excluding specimen handling errors) is well-recognized during the window period. It is otherwise very rare and identified only when clinical presentation suggests HIV/AIDS with a negative HIV antibody test but positive PCR for HIV RNA/DNA (or viral culture). Possible causes:

- profound hypogammaglobulinaemia
- seroreversion—extremely rare
- HIV group O infection
- unknown.

Medical situations to consider HIV infection

- Reticulo-endothelial abnormalities:
  - impaired immunity
  - unexplained lymphadenopathy
  - thrombocytopenia
- Infections:
  - tuberculosis or atypical mycobacterial infection
  - *Pneumocystis jiroveci (carinii)* pneumonia
  - cerebral toxoplasmosis
  - oral or oesophageal candidiasis
  - herpes zoster (in younger people)
  - cytomegalovirus retinitis
- Tumours:
  - non-hodgkin's lymphoma
  - cerebral lymphoma
- General:
  - symptoms suggesting seroconversion illness, especially if associated with another STI
  - oral hairy leukoplakia
  - unexplained weight loss
  - unexplained diarrhoea
  - night sweats
  - pyrexia of unknown origin

Assessment of an HIV positive patient

Initial assessment

Objectives

- Reinforce the patient's understanding of HIV infection and how to avoid further transmission.
- Identify medical, socio-economic, and legal problems.
- Establish stage of disease.
- Establish a rapport with patient (essential to ensure efficient follow up).

Full history, medical examination, and baseline investigations to plan future management and drug therapy. Further tests depend on the circumstances and stage of disease.

History

- Sexual history including, sexual partners/practices, condom use, and contraception.
- Current and previous medical (especially, tuberculosis, STIs, or hepatitis), surgical, gynaecological, and obstetric history.
- Current medication and allergies.
- Drug, substance, and alcohol use.

Clinical examination

- General: weight, temperature, pulse, BP, respiratory rate, pallor, and jaundice.
- Lymph glands: lymphadenopathy—site, size, symmetry, tenderness, and consistency.
- Mouth and throat: gum and tooth disease, oral ulceration, hairy leukoplakia, candidiasis, and enlarged pharyngeal lymphoid tissue.
- Cardiovascular: routine examination.
- Respiratory: routine examination.
- Abdomen: routine examination.
- Neurological: routine examination. Specifically assess eyes checking visual acuity, visual fields, pupil size, pupil reactivity, and extra-ocular movements. Examine retinae ideally with pupils dilated.
- Genital/pelvic examination: discharges, ulcers, condylomata, testicular enlargement or atrophy, cervical abnormalities, pelvic masses, and STI screening.
- Cervical cytology: annual review with close follow up if abnormal.
- Perianal and rectal examination: anal/rectal discharge, condylomata, ulcers, prostate assessment, and tests for STIs as appropriate.
- Skin: general skin examination specifically checking for seborrhoeic dermatitis, fungal nail infection, warts, Kaposi's sarcoma, molluscum contagiosum, and abnormal pigmentation.

Laboratory investigations

- Full blood count, urea, electrolytes and liver function tests, glucose, triglycerides, and cholesterol.
- Serological tests: hepatitis A, hepatitis B (surface antigen and core antibody), hepatitis C, cytomegalovirus (CMV) IgG, toxoplasma, varicella zoster virus (VZV) IgG and syphilis.

- Viral load (VL): informs on likely rate of disease progression and monitors response to therapy.
  - Undetectable VL indicates level <25/50copies/mL (depending upon test used).
  - <5000copies/mL generally suggests low rate of progression in the coming 5 years.
  - >55,000copies/mL are associated with ↑ rate of progression
- CD4 count: usually measured as part of lymphocyte subsets.
  - Main indicator of risk of opportunistic infection and possible need for prophylactic treatment in the asymptomatic patient.
  - Individual results may be influenced by other factors, e.g. intercurrent infections.
  - Repeat if unexpectedly low or high count.
  - Trend is more useful than single readings.
- Plasma samples for viral resistance testing.

Frequently asked question

Do I have to tell people that I am HIV positive?

When you are diagnosed you will speak to a health adviser who will discuss this and similar issues with you. You should be careful who you tell as once it's done, there's no going back. Although safety precautions are taken you should inform anyone who could come into contact with infected body fluids (e.g. dentists, surgeons) and your doctor especially if you develop unusual symptoms which may be related to or altered by the HIV infection. If you are a healthcare professional (HCP) you should seek appropriate counselling as certain invasive procedures cannot be performed by HIV positive HCP.

It is important to act responsibly where others are concerned, especially sexual (or drug-sharing) partners. There are court cases where HIV positive individuals have been prosecuted for infecting partners without informing them that they are HIV positive.

Further investigations and follow-up

- Estimate stage of HIV infection from initial assessment and baseline investigations.
- Assess disease progression: HIV-related infections and malignancies, response to therapy and signs of drug toxicity.
- Monitor VL and CD4 count at regular intervals, frequency depends on the patient's clinical status. Asymptomatic patients with stable disease may have their VL and CD_4 count measured every 3–6 months but shorter intervals may be necessary for those with more advanced disease.

Drug prophylaxis

- *Pneumocystis jiroveci* (*carinii*) pneumonia (PCP): when CD4 count <200cells/μL, first choice is trimethoprim/sulfamethoxazole (co-trimoxazole) orally 960mg 3 times a week. If allergic consider desensitization (see Table 38.1). Alternatives are: dapsone 50–100mg daily, dapsone 50mg plus pyrimethamine 50mg 3 times a week, atovaquone 750mg 3 times a week or nebulized pentamidine 300mg once a month.
  Azithromycin 500mg 3 times a week may be effective as 1° prophylaxis.
- Tuberculosis (TB): prior BCG vaccination provides unreliable protection. A negative tuberculin test may be due to anergy and does not exclude TB. Chemoprophylaxis is recommended for close contacts of smear positive pulmonary TB. 6 months of isoniazid 300mg daily or 3 months of isoniazid 300mg daily plus rifampicin 600mg daily are effective.
- Toxoplasmosis: if CD4 count <100cells/μL and toxoplasma IgG positive. Co-trimoxazole and maloprim (as for PCP prophylaxis).
- VZV: varicella zoster immunoglobulin (5 vials IM) if seronegative for VZV antibodies within 72 hrs of significant exposure.
- *Mycobacterium avium* complex prophylaxis may be considered with CD4 counts <50 cells/μL (see p.460).

Vaccination

Inactivated rather than live vaccines should be used (e.g. polio). If travelling abroad additional vaccination may be required (see p.546). Those immuno-deficient may not mount a good response to vaccination. Vaccination can be delayed until immune reconstitution ensues although unnecessary delay should be avoided if there is a specific infection risk.

- Pneumovax: can be given to all patients.
- Hepatitis A: if immuno-naïve.
- Hepatitis B: if immuno-naïve.
- Influenza vaccination: controversial, but safer if given to those whose HIV infection is suppressed by antiviral therapy.

Table 38.1 Suggested desensitization schedule for trimethoprim/sulfamethoxazole (T/S)

Day	Dose	T/S
1	1mL of 1:20 paediatric suspension	0.4mg/2mg
2	2mL of 1:20 paediatric suspension	0.8mg/4mg
3	4mL of 1:20 paediatric suspension	1.6mg/8mg
4	8mL of 1:20 paediatric suspension	3.2mg/16mg
5	1mL of paediatric suspension	8mg/40mg
6	2mL of paediatric suspension	16mg/80mg
7	4mL of paediatric suspension	32mg/160mg
8	8mL of paediatric suspension	64mg/320mg
9	1 tablet	80mg/400mg
10	1 double strength tablet	160mg/800mg

Thereafter 1 double strength tablet three days a week until CD4 count is >200cells/μL for at least 3 months.

Reprinted from N. Absar, H. Daneshvar, G. Beall (1994). *J Allergy Clin Immunol*, **93**, 1001–5. With permission from American Academy of Allergy, Asthma and Immunology.

Chapter 39

HIV: primary infection

Definitions

Primary HIV infection (PHI)

The period of time from the onset of infection until the immune system establishes a balance with viral replication. Characterized by rapidly increasing viraemia with transient immune suppression and usually takes weeks–months to stabilize.

Acute seroconversion illness—acute retroviral syndrome (ARS)

The symptomatic development of HIV specific antibodies.

Prevalence of acute seroconversion illness

Difficult to determine due to the wide spectrum of clinical presentations which may be mild and non-specific. These explain the wide range of reported prevalence of 30–93% in those recently infected. Clinician awareness, experience, and high index of suspicion ↑ diagnostic rate. It is unclear what determines the severity of symptoms. The inoculum size, HIV strain virulence, and patient's immune status may be factors. Almost all reports of ARS are in adults with HIV-1 but it may occur in children or those with HIV-2 infection.

Clinical features of acute seroconversion illness

Symptoms usually begin 2–6 weeks after infection typically lasting 5–10 days and rarely >14 days. Subjective symptoms such as fatigue may continue for several weeks or even months but eventually almost all patients enter an asymptomatic phase that may last for years. Within 2–4 weeks of infection very high levels of free HIV and p24 antigen can be detected in the peripheral blood. Symptoms coincide with peak levels of plasma viraemia.

Usual clinical features

Fever followed by lymphadenopathy, pharyngitis, and skin rash.

Others

- Dermatological manifestations (involving face, neck, and trunk >limbs):
  - maculopapular skin rashes
  - mucosal ulceration of genitals, mouth, and oesophagus
  - additional skin lesions include pustules, urticaria, erythema multiforme, and alopecia
- Infectious mononucleosis-like illness:
  - fever, pharyngitis, myalgia, arthralgia, and lymphadenopathy
  - oral ulceration (highly suggestive of acute seroconversion illness)
  - no prominent tonsillar involvement (unlike in infectious mononucleosis)

- Evidence of immune deficiency:
  - oral and oesophageal candidiasis
  - *Pneumocystis jiroveci* (*carinii*) pneumonia
- Neurological manifestation:
  - meningitis, peripheral neuropathy, brachial neuritis, Bell's palsy, myelopathy, encephalitis, Guillain–Barré syndrome.

Severe and prolonged illness, especially with neurological manifestations, is associated with a poorer prognosis. Resolution of symptoms coincides with ↓ in plasma viraemia and the development of a CD8 cell-specific immune response with the later emergence of HIV-specific antibodies (usually within 4–6 weeks of infection but may be up to 3 months).

Acute retroviral syndrome—frequency of clinical features

Fever	80–97%
Lymphadenopathy	40–77%
Pharyngitis	44–73%
Skin rashes	51–70%
Myalgia or arthralgia	49–70%
Thrombocytopenia	45–51%
Leucopenia	35–40%
Diarrhoea	32–33%
Headache	30–70%
↑ serum transaminases	21–23%
Nausea and vomiting	20–60%
Hepatosplenomegaly	14–17%
Weight loss	13–32%
Oral candidiasis	10–12%
Encephalopathy	8%
Neuropathy	8%

Immune responses in primary HIV infection

Cellular response

More important than humoral immunity in containing HIV infection and develops earlier. HIV-specific immune responses, particularly cytotoxic CD8 cells, influence the natural history of HIV infection.

1° infection is characterized by active viral replication and very high levels of plasma viraemia. The virus disseminates throughout the body, particularly to the lymphoid system where its replication is never completely suppressed. During the first few days of infection both CD4 and CD8 cells are suppressed resulting in lymphopenia approaching levels seen in patients with advanced disease. This is followed by relative lymphocytosis, predominantly CD8 cells, normalizing when acute sero conversion is complete. However, CD4 count, though increasing, does not return to baseline values. These changes result in reversal of the CD4/CD8 ratio to <1.

HIV viraemia ↓ with HIV-specific immune responses, gradually stabilizing within 6–12 months to reach a 'viral set point'. Higher set points indicate ↑ risk of disease progression.

Humoral response

Antibody response usually becomes detectable within 10–21 days of the onset of symptoms but may take up to three months from infection. Antibodies to gp160 and p24 develop first, followed by gp120 and gp41. Anti-p24 diminishes with time and may disappear with advanced disease. However anti-gpl20 and anti-gp41 persist for life. Poor prognosis if inadequate HIV antibody response. Neutralizing antibodies are usually detected 4–8 weeks after resolution of the viraemic peak. Non-neutralizing antibodies to envelope and p24 antigens develop much earlier, coinciding with seroconversion.

Diagnosis

PHI usually presents before the development of antibodies and is therefore diagnosed by finding p24 antigen or HIV RNA in the appropriate clinical setting. Although p24 antigen detection tests are ~100% specific they can be falsely negative during PHI. HIV RNA levels are usually extremely high, often $>10^6$ copies/mL.

Atypical lymphocytes are commonly seen in the peripheral blood with levels up to 30%. Anaemia, thrombocytopenia, abnormal liver function tests, or ↑ inflammatory markers may also be found.

Management of primary HIV infection

PHI is the time of highest infectivity in HIV infection. Plasma level of HIV RNA strongly predicts progression rate. Early intervention has theoretical advantages as the virus is likely to be homogenous and the immune system intact. Antiretroviral treatment may ↓ the number of infected cells, preserve HIV-specific immune responses and possibly ↓ the viral set point. However, the long-term benefit of early therapy has not been demonstrated.

It is unusual for PHI to be identified unless patients present with symptoms (ARS), the nature and severity of which may influence the decision to treat. If treatment is considered it is common practice for them to be offered entry into controlled clinical trials. Failing this standard 1st line treatment may be the option (see p. 514). Possible benefits of treatment should be weighed against drug toxicity, adherence, and potential for resistance in discussion with the patient. The optimum duration of treatment is not yet established. Benefit from structured treatment interruptions in stimulating host immune response has not been conclusively demonstrated. The role of drugs that inhibit activation of CD4 cells, e.g. hydroxyurea and cyclosporin A, in boosting cellular responses is not known.

Other possible benefits of diagnosing PHI:
- early identification of partners most at risk
- advice on reduction/prevention of infection
- if treated ↓ viral load may ↓ infectivity.

Main differential diagnoses of the acute seroconversion illness

- Epstein–Barr virus infectious mononucleosis
- Cytomegalovirus infection
- Toxoplasmosis
- Viral hepatitis
- 2° syphilis
- Rubella
- 1° herpes simplex virus infection
- Drug reaction
- Aseptic meningitis
- Streptococcal pharyngitis

Chapter 40

HIV: gastrointestinal disorders

Oral diseases

Very common in HIV infection and oral disease may indicate the diagnosis. Detailed oral examination should be part of the assessment of the newly diagnosed HIV +ve individual. Various lesions of ulcerative, raised, white, or pigmented appearance may be encountered. Advice from oral or maxillofacial surgeon should be obtained when necessary.

Viral infections

Herpes simplex virus (HSV)

HSV infection is very common, with seropositivity rates approaching 80% in HIV +ve homosexual ♂. Oral HSV, like herpes infection elsewhere, is characterized by latency (in the trigeminal ganglia).

1° episodes: vesicles normally appear on lips, gingiva, hard palate, or rarely the dorsal aspect of the tongue. Unlike herpes zoster, primary HSV infection is not associated with viraemia. Lesions are initially vesicular followed by ulcers, crusting, and then healing. It may take up to 3 weeks for 1° HSV lesions to heal. The duration is longer in the severely immunocompromised.

Recurrent HSV: tend to localize to the vermilion border of the lips. Some patients experience pain or tingling sensation before the appearance of the lesions. It may take 7–10 days for oral HSV lesions to heal. Recurrent HSV infection may be more common in patients with symptomatic HIV disease and severely immunocompromised patients tend to have more frequent and more severe attacks.

Complications:

- ocular keratitis occurs with the same frequency as in HIV –ve individuals.
- herpes oesophagitis occurs more frequently in patients with late HIV disease but not necessarily associated with concomitant oral herpes.

Management: see p. 398.

Cytomegalovirus (CMV)

Seroprevalence rates rise with age. >90% prevalence rates have been found in HIV +ve homosexual ♂.

CMV oral ulcers:

- are difficult to differentiate from those of other aetiology but they are typically solitary, deep, necrotic ulcers with a red margin and a white halo
- arise when the CD4 count is <50cells/μL
- usually occur as part of disseminated CMV disease and attempts must be made to exclude infection of other organs such as the retina
- diagnosis is established by the biopsy finding of typical owl's eye inclusions.

Management: see p. 436.

Varicella zoster virus (VZV)

Reactivation of VZV causes herpes zoster (HZ)/shingles in the immunocompromised host, including HIV infection at any stage. Rarely found as 1° infection in those without previous exposure to the virus. People with HIV infection are 15 times more likely to have HZ than age-matched controls. Oral HZ is latent in the trigeminal nerve. Mandibular branch

involvement results in lesions in the lower lip and lateral border of the tongue and maxillary branch involvement results in lesions of the hard palate. Oral vesicles only last for a few hours followed by painful ulcers, while the concomitant skin lesions may last for 2–4 weeks.
Diagnosis and management: See pp. 442–3.

Oral hairy leukoplakia (OHL)

White adherent vertically corrugated lesion seen only in the mouth, most commonly found on the lateral aspect of the tongue (Plate 16). The affected area may fluctuate in size.

Caused by Epstein–Barr virus (EBV), demonstrated by finding EBV DNA, RNA, and proteins in biopsies of OHL. Usually asymptomatic but a few patients may complain of pain, altered sensation, and taste. Reported in all risk groups but more common in adults, ♂, and smokers. It is not pathognomonic and occurs in HIV –ve immunocompromised individuals such as bone marrow and renal transplant recipients. Incidence and persistence increase with advancing HIV disease and declining CD4 counts. Its occurrence is associated with faster progression towards AIDS even after adjustment for CD4 count. It is not premalignant and does not need specific treatment but regresses with improved immune function associated with highly active antiretroviral therapy (HAART).

Human papilloma virus (HPV)

Most commonly identified HPV types associated with oral warts in HIV +ve individuals are 7, 13, 18, and 32. Mutant strains are frequently reported. Oral warts are more common in HIV +ve individuals than the general population but there is no association with the stage of infection and malignant transformation has not been found. Although mostly localized to the oral cavity, laryngeal warts may occur and may be solitary or multiple, pedunculated or sessile with small papilliferous or cauliflower-like projections.
Management: Surgical excision, laser, or cryotherapy.

Bacterial diseases

Periodontal disease

Dental hygiene is very important in HIV infection because of the high incidence of gum and periodontal disease. Periodontal disease should be managed in consultation with maxillofacial or dental surgeon. Mild gingivitis and dental abscesses are common at all stages infection. Linear gingival erythema (LGE), necrotizing ulcerative periodontitis (NUP) and necrotizing stomatitis (NS) occur more frequently in HIV infection. They are characterized by rapid onset, increased severity, and poor response to conventional treatment.

- Linear gingival erythema (LGE): Patients present with spontaneous painless gum bleeding. Examination reveals an oedematous erythematous band parallel to the free gingival margin, which may be a precursor of NUP. Commonly isolated organisms include *Bacteroides gingivalis*, *Fusobacterium nucleatum*, and Actinobacilli. The response to treatment is poor but attention to oral hygiene and chlorhexidine mouthwash is helpful although systemic metronidazole may be required.
- Necrotizing ulcerative periodontitis (NUP): An acute onset severe and rapidly progressive condition, usually seen in patients with advanced HIV disease, that tends to occur in clean mouths with little plaque. A few teeth may be affected but in severe cases all may be involved. Severe gum pain precedes the appearance of signs which include soft tissue necrosis with destruction of periodontal ligament and bone. NUP may resemble intraoral lymphoma.
- Necrotizing stomatitis (NS): NS also called necrotizing ulcerative stomatitis. Very difficult to differentiate from NUP although usually localized and less severe. It is a rapidly progressive process involving the gingiva, alveolar bone, and palate causing severe deep pain. Bone sequestration may occur and management includes oral hygiene, chlorhexidine mouthwashes, and systemic antibiotics such as metronidazole and amoxicillin together with gentle debridement.

Tuberculosis

The most common oral manifestation is irregular ulceration of the tongue or palate. Culture has been shown to be insensitive in its detection from this site (2–17%) so polymerase chain reaction should also be considered.

Fungal diseases

Oral and pharyngeal candidiasis

Probably the most common opportunistic infection (OI) in HIV disease. >90% would have oro-pharyngeal candidiasis at some stage. Commonly caused by *Candida albicans* but other species such as *Candida glabrata* and *Candida tropicalis* are implicated. Though oro-pharyngeal candidiasis may occur at acute seroconversion, it becomes more frequent as the CD4 count ↓.

Clinical features

- *Pseudomembraneous candidiasis.* The pseudomembraneous appearance results from overgrowth of candidal hyphae mixed with desquamated epithelium and inflammatory cells. Appears as white plaques at any site of the mouth or pharynx and leaves an erythematous raw bleeding mucosa on scraping. Patient may complain of soreness and altered taste (Plate 15).
- *Erythematous candidiasis.* Appears as flat, red patches of varying morphology that can be difficult to recognize and therefore diagnosis may be delayed. The most common sites are the palate and the dorsal surface of the tongue. Usually asymptomatic but soreness and burning sensation may be reported.
- *Angular cheilitis.* Appears solely or in conjunction with other forms of oro-pharyngeal candidiasis resulting in redness, ulcers, and fissuring of one or both corners of the mouth.
- *Hyperplastic candidiasis.* This the rarest form of candidiasis in *HIV* positive individuals. Lesions appear as white and hyperplastic but are more easily removed than in the pseudomembraneous form.

Diagnosis

Can be made on the clinical appearance. Candidal hyphae can be demonstrated on Gram or periodic acid Schiff staining of smears from the lesions. Culture may be used to identify the candidal type which may guide treatment as sensitivities may be difficult to interpret. It does not help in making the diagnosis, as candida is a commensal of the oropharynx.

Management

- Systemic antifungal (standard mode of therapy):
  - fluconazole: 50–100mg once daily for 7–14 days
  - itraconazole: 100–200mg once daily for 7–14 days

⚠ Avoid terfenadine as risk of arrhythmias.

- Topical antifungal (consider in mild cases):
  - nystatin (as pastilles or as suspension): 100,000–500,000 units 4 times a day after food for 7 days or continue for 48 hours after lesions have resolved.
  - amphotericin (lozenges and suspension): dissolve 1 lozenge (10mg) slowly 4 times a day after food for 10–15 days or continue for 48 hours after lesions have resolved.
  - miconazole oral gel: 5–10mL after food and retained near lesions 4 times a day, continue treatment for 48 hours after lesions have resolved.

Topical treatment must be retained in the mouth in contact with lesions for sufficient time.

Prognosis

Relapses are common and may be the result of poor compliance rather than resistance to antifungals. Consider prophylactic therapy (fluconazole 50mg daily) when recurrences are common but risk of resistance ⚠.

Differential diagnosis of white lesions in the oral cavity

- Candidiasis
- Frictional keratosis
- Tobacco induced leukoplakia
- Lichen planus
- White sponge naevus
- Geographical tongue
- Primary syphilis and syphilitic mucous patches
- Squamous cell carcinoma

Neoplasia

***Kaposi's sarcoma (KS)**—see p. 498*

Oral KS was among the first recognized features early in the AIDS epidemic. More common in homosexual/bisexual ♂. Usually presents as a blue, purple, or red lesion that may be flat, papular, nodular, or rarely a large tumour (Plate 17). Large nodular lesions may ulcerate and be secondarily infected. Occasionally the adjacent mucosa is yellow stained (due to haemosiderin). Commonest site is the hard palate but may be seen on the gingiva, tongue, soft palate, and buccal mucosa. Local pain may be a feature in secondarily infected, ulcerative KS lesions.

Management: see p. 502

- Immune reconstitution achieved by HAART may result in KS resolution, improves survival and response to therapy.
- Small lesions respond to local therapy such as surgical excision, laser excision, and intralesional chemotherapy.
- Larger lesions may be treated with radiation therapy, which may be complicated by mucositis.

Oral lymphoma

Caused by Epstein–Barr virus. The vast majority are B-cell non-Hodgkin's lymphomas. Oral lymphoma may precede the development of lymphomas at other sites. Presents as a rapidly growing tumour at any site in the mouth (Plate 18). May be diffuse or discrete nodules or may present as ulcers of variable morphology. Diagnosis must be confirmed by tissue biopsy.

Management

Once the diagnosis is established lymphoma must be staged by appropriate imaging. Systemic chemotherapy and local radiation are the main stay of therapy in collaboration with the maxillofacial surgeons to minimize oral side-effects. The intensity of chemotherapy used is dependant on the degree of immune suppression.

Idiopathic aphthous ulcers

Recurrent oral ulceration resembling aphthous ulcers is a common phenomenon in HIV +ve individuals, usually well circumscribed, superficial, and varying in size:

- herpetiform—appear as clusters of 1–2mm ulcers, usually in the mouth and soft palate.
- minor—usually solitary, 0.5–1.0cm in diameter.
- major—2–4cm in size and necrotic. Usually found on the tonsils and tongue base and rarely the pharynx and nasopharynx. Typically very painful, persisting for several weeks.

Management

- Topical steroids: clobetasol in orabase or adocortyl in orabase 3–4 times a day is usually effective.
- Systemic steroids may be used if associated with oesophageal ulcers 40–60mg daily for 7–10 days.
- Thalidomide (50–200mg/day) produces an excellent response in resistant cases. Prescribing thalidomide needs fulfilment of special requirements, especially the avoidance of pregnancy ⚠.

Salivary gland disease

In HIV infection the salivary glands may become infiltrated with lymphocytes, predominantly CD8 cells, resulting in enlargement especially affecting the parotids. Xerostomia may be caused by drugs such as didanosine, antihistamines, and antidepressants but also as a manifestation of HIV infection where the precise aetiology is unclear. Salivary amylase levels may be raised in drug-related cases.

Management

- Salivary stimulants such as sugarless sweets and chewing gum for symptomatic relief.
- Artificial saliva as necessary.
- Careful dental hygiene.

Differential diagnosis of oral–pharyngeal ulcers

Viral

- Herpes simplex virus
- Cytomegalovirus
- Herpes zoster virus

Bacterial

- Necrotizing ulcerative periodontitis
- Necrotizing stomatitis
- *Mycobacterium tuberculosis*
- *Mycobacterium avium* complex
- *Treponema pallidum*

Fungal

- Histoplasmosis

Tumours

- Lymphoma
- Kaposi's sarcoma

Other causes

- Aphthous ulcers
- Behçet's disease

Oesophageal diseases

Dysphagia ± odynophagia are the main symptoms of oesophageal disease. Symptoms and signs are not discriminative enough to establish the underlying aetiology. Assessment of the nutritional status and hydration is essential in managing such patients.

Dysphagia investigations

- Endoscopy and biopsy are required to establish a definitive diagnosis.
- Double contrast barium swallow may differentiate between infection and neoplasm but rarely diagnostic.
- More than one pathology may coexist and therefore multiple biopsies (>6) from different sites are advisable.
- Generally culture of oesophageal specimens is not helpful as does not differentiate between colonization and actual tissue invasion but may be useful in identifying viral and mycobacterial pathogens.

Candidal oesophagitis

Most common cause of oesophagitis in HIV infection. A patient with oral candidiasis and odynophagia can be treated empirically for oesophageal candidiasis and investigated if it fails to respond. It usually occurs when the CD4 count <200cells/μL and is rarely asymptomatic. Candidal exudate can be seen during upper gastrointestinal endoscopy.

Management

- fluconazole 100–200mg or itraconazole 200mg once daily for 7–14 days.
- itraconazole suspension 200mg twice daily (the suspension formulation of itraconazole has a better bioavailability than the capsular form). This is especially useful in fluconazole-resistant candidiasis (rare and seen in those with very low CD4 count who have had repeated courses of fluconazole).
- liposomal amphotericin B (e.g. Amphocil, AmbiZone) or voriconazole, in refractory cases.

CMV oesophagitis

CMV causes large distal oesophageal ulcers. Biopsy required to confirm diagnosis and exclude other or concomitant causes of oesophagitis.

Management

CMV disease is treated with ganciclovir, cidofivir, or foscarnet until clinical improvement. Patients may be given maintenance oral valganciclovir to prevent CMV retinitis. See p. 436.

Causes of oesophagitis

Infections

- *Candida* spp.
- Cytomegalovirus
- Herpes simplex virus
- *Mycobacterium avium* complex

Malignancies

- Kaposi's sarcoma
- Lymphoma

Idiopathic oesophageal ulceration

Non-HIV related

- Reflux oesophagitis
- Pill-induced oesophagitis, e.g. zalcitabine and zidovudine

Enteric diseases

Diarrhoea is an extremely common symptom in HIV infection. It may be debilitating and require extensive and invasive investigation techniques. In patients with CD4 >200cells/μL it is usually caused by virulent organisms and managed as in the immunocompetent. When CD4 <200cells/μL it is usually more severe, more likely to be caused by OIs, more difficult to diagnose and is less responsive to treatment. Large bowel diarrhoea is typically of small volume, may be blood stained, and is associated with lower abdominal pain and tenesmus. Small bowel diarrhoea is characteristically of large volume, offensive, and of pale colour. Diarrhoea is described as being chronic when it persists >1 month.

Although infection with campylobacter, shigella, and other enteric pathogens occur (see p. 228), particularly important organisms are cryptosporidium, microsporidium, isosopora, and salmonella.

Cryptosporidiosis

Cryptosporidium parvum (4–6μm intracellular protozoon) has a complete life cycle (with a sexual and an asexual stage) in the intestinal mucosa of a single host. It is a common cause of diarrhoea in young calves. The infected animal excretes large numbers of cysts in the environment. The oocyst can survive in the environment for >3 months. As it is small it may bypass water filtration systems and standard home and hospital disinfectants are ineffective in its killing. The infectious dose for human is around 130 oocysts. Infection is self-limiting and usually asymptomatic in the immunocompetent host but can cause debilitating symptoms in patients with advanced HIV disease. Human disease is limited to the jejunum but may involve all the gastrointestinal and respiratory epithelium in the immunocompromised.

Important factors in transmission

- Zoonotic infection e.g. rural communities
- Contaminated water and food
- Travellers to countries with poor sanitation systems
- Human to human transmission which may include sexual
- Oocysts may be excreted for 2 weeks after recovery.

Postulated mechanism of diarrhoea in cryptosporidiosis

- Osmotic
- Cholera-like cryptosporidial toxin production resulting in cyclic adenosine production
- Villous atrophy resulting in malabsorption.

Clinical features

- HIV +ve with preserved immune function—similar to HIV –ve immunocompetent.
- In advanced HIV disease—persistent watery diarrhoea of variable frequency and volume (1–15L/day). This is commonly associated with nausea, abdominal cramps, malabsorption, weight loss, and electrolyte disturbances. Intrahepatic and extrahepatic biliary duct strictures, interstitial lung disease, chronic sinusitis, and otitis media are rare features.

Diagnosis

The parasite can be easily missed on routine stool analysis. Special staining techniques such as phenol auramine (fluorescent stain) are required. Intestinal mucosal biopsies may identify the organism.

Management

Attention to fluid and nutrition is important. No proven effective regimens though paromomycin, azithromycin, and other antibiotics are used with variable degrees of success.

- Best response is achieved by improving the immune function with specific treatment of HIV itself by HAART.
- Antidiarrhoeal agents
  - Loperamide
  - Opiates
  - Diphenoxylate
- Octreotide (somatostatin analogue)—effective in secretory diarrhoea.

Prevention

- Raising awareness of modes of transmission
- Boiled water is advisable especially for those with advanced disease
- Use of fine filters to the mains water supplies

Microsporidiosis

Caused by small (1–7μm) obligate intracellular protozoa of which several hundred species identified but only a few cause disease in humans, rarely in immunocompetent. The commonest microsporidia causing disease in patients with advanced HIV infection are:

- *Encephalitazoon intestinalis*—accounts for 80% of microsporidial diarrhoea. Infects the small intestinal epithelium and biliary tract and presents with chronic watery diarrhoea (usually less severe than that of cryptosporidiosis), cramps, weight loss, and cholangiopathy. May infect macrophages leading to dissemination with pulmonary, sinus, renal, and conjunctival disease.
- *Enterocytozoon bieneusi*—accounts for most of remainder of microsporidial diarrhoea. Infects enterocytes (jejunum) and causes abdominal symptoms, as above, but does not disseminate.

Diagnosis

Identification of the organism in the stools with immunofluorescent stains or modified trichrome stain. Transmission electron microscopy of intestinal biopsies considered as gold standard if available. Various staining methods are used to visualize the organism in tissue biopsies. Serological tests are unreliable and PCR of limited use.

Management

- Albendazole 400mg twice daily for 4 weeks produces best results for *Encephalitazoon* infection.
- Some relief of symptoms have been described with metronidazole, co-trimoxazole, erythromycin, octreotide but all fail to eradicate the organism.
- Significant symptom improvement has been achieved with HAART.

Isospora belli

A common cause of epidemic diarrhoea in tropical countries and travellers. Infection is caused by ingestion of the 25μm oocysts contaminating food and water. Infection is usually confined to the small intestine but may cause acalculous cholecystitis and may disseminate in patients with advanced HIV disease.

Clinical features

Crampy abdominal pain, watery diarrhoea, and weight loss similar to cryptosporidiosis.

- Steatorrhoea (involvement of the pancreatic and biliary tracts)
- Eosinophilia
- Rarely involves the spleen, liver, and abdominal lymph nodes.

Diagnosis

Oocysts are visualized in the stools by using a modified Kinyoun stain (an acid fast stain) or in duodenal aspirate or biopsy.

Management

- Co-trimoxazole 960mg 2–4 times a day for 2–4 weeks gives good results.
- 2° prophylaxis recommended because relapses are common, e.g. co-trimoxazole as for *Pneumocystis jiroveci* (*carinii*) pneumonia (PCP).
- HAART results in significant improvement of symptoms.

Management of chronic diarrhoea in HIV infection

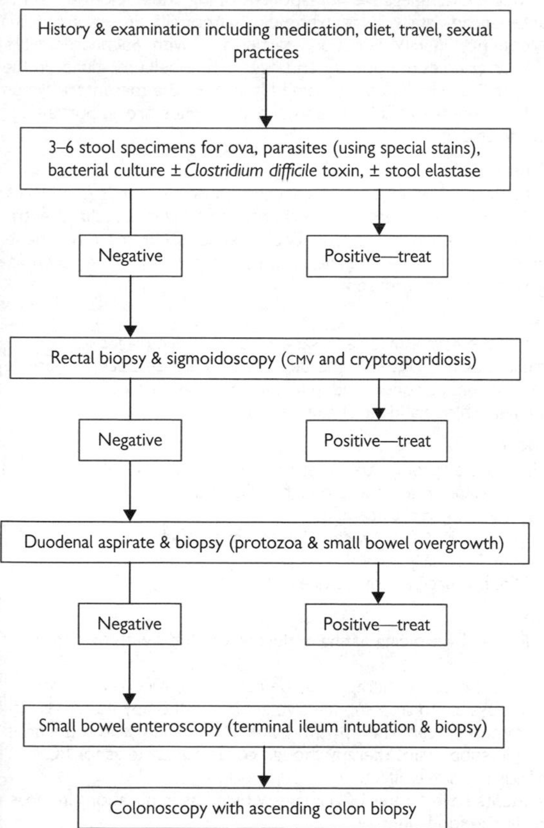

Salmonellosis

Salmonellae are Gram-negative non-spore-forming rods belonging to the Enterobacteriaceae family. Non-typhoidal salmonella infections occur with ↑ frequency in HIV infection, particularly with *Salmonella typhimurium*. Major sources are poultry and eggs. Salmonella multiplies in the intestinal epithelium, and if not contained it invades the mesenteric lymph nodes and disseminates. Cellular immune responses are important defence mechanisms.

Clinical features

In HIV infection salmonella tends to cause more systemic symptoms. A common feature is severe gastroenteritis and fever. Localized extra-intestinal focal infection may occur. Bacteraemia is common in patients with advanced HIV disease, may be recurrent and may not be accompanied by gastrointestinal symptoms.

Diagnosis

- Isolation of the organism is necessary for a definitive diagnosis
- Salmonella may be isolated in the blood before stools become positive
- Diagnosis should be considered in all HIV +ve patients with ± diarrhoea and blood and stool cultures taken.

Management

Salmonella requires prompt treatment in HIV +ve individuals because of severity, high relapse rates, and the higher dissemination risk

- Fluid and electrolyte replacement
- Oral ciprofloxacin 750mg twice daily (the drug of choice)
- Ceftriaxone 1–2g daily
- Amoxicillin, but bacterial resistance is ↑.

Prevention

- Risk reduction by avoiding eating undercooked food with particular care during travel.
- Long-term suppressive therapy may be required if recurrent episodes. It may be possible to stop suppressive antibiotic therapy if there is significant immune reconstitution with HAART. Ciprofloxacin is the drug of choice in suppressive therapy though co-trimoxazole as for PCP prophylaxis has some effect.
- AIDS patients have ↑ rates of carriage, which has implications in those working in the food industry.

HIV enteropathy

HIV has been found in the macrophages of the lamina propria and enterochromaffin cells. HIV can also affect the local humoral immunity and gut motility because of autonomic dysfunction. Villous atrophy with variable degrees of compensatory crypt hyperplasia is a common finding. This leads to rapid cell turnover and functional immaturity of intestinal epithelium with a resultant reduction in enzyme production leading to impaired absorption of sugars and peptides. Evidence of malabsorption such as abnormal D-xylose test, low vitamin B12 levels, and impaired triolein breath tests are described in patients with advanced HIV disease.

These abnormalities may occur in the absence of intestinal disease. HIV enteropathy is a diagnosis only entertained after exclusion of other pathogens.

Management

There are no agreed criteria for the diagnosis of HIV-related enteropathy. Every attempt should be made to find an underling cause especially infection. Principles of therapy are attention to nutrition and symptomatic control of diarrhoea.

Factors contributing to diarrhoea such as alcoholism and drugs must be addressed.

Anal diseases

Anal complaints and anal lesions are frequent presentations in those with HIV infection, especially homosexual ♂. Anal pain, pruritus, discharge, and bleeding should be assessed by enquiring about sexual practices, followed by anal and rectal examination by proctoscopy. Gonorrhoea, chlamydia, syphilis, and anogenital warts are common and must be excluded.

Anal HSV infection

Although HSV2 causes the majority of infection, HSV1 is increasing in frequency. Patients with advanced HIV disease tend to have more recurrences and prolonged episodes that are less likely to resolve spontaneously.

Typical painful vesicles and ulcers occur in the anal and perianal region. Severe disease may result in diffuse perianal ulceration. The distal rectum may be involved resulting in anal discharge, painful defecation, rectal bleeding, and tenesmus. Fever and painful inguinal adenopathy occur more commonly in primary attacks.

Diagnosis: see p. 242.

Management

Prompt treatment with specific antiviral drugs reduces the duration of symptoms and viral shedding. Chronic episodes (>4 weeks) occur more frequently in patients with advanced HIV disease. Aciclovir-resistant HSV has been reported, usually in association with HIV infection. Valaciclovir and famciclovir have better bioavailability.

Recommended initial treatment in the immunocompromised:
- aciclovir 400mg 4 times a day for 10 days
- famciclovir 500mg twice daily for 7 days
- valaciclovir 500mg twice daily for 5 days (up to 10 days if severe)—similar regimen to immunocompetent.

Suppressive treatment (interrupted and reviewed every 6–12 months):
- aciclovir 200mg 4 times a day (or 400mg twice daily)
- valaciclovir 500mg twice daily
- famciclovir 500mg twice daily

Human papilloma virus (HPV) infection

Anal warts are common in HIV +ve individuals especially so in homosexual men. HPV6 and 11 are the most frequently found types but others including 16, 18, 31, and 33 have been detected. Patients with advanced HIV disease may have exuberant plaques in the perianal region as well as flexural areas. Extensive anal and perianal warts may present with rectal bleeding and constipation.

Management: see p. 254.

No treatment ensures HPV eradication and is similar to those HIV –ve although persistence and recurrences are more common but may improve with immune reconstitution produced by HAART.

Anal intraepithelial neoplasia (AIN)

The epithelium of the transitional zone between the anus and colonic mucosa has the same embryonic origin as the cervix and is susceptible to intraepithelial neoplasia and invasive cancer similar to those seen in the cervix. AIN1–3 precedes the development of anal cancer similar to cervical cancer. HPV (type 16 and 18) infection, receptive anal intercourse, and HIV infection are co-factors associated with the development of these changes.

Anal carcinoma may be prevented by the early detection and treatment of AIN3. Anal cytology can be used to detect dyskaryosis, although this is not routine clinical practice. It is anticipated that the incidence of AIN and anal carcinoma will increase as life expectancy rises with the introduction of HAART (which does not appear to be protective).

Low grade AIN lesions can be treated conservatively by regular monitoring and high grade lesions (AIN3) by ablative surgical techniques.

Pancreatic diseases

Pancreatic involvement in HIV infection is common but is usually asymptomatic. Drugs, alcohol, and OIs are the usual causes. Pancreatic disease tends to occur in conjunction with hepatic and hepatobiliary disease.

Clinical presentation may be with acute or chronic pancreatitis though elevation of serum amylase or lipase may predate the development of symptoms.

Acute pancreatitis

Patients usually severely ill, in shock, with acute abdominal pain, nausea, and vomiting. It is associated with OIs including:

- CMV—most common infective cause
- cryptococcus and toxoplasmosis
- cryptosporidiosis, HSV, non-Hodgkin's lymphoma and KS (less common).

Drugs such as didanosine, zalcitabine, co-trimoxazole, and pentamidine are probably the most common cause of acute pancreatitis. Very high levels of triglycerides associated with protease inhibitors may also cause pancreatitis. The serum amylase is elevated and computerized tomography (CT) scanning demonstrates an oedematous, enlarged pancreas with surrounding fluid. Admission to a high dependency unit for cardiovascular and electrolyte support is usually required.

Chronic pancreatitis

Typically presents with pancreatic exocrine deficiency. Chronic diarrhoea and malabsorption are the usual presenting features. As with HIV –ve patients, the discontinuation of any offending drugs and alcohol may result in symptomatic improvement. Associated HIV-related cholangiopathy is a recognized underlying cause.

Diagnosis

Chronic abdominal pain (especially if there is history of acute pancreatitis) is suggestive of chronic pancreatitis. This may be accompanied by pancreatic insufficiency symptoms e.g. steatorrhoea, weight loss, and other evidence of malabsorption. Screen by measuring faecal elastase and triolein breath tests (serum amylase and lipase are usually normal). The best diagnostic test is endoscopic retrograde cholangiopancreatography (ERCP).

Management

- Pain control
- Pancreatic enzyme supplement

Hepatic and biliary tract diseases

Hepatic disease

Biliary tract disease

Hepatic and biliary tract diseases

HIV itself has been found in Kupffer cells, hepatic macrophages, and hepatocytes. The liver in those with HIV infections is a target of specific viral, bacterial, fungal, and protozoal infections. Infection with hepatitis B or C viruses may pre-date HIV infection. With improved life expectancy and the effect of drugs more liver-related problems are being identified.

Hepatic disease

>80% of those with HIV infection are estimated to have abnormal liver function tests (LFTs) at some time during the course of their infection. This does not necessarily indicate the presence of liver disease. The presence of fever, hepatomegaly, and right upper quadrant abdominal pain warrant further investigation. Important causes of abnormal LFTs and liver disease are viral co-infections, drugs, and alcohol. Bacterial, fungal, and protozoal infections and neoplasms occur much less frequently. The pattern of LFTs and the clinical stage of HIV infection may help to narrow the diagnostic options.

History: prior infection with viral hepatitis, alcohol intake, prescribed and recreational drug use and recent travel.

Examination: fever, hypotension, signs of chronic liver disease and nutritional status (obesity and malnutrition).

Abnormal LFTs: mixed hepatitic and obstructive liver enzyme abnormalities are common but rarely diagnostic in isolation.

- Predominant ↑ of serum transaminases usually indicate hepatitis but lacks sensitivity and specificity. A new hepatitis viral infection or reactivation of hepatitis B and/or C infection with immune reconstitution should be excluded. Consider drug hepatotoxicity and investigate for other infections.
- Predominant ↑ of serum alkaline phosphatase usually indicates biliary obstruction. Initial assessment is by ultrasound scan or CT of the liver and abdomen. Lesion identified can be targeted by image-guided biopsy. ERCP must be considered if imaging techniques reveal intrahepatic and/or extrahepatic duct dilatation.

Biliary tract disease

Presents with right upper quadrant abdominal pain, weight loss. Investigations to exclude common biliary conditions such as cholelithiasis should proceed before attributing to HIV infection.

HIV-associated cholangiopathy

Similar to sclerosing cholangitis presenting with right upper abdominal pain associated with nausea, vomiting, fever, and marked elevation of serum alkaline phosphatase. Ultrasound shows dilated intra and/or extrahepatic bile ducts. ERCP provides further structural delineation. Some cases are associated with cryptosporidial and cytomegalovirus infections.

Acalculous cholecystitis

Presents with similar symptoms to HIV-associated cholangiopathy. Ultrasound of the abdomen normally shows thickened dilated gall bladder but may be normal. Can be complicated by recurrent cholangitis. Associated with CMV, *Cryptosporidium parvum*, microsporidia, and MAC infection but no cause in >50%.

Diagnosis by ultrasound or technetium scintigraphy. Treatment is cholecystectomy.

Main causes of HIV-related liver disease

Viral

- Hepatitis B virus
- Hepatitis C virus
- Cytomegalovirus

Alcohol

Drugs

- Recreational
- Therapeutic (e.g. antiretroviral and antituberculous)

Other infections

- Mycobacteriosis

Neoplasia

- Lymphoma
- Kaposi's sarcoma

HIV: hepatitis virus co-infection

Introduction

Since the introduction of HAART mortality of HIV has markedly ↓ especially from opportunistic infections (OIs). However, liver related deaths have ↑. As hepatitis B, C, and HIV share blood-borne and sexual transmission, co-infection is common.

Co-infection requires the multidisciplinary assessment of ongoing drug and alcohol use, psychiatric illness, progressive liver disease, and degree of HIV immune-suppression. Alcohol should be strongly discouraged. IDUs should enter a maintenance programme.

If immuno-naïve hepatitis A/B vaccination should be provided.

HIV/hepatitis B virus (HBV) co-infection

Epidemiology

In high endemic areas of sub-Saharan Africa, E. Europe, S., and S.E. Asia co-infection rates of 10–15% are found. In the UK, HBV is associated with HIV infection in 5–8% with co-infection more common in haemophiliacs, injecting drug users (IDUs), and those from high prevalence areas. Co-infection rates vary regionally within the UK.

Natural history and clinical features

Co-infection is usually associated with a higher HBV viraemia and a more rapid progression to cirrhosis. Although HBV does not appear to influence the natural history of HIV there is ↑ rate of hepatotoxicity in relation to antiretroviral therapy. HBV reactivation can occur in those who appear to have cleared their HBV infection. This can lead to transient HB surface-antigenaemia or chronic HBV infection and may occur more frequently when CD4 counts are ↓. In addition the natural clearance of HBe antigen is ↓ but spontaneous recovery from chronic HBV infection may occur in those whose CD4 count ↑.

Diagnosis and investigations

- As for HBV and HIV (see p. 270, p. 366).
- It is important to repeat HBV serology regularly in immuno-naïve patients with HIV infection. Other factors causing liver disease/infection require exclusion.
- Liver biopsy is important when active HBV replication (high HBV–DNA, abnormal liver function, or advanced liver disease). Serum fibrosis markers may be introduced. HBV-genotyping is currently rarely available and testing for lamuvidine resistance (e.g. YMDD motif codon substitution) is not readily available.
- More frequent monitoring of liver function on HAART (due to enhanced hepatotoxicity of most antiretroviral drugs).

Management

General advice: as for HBV mono-infection (see page p. 270).

In chronic HBV/HIV co-infection the aim of HBV treatment is to suppress viral replication. Only rarely is it curative (loss of surface antigen).

Available treatment options include lamivudine, tenofovir, adefovir, and interferon (pegylated), emtricitabine and most recently, entecavir.

HBe-antigen negative patients with normal liver function and low viral load do not require treatment. It should be considered for patients with HBV–DNA >10^5copies/mL and abnormal liver function.

The optimum time to initiate treatment is unknown. Early intervention may be aided by higher CD4 counts but the risk of emergence of HIV drug resistance must be considered. If treatment prior to HAART is provided interferon (pegylated) or adefovir should be considered. Lamivudine, tenofovir or emtricitabine should only be used as part of HAART. If HAART regimens containing lamivudine or tenofovir need to be changed, despite good HBV response, then these agents should be maintained in addition to the new HAART combination. The dose for lamivudine in co-infected patients should be 150mg twice daily or 300mg daily not 100mg daily as in HBV mono-infection.

Assessment for liver transplantation if cirrhosis develops should not be denied.

HIV/hepatitis C virus (HCV) co-infection

Epidemiology

HCV infection is a major factor in end stage liver disease (ESLD) in HIV infection. HCV prevalence is much higher in those HIV infected than the rest of the population (in the UK 5–15% compared with 0.4% respectively). Higher rates are found in HIV positive haemophiliacs, IDUs, and those from S. or E. Europe.

Heterosexual HCV transmission is infrequent but may be more likely with anal sex or co-existing STIs.

Natural history and clinical features

Effect of HCV on HIV: it is not clear whether HCV itself leads to a worsening of HIV disease although it may ↓ CD4 response to HAART.
Effect of HIV on HCV: if untreated there appears to be a faster progression to cirrhosis ↓ the median time from 32 to 23 years with death from ESDL more common (most studies on haemophiliacs or IDUs). Vertical transmission of HCV ↑ to 14–17%.

Otherwise clinical features as for mono-infection (see p. 274).

Diagnosis and investigations

- As for HCV and HIV (see p. 274, p. 366) including HCV genotype testing.
- Liver biopsy currently recommended—all genotypes except if bleeding disorders. Serum fibrosis markers may be introduced in the future.
- Regular monitoring of progression of liver disease i.e. alpha-fetoprotein, abdominal ultrasound and Doppler scan of portal vein.
- More frequent monitoring of liver function on HAART (due to enhanced hepatotoxicity of most antiretroviral drugs).

Management

Guidelines for management of patients with HCV mono-infection are applicable for patients with co-infection (see p. 275) and recommend combined pegylated α-interferon and ribavirin. If possible HCV should be treated before there is a need for HAART. A temporary CD4 drop of up to 150cells/μL while on interferon (pegylated)/ribavirin may occur and ribavirin induced haemolytic anaemia may require dose ↓ or its cessation. Interaction between ribavirin and antiretroviral drugs is common. Cirrhotic co-infected patients who are decompensated should not be treated with these drugs and require specialist input.

Interferon may have a protective effect on the progression of liver disease (currently under evaluation). The response to treatment with interferon (pegylated)/ribavirin in co-infected patients is ↓. Patients with genotypes 2 and 3 and mild/moderate liver disease have a sustained viral response of ~60% and should be offered a 48-week treatment regimen. Patients with genotype 1 have a sustained viral response of ~30% at best (48 week regimen). When the treatment response has been successful regular HCV monitoring is required to detect relapse. Those with a CD4 count <200cells/μL have a poorer response to HCV treatment and are also at ↑ risk of OIs.

Those with stable HIV disease requiring liver transplantation should not be denied assessment although current experience is small.

Chapter 42

HIV: respiratory disorders

Introduction

Respiratory symptoms are common in HIV infection with a wide disease spectrum. These include processes not directly related e.g. bronchogenic carcinoma, smokers' bronchitis, or intravenous drug use associated pulmonary vascular disease.

In HIV infection

- HIV itself, without pulmonary opportunistic infection (OI), leads to ↓ lung function.
- Respiratory disease ↑ in frequency with falling CD4 counts ↑ duration of HIV infection.
- Risks of OI ↑ by other factors e.g. cigarette smoking (further damages lung defences).
- The advent of HAART (where available) has significantly ↓ the burden of HIV associated respiratory disease.

Pathology varies with

- Age e.g. lymphocytic interstitial pneumonitis (LIP) occurs predominantly in children.
- Exposure (travel to or residence in endemic areas for specific pathogens) e.g. histoplasma.
- Level of immune function.
- Specific immune defects e.g. failure to produce antibodies against pneumococcal capsular antigen (independent of CD4 count).
- HIV infection—by modifying typical clinical presentations and influencing results of investigations e.g. ↓ rate of sputum smear positivity in pulmonary tuberculosis (TB).

Considerable overlap of symptoms and signs in different conditions and dual infections may occur. Uncommon for a particular constellation of symptoms, clinical findings, and radiological abnormalities to be absolutely diagnostic a full investigation is always required. However, radiological appearances may suggest different groups of conditions.

Chest X-ray appearances

Interstitial	*Pneumocystis jiroveci* (*carinii*) pneumonia (PCP), LIP (in children), rarely CMV
Lobar	Bacterial infection
Nodular	Kaposi sarcoma (KS), septic emboli, fungal infection, non-Hodgkin's lymphoma
Miliary	Tuberculosis (TB)
Pneumatocoel	PCP, staphylococcal pneumonia
Pleural effusion	KS, TB, lymphoma
Mediastinal and/or hilar lymphadenopathy	Mycobacteriosis, lymphoma, fungal infection

As deterioration can sometimes be rapid it is important that 'best guess' therapy is initiated while awaiting the result of microbiology.

Spectrum of respiratory illnesses in HIV-infected patients

Infections (organisms identified most commonly)

- Bacteria
  - *Streptococcus pneumoniae*
  - *Haemophilus influenzae*
  - Gram-negative bacilli (*Pseudomonas aeruginosa, Klebsiella pneumoniae*)
  - *Staphylococcus aureus*
  - *Mycobacterium tuberculosis*
  - Atypical mycobacteria (*Mycobacterium kansasii, Mycobacterium avium complex*)
  - *Rhodococcus equi*
- Fungi
  - *Pneumocystis jiroveci (carinii)*
  - *Cryptococcus neoformans*
  - *Histoplasma capsulatum*
  - *Aspergillus* spp.
  - *Candida* spp.
  - *Coccidioides immitis*
- Viruses
  - Cytomegalovirus
  - Herpes simplex virus
- Parasites
  - *Strongyloides stercoralis*
  - *Toxoplasma gondii*
- Neoplasia
  - Kaposi's sarcoma
  - Non-Hodgkin's lymphoma
  - Bronchogenic carcinoma
- Other respiratory illnesses
  - Upper respiratory tract infection (sinusitis, pharyngitis)
  - Lymphocytic interstitial pneumonitis
  - Non-specific interstitial pneumonitis
  - Acute bronchitis
  - Obstructive lung disease (asthma, chronic bronchitis)
  - Bronchiectasis
  - Emphysema
  - Pulmonary vascular disease
  - Illicit drug-induced lung disease
  - Medication-induced lung disease
  - 1° pulmonary hypertension
  - Bronchiolitis obliterans organizing pneumonia

Bacterial pneumonia

Before HAART bacterial pneumonia was the most frequent pulmonary complication of HIV occurring in up to 42% in autopsy studies. An episode of bacterial pneumonia is associated with subsequent ↑ morbidity and ↓ survival time.

Aetiology

Most common pathogens are *Streptococcus pneumoniae*, *Haemophilus influenzae*, and *Staphylococcus aureus* occurring more frequently in the general population as a cause of pneumonia. In pneumococcal infection rate of bacteraemia is ↑ and there may be ↑ incidence of penicillin resistant isolates. Intravenous drug use further ↑ the risk of bacterial pneumonia. Less common causes include *Rhodococcus equi* which produces a cavitatory pneumonia of insidious onset.

Clinical and diagnostic features

Most bacterial pneumonias present acutely with symptoms and radiological patterns similar to that seen in HIV negative patients (lobar or broncho-pneumonic consolidation). However the radiological presentation may be indistinguishable from other OIs and *H. influenzae* has been reported to present with diffuse opacities mimicking PCP. As immunodeficiency becomes more advanced pneumonias due to *Staph. aureus* and *Pseudomonas aeruginosa* become more important and may produce cavitation.

Management

In patients presenting with a clinical diagnosis of bacterial pneumonia:

- assess and correct hypoxia, volume depletion and hypotension.
- gauge severity by presence of confusion, ↑ blood urea, ↑ respiratory rate, ↓ blood pressure, older age group, and co-pathologies.
- obtain sputum and blood cultures and baseline atypical pneumonia serology. Consider urine testing for legionella antigen.
- check inflammatory markers and white cell count, although white cell response may be ↓ if there is HIV induced marrow suppression
- commence intravenous antibiotic therapy with—
  - either cefuroxime 1.5g three times a day plus a macrolide (e.g. clarithromycin 500mg twice daily)
  - or amoxicillin 1g three times a day plus a macrolide.
- consider modification to these combinations if there are features to suggest involvement with *Staph. aureus*, *Pseudomonas aeruginosa* or atypical organisms such as *Rhodococcus equi.*
- if recurrent and evidence of ↓ antibody production consider intravenous immunoglobulin therapy or prophylactic antibiotics.

Comparison between bacterial pneumonia and *Pneumocystis jiroveci* pneumonia (PCP)

	PCP	**Bacterial pneumonia**
CD4 cell count	<200cells/μL	Any
Symptoms	Non-productive cough	Productive cough (purulent sputum)
Duration	Typically weeks	Typically 3–5 days
Signs	50%—clear lungs	Focal lung abnormalities
Laboratory tests		
White blood count	Varies	Frequently ↑
Serum lactic dehydrogenase	↑	Varies
Chest radiograph		
Distribution	Diffuse > local	Focal > diffuse
Location	Bilateral	Unilateral, segmental/lobar
Pattern	Reticular, granular	Alveolar
Cysts	15–20%	Rarely
Pleural effusions	Very rarely	25–30%

Pneumocystis jiroveci (carinii) pneumonia (PCP)

The AIDS indicator disease in ~65% of patients before the initiation of 1° prophylaxis programmes and effective antiretroviral therapy. Initially thought to be protozoan but genetic analysis indicates that this organism is a yeast. Infection usually occurs when CD4 counts <200cells/μL. Although natural colonization/infection occurs frequently in early life it is thought that clinical pneumonitis represents new infection rather than reactivation of latent organisms.

PCP is almost completely preventable using 1° prophylaxis. The gold standard is co-trimoxazole. Dapsone, dapsone and pyrimethamine, atovaquone and pentamidine are alternatives (see p. 372). 80% of those with HIV infection and cutaneous hypersensitivity reactions to co-trimoxazole can be desensitized by the use of gradually ↑ doses (see p. 373).

Clinical features

Usually presents sub-acutely with symptoms ↑ over weeks with night sweats, systemic symptoms and weight loss, dry cough, progressive dyspnoea initially on exertion and eventually at rest, occasionally with a spontaneous pneumothorax. Abnormalities on respiratory examination often minimal or absent and significant ↓ of pulmonary function may occur despite minimal chest X-ray changes.

Diagnosis

Radiology

- High resolution computerized tomography shows ground glass appearance of interstitial pathology.
- In severe PCP typical chest X-ray pattern is bi-basal perihilar interstitial consolidation (Plate 19).
- Atypical upper lobe involvement may be seen if patient has been on nebulized pentamidine prophylaxis. They may also develop extra pulmonary involvement of various organs including eyes, spleen, and skin (due to lack of systemic effect).

Oximetry

If history suspicious but normal resting oxygen saturations, exercise oximetry showing ↓ in oxygen saturation by 5% or to <90% highly suggestive of PCP.

Respiratory secretions/lung tissue

Specific diagnosis requires demonstration of *Pneumocystis jiroveci* cysts in respiratory secretions or lung tissue. Patients with borderline lung function may require sputum induction and bronchoscopy.

- Sputum should be induced by 3% saline using an ultrasonic nebulizer. When stained with fluoroscene linked monoclonal antibodies—sensitivity up to 77%, negative predicted value up to 64%.
- Fibre optic bronchoscopic alveolar lavage (BAL)—sensitivity ~90%.
- Transbronchial biopsy with histology of fixed tissue—sensitivity up to 98%.

Management

Prior to initiating investigations in those presenting with a history suggestive of PCP, it is essential to assess pulmonary impairment and the need for oxygen supplements by pulse oximetry and arterial blood gases.

► If there is pulmonary impairment, delays in initiating PCP therapy should be kept to a minimum. Initiation of HAART should be deferred until completion of the acute PCP treatment to avoid the potential of synergistic toxicities.

Gold standard antibiotic therapy is co-trimoxazole 120mg/kg in 4 divided doses daily for 21 days. Haematology, liver function tests and the skin must be monitored carefully for evidence of toxicity or developing hypersensitivity. Folinic acid supplements may be considered if there is evidence of impaired marrow function. For non-responders or hypersensitive patients alternative regimens include clindamycin (600mg 4 times a day) and primaquine (15mg/day), dapsone (100mg/day) and trimethoprim (5mg/kg every 4–6 hours), atovaquone (750mg 3 times a day), intravenous pentamidine (600mg/day), and trimetrexate (45mg/m^2/day IV plus folinic acid).

In patients with arterial oxygen pressures <9.3kPa steroid therapy is recommended as it ↓ risk of respiratory failure and mortality. Conventional regimen is prednisolone, or equivalent, 40mg twice daily for 5 days, 40mg once daily for 5 days followed by 20mg daily for 5 to 10 days. There is no significant ↑ in risk of other OIs except *Candida* spp. and local herpes simplex virus.

Patients with severe PCP may progress to respiratory failure requiring ventilatory support with constant positive airways pressure (CPAP) or intubation and ventilation. Pneumothorax may require chest drain insertion. Adverse prognostic indicators include ↑ serum lactic dehydrogenase (LDH) levels, need for high ventilatory pressures and prolonged intensive therapy unit (ITU) stay.

Maintenance and withdrawal of 2° prophylaxis

Following successful treatment 2° prophylaxis, with the same regimens for 1° presentation, should be continued.

- For patients receiving 1° PCP prophylaxis discontinue when the CD4 count has been >200 cells/µL for at least 3–6 months (rate of OIs do not ↓ until after 2 months of HAART).
- Careful consideration is needed before stopping prophylaxis in patients who have had PCP or other AIDS defining illness, perhaps deferring interruption until complete viral suppression and sustained CD4 count ↑ present for 6 months.

Tuberculosis (TB)

On a world-wide scale TB is the most important HIV-associated OI and as a result the prevalence of TB in the developed world has ↑. In sub-Saharan Africa up to 65% of patients with extra-pulmonary TB have HIV infection. Patients presenting primarily with TB should have their risk profile for HIV infection assessed and be offered HIV testing as appropriate. Those with known HIV infection and pulmonary disease should have TB excluded. Proven or suspected TB should be notified and contact tracing with assessment initiated.

Clinical features

TB can occur at any stage of HIV infection. Classic presentation of pulmonary TB is night sweats/fever, cough, pleuritic chest pain, haemoptysis, and weight loss. Less typical presentations occur as CD4 count ↓. Lobar distribution of pulmonary infection may be atypical and mimic community acquired pneumonia. Disseminated and extra-pulmonary diseases are more common with ↓ CD4 count. Although most cases are caused by reactivation of latent infection, 1° infection with rapid progression to active TB can occur when CD4 counts are <100cells/μL. TB has an additional immunosuppressive effect in HIV infection.

Diagnosis

- Radiology: in patients with preserved immune function typical upper lobe cavitatory changes occur. In those with lower CD4 counts appearances may be more extensive mimicking other infections.
- Examination of at least 3 sputum samples by microscopy of Ziehl–Neelsen or auramine stained samples and culture. Induced sputum or BAL samples are important if patients cannot produce sputum. Careful control of infection precautions are required to avoid nosocomial transmission of TB during such procedures. Smear positivity ↓ if advanced immunodeficiency.
- If extra-pulmonary findings (e.g. lymphadenopathy, bone marrow abnormalities) tissue cultures may be diagnostic.
- Molecular methods, e.g. interferon gamma production from peripheral blood mononuclear cells in response to antigenic stimulation, have an undefined role in diagnosis. However, detection of mutations by gene probing may allow identification of resistance against some agents.

Management

If TB is strongly suspected, empirical therapy with 4 drugs should be initiated immediately. Even if cultures are negative a full course may be required if there is clinical response despite negative cultures. Treatment of active TB may lead to ↑ in CD4 counts.

For fully sensitive organisms 6 month short course of anti-TB therapy is sufficient. Treatment should preferably start with quadruple therapy using isoniazid (300mg daily), rifampicin (600mg daily), pyrazinamide (1.5–2g daily), and ethambutol (15mg/kg/day) with standard monitoring precautions until mycobacterial drug sensitivities are known. After 2 months switch to rifampicin and isoniazid for a further 4 months.

► Check visual acuities prior to starting ethambutol. Monitor visual symptoms and liver function tests regularly.

► There are very important drug–drug interactions between anti-TB and anti-HIV therapies because of their varying enzyme inducing and enzyme inhibiting effects (see p. 521). Joint management involving physicians experienced in TB and HIV therapy is important.

The effects of HAART on TB medication are maximal with protease inhibitors which increase rifampicin and rifabutin levels significantly. Rifampicin produces across-the-board ↓ in HAART levels.

Drug interactions may be minimized by:

- deferring HAART until after completion of anti-TB drugs, particularly if CD4 count ↑ on anti-TB medication
- if CD4 count of >100/μL, defer HAART until anti-TB medication is reduced to dual therapy
- careful choice of HAART and anti-TB drugs to reduce interactions. This may reduce anti-TB efficacy.

TB treatment regimens with declining evidence of efficacy

- Standard short course of rifampicin containing regimen for 6 months
- Standard short course of induction with rifabutin/rifampicin substitution at 2 months
- Rifabutin/rifampicin substitution throughout 6 month course
- Standard induction followed by non-rifamycin continuation, total duration of 8 months
- 8 month non-rifamycin regimen.

► If CD4 counts <100/μL there is significant risk of developing additional OIs and the initiation of HAART should not be deferred.

Where there is no suspicion of resistant organism the patient would be regarded as no longer an infection risk, after 2 weeks of therapy.

Immune reconstitution syndrome (see p. 524)

A further complication of anti-TB with HAART is the development of an immune reconstitution syndrome with high fevers and malaise as a result of improved immune function directed at mycobacteria. This may require steroids for its control or interruption of HAART until the TB is better controlled.

Opportunist mycobacterial infections

Mycobacterium avium complex infections occur in HIV infected individuals in CD4 counts of <100/μL and characteristically produce generalized bacteraemic disease. Colonization of the respiratory tract can occur without evident morbidity but this presages the occurrence of disseminated disease. During immune reconstitution as a result of HAART, previously subclinical infection in the lungs may become apparent as an inflammatory response develops, leading to pulmonary inflammation and X-ray changes.

Other fungal infections

Pulmonary cryptococcosis

Pulmonary disease is diagnosed less frequently than meningitis in patients with AIDS although the lung is the most likely portal of entry. Pulmonary involvement can be asymptomatic but precedes the onset of disseminated disease in the majority of patients. Pulmonary involvement can produce cough, fever, malaise, shortness of breath, and pleuritic pain.

Diagnosis

- Chest X-rays show focal or diffuse infiltrates that may mimic PCP. Less commonly mass lesions, hilar, and mediastinal adenopathy and pleural effusions occur.
- Organism are more likely to be isolated from BAL samples than sputum.

Management

Treating the pulmonary lesion can prevent disseminated disease. Consists of amphotericin B combined with flucytosine as induction therapy, followed by fluconazole or itraconazole.

Pulmonary aspergillosis

Aspergilla infections in advanced HIV disease are uncommon and occur in conjunction with other OIs. Invasive disease occurs predominantly in patients with severe neutropenia as an additional risk. In HIV disease the lung is the most important site of invasive aspergillosis. Symptoms include fever, dyspnoea, cough, chest pain, and haemoptysis. ~20% have unilateral or bilateral diffuse or nodular infiltrates.

Diagnosis

- Chest X-ray
  - ~30% have thick walled upper lobe cavities.
  - ~20% have unilateral or bilateral diffuse or nodular infiltrates.
- Microbiology
  - Sputum, BAL, blood, bone marrow, and tissue biopsies should be examined by microscopy and cultured for fungi. Only 10–30% have positive findings on sputum culture. BAL has a higher yield.
  - Culture is required as microscopy alone cannot distinguish aspergillus from other fungal species.

Management

- Amphotericin B 1mg/kg/day or higher doses in liposomal form.
- Itraconazole or voriconazole.

In patients with severe neutropenia granulocyte macrophage colony stimulating factor may have an adjunctive role.

Other conditions

Cytomegalovirus (CMV) pneumonitis

Patients with PCP often have CMV isolated from bronchial washings or lung biopsy. In most cases this represents viral replication without pneumonitis and the patient responds to PCP therapy alone. Active pneumonitis occurs much less frequently than in patients taking immunosuppressive therapy post transplant. Hypoxia is usual.

Diagnosis

Chest X-ray shows diffuse interstitial infiltrates.
Identification of CMV in lung tissue.

Management

Patients with interstitial pneumonia and positive CMV identification in lung tissue should be treated with anti-CMV therapy using ganciclovir or foscarnet (see p. 436). A role for CMV immune globulin is not proven in the HIV setting.

Mediastinal and hilar lymphadenopathy

Patients with HIV related persistent generalized lymphadenopathy have sub-diaphragmatic lymphadenopathy but do not have significant hilar or mediastinal node enlargement. Hilar or mediastinal adenopathy implies significant pathology. The differential diagnosis includes:

- lymphoma
- Kaposi's sarcoma
- TB
- fungal disease.

May occasionally be seen in active PCP, but other pulmonary radiological abnormalities will be present. A careful search for peripheral lymphadenopathy, skin lesions and other abnormalities that could be subjected to histological and microbiological examinations should be sought.

Pulmonary vascular disease

1° pulmonary hypertension can occur as a consequence of HIV infection. Intravenous drug users may develop pulmonary small vessel obstruction due to injection of particulate material or may suffer recurrent pulmonary emboli.

Intense fatigue, breathlessness, and faintness on exertion are features of severe pulmonary hypertension. Clinical features of right ventricular hypertrophy include a heave, prominent A wave in the jugular pulse and a third heart sound.

Diagnosis

- Echocardiography
- Ultrasonography of the deep veins
- Pulmonary angiography

Management

Anticoagulants and pulmonary vasodilators.

Chapter 43

HIV: neurological disorders

Introduction

HIV enters the central nervous system (CNS) soon after 1° infection, carried by infected mononuclear cells or by cell free transfer across the blood brain barrier. Macrophages and microglial cells are the predominant cell types infected and the main sites of HIV replication in the brain.

Neurological disease is common and may be the presenting clinical syndrome in 30% of HIV infections occurring at any stage but most often following seroconversion or with severe immunodeficiency. Pre-HAART 10–20% of patients developed cognitive impairment and neurological features were reported in 40–70% of patients with AIDS ↑ to 90% at postmortem examination. Abnormal cerebrospinal fluid (CSF) findings including ↑ lymphocytes, protein, immunoglobulin, and oligoclonal bands may be found in patients with no neurological symptoms or signs. Presence or absence of neurological disease is independent of CSF viral load.

Mechanisms of CNS injury and spectrum of neurological disease vary with the stage of HIV infection and the degree of immune deficiency.

- At seroconversion—viraemia and inflammation resulting from the initial immunological response to HIV infection predominate, inducing aseptic meningitis, meningoencephalitis, ataxic neuropathy, Guillain–Barré syndrome, acute myelopathy, a multiple sclerosis like syndrome, acute brachial neuritis, Bell's palsy, and acute meningoradiculitis. ►Patients presenting with these syndromes should have their HIV risk assessed and be offered HIV screening.
- During the asymptomatic phase—neurological disease reflects that of the general population.
- As HIV progresses—altered CNS cytokine production and direct neurotoxic effects of HIV components such as gp120 are pathogenic.
- With immunodeficiency—opportunist infections (OIs)/tumours and complications of treatment predominate.

HAART has changed the epidemiology of the neurological manifestations of HIV resulting in ↓ CNS OIs, ↓ incidence of HIV dementia complex, and improved prognosis for some previously difficult-to-treat infections, such as progressive multifocal leukoencephalopathy (PML). However, there has been ↑ occurrence of drug induced CNS and peripheral nerve disease.

HIV-related neurological and neuromuscular disease may present with a number of symptom complexes

Headaches. May be an important symptom of neuropathology, such as primary or opportunist meningitis, intracerebral opportunist pathologies, or the side-effects of drugs such as zidovudine or co-trimoxazole. Non-HIV-related problems such as migraine or psychogenic headache may occur.

Altered peripheral sensation. May occur with or without motor abnormalities and a significant symptom in peripheral neuropathy.

Leg weakness. May result from muscular weakness due to myopathic processes but intrinsic or extrinsic spinal cord disease should be considered and sensory levels searched for.

Seizures. ↑ risk. First seizure is a presenting manifestation of an HIV associated disease in ~20% of patients. Seizures may result from:

- metabolic encephalopathy
- cerebrovascular disease
- OIs such as toxoplasmosis, cryptococcosis, and PML
- CNS lymphomas.

Focal neurological signs and symptoms. Particularly with cerebral toxoplasmosis, 1° cerebral lymphoma, and PML.

Cerebral disorders

HIV-associated dementia complex

Cognitive impairment usually occurs when CD4 counts are <200cells/μL in patients with systemic symptoms of HIV disease. Pathogenesis may include altered cytokine levels, free radicals, and the neurotoxic effects of gp120. Histological abnormalities include perivascular infiltrates, microglial nodules, multinuclear giant cells, and pruning of dendritic processes in the white matter and subcortical grey matter with relative sparing of the cortex.

Presentation: poor concentration, impaired short-term memory, and slowed thought and reaction times. Clumsiness and gait disturbance may follow with corticospinal tract abnormalities. Psychiatric illness and personality change may also be presenting features. Depression, effects of substance abuse, cerebrovascular disease, and neurosyphilis should be excluded.

Diagnosis: magnetic resonance imaging (MRI)—preferred option, or computerized tomography (CT) brain scan reveal cerebral atrophy with abnormality of the periventricular white matter. Neuropsychological examination reveals ↓ thought processes and ↓ short-term memory. CSF should be examined to exclude other pathologies and OIs. Electroencephalogram (EEG) may reveal encephalopathic changes. Blood and CSF serological tests for syphilis should be carried out and vitamin B12 deficiency excluded.

Management: HAART, if possible including zidovudine (proven efficacy) or other drugs that cross the blood brain barrier, can produce marked improvement in intellectual function and return to independent living. The patient may require psychological and social support.

Viral encephalitis

Varicella zoster virus (VZV) is an important cause of meningoencephalitis which may be complicated by cranial nerve palsies and cerebral vasculitis leading to cerebral infarction. Consider in patients with stroke or transient ischaemic attacks, even in the absence of a vesicular rash. CSF should be examined by PCR and culture for VZV. CT or MRI may show evidence of ischaemia or haemorrhage. Treatment with aciclovir 10mg/kg 8 hourly should be given for at least 14 days.

CMV encephalitis occurs in advanced immunodeficiency and may be suspected when there is evidence of CMV disease in other organs or blood and CSF PCR are positive.

Herpes simplex virus (HSV) is an uncommon cause.

Progressive multifocal leukoencephalopathy (PML)

Unlike other OIs its prevalence has not significantly declined with HAART. A demyelinating disease caused by the JC polyoma virus and occurs in 4–8% in patients with advanced HIV infection. Fulminant disease with dementia and coma can occur but the usual picture is of subacute or chronic progressive disease with focal deficits. These include personality change, hemiparesis, dizziness, gait disturbance, visual field defects, and epilepsy. CT or MRI scans usually reveal lesions (single or multiple) in the white matter, particularly in the parieto-occipital region (Plate 20). Treatment options include immune reconstitution with HAART and specific antiviral therapy with cidofovir (does not alter survival).

Cerebral toxoplasmosis (*Toxoplasma gondii*)

The most common cause of mass lesions in HIV prior to the introduction of 1° PCP prophylaxis which has ↓ incidence.

Presentation: typically includes confusion, headache, personality change, hemiparesis, focal sensory disturbances, fits, and fever.

Diagnosis: MRI or CT scanning reveal ring enhancing lesions, usually multiple, particularly in the cortex and deep grey matter. The differential diagnosis, particularly if lesions are single, includes 1° cerebral lymphoma, cryptococcal cerebritis, and tuberculomas. CSF changes are non-specific. Positive toxoplasma serology in 90%.

Management: standard therapy for cerebral toxoplasmosis is sulfadiazine 100mg/kg/day in divided doses and pyrimethamine 200mg loading dose followed by 50–100mg/day with folinic acid to reduce bone marrow toxicity. High dose clindamycin 1.2g intravenously 4 times daily if allergic to sulfonamide. Neuro-imaging should be repeated after 2 weeks followed by brain biopsy to exclude other pathologies if no improvement.

Meningitis

Cryptococcal meningitis

Cryptococcus neoformans (an encapsulated yeast)—most common fungal pathogen in the CNS.

Presentation: usually as subacute meningitis (but symptoms may initially be surprisingly mild) with headache and fever. Evidence of meningism occurs in only 30%. A high index of suspicion must be maintained to avoid delays in diagnosis. Other presentations include acute confusional state and cranial nerve palsies.

Diagnosis: CSF pressures can be markedly raised but pleocytosis may be absent and protein and sugar levels normal. The organism may be visualized by India ink staining but relatively insensitive. Mainstay of diagnosis is detection of CSF and serum cryptococcal antigen, which is highly sensitive. Neuro-imaging is usually normal but cryptococcomas can occur usually in the basal ganglia.

Management: daily lumbar punctures may be required until CSF pressures normalize to avoid cranial nerve lesions. Antifungal therapy with intravenous amphotericin B 1mg/kg/day intravenously in combination with flucytosine 100mg/kg/day or liposomal amphotericin 3mg/kg/day plus flucytosine for 2 weeks followed by fluconazole 400mg daily. A test dose of amphotericin 25mg should be given before commencing full therapy to detect hypersensitivity. Renal function should be monitored. Ongoing suppressive therapy with fluconazole is required to minimize significant relapse rates. Continue until immune reconstitution is achieved with HAART.

Aseptic meningitis

Most commonly presents at seroconversion but may be recurrent or become chronic. Usually presents with headache. Cranial nerve palsies and altered mental state can occur. Lumbar puncture, following neuro-imaging when focal deficits are present, needed to exclude other pathologies. Mildly ↑ CSF lymphocyte counts and protein level with normal glucose are typical findings.

Autonomic neuropathy

Evidence of autonomic dysfunction can be found at various stages of HIV infection. Measurement of pulse rate variation in response to standing, deep breathing, Valsalva manoeuvre and cold exposure reveal autonomic dysfunction in ~15%. Frequency related to the level of immune function but, unlike sensory neuropathy, not the use of nucleoside reverse transcriptase inhibitors. Symptomatic autonomic neuropathy occurs in advanced immunodeficiency and may result in severe postural hypotension and syncope. Cardiac denervation may lead to serious cardiac dysrhythmias. Those developing postural dizziness or syncope should have postural blood pressure recordings, tests of autonomic function, and assessment of sodium intake. Adrenal insufficiency should be excluded by carrying out a short synacthen test. Therapy with mineralocorticoid (fludrocortisone 50–200μg daily), sodium supplements, compression stockings, and alpha-adrenergic agents, such as midodrine, may reduce postural blood pressure falls and alleviate symptoms. There may be improvement in autonomic function with HAART.

Spinal cord disease

Vacuolar myelopathy

Postmortem studies have shown vacuolar myelopathy in up to 30% but clinically it is far less common. Pathological mechanisms are probably the same as in HIV dementia complex and the clinical picture mimics that of a vitamin B12 deficiency spinal cord disease.

Presentation: typically with subacute progressive motor and sensory deficits with paraesthesiae, but brisk tendon reflexes. Uncharacteristic findings may occur if there is concomitant peripheral neuropathy or other cause.

Diagnosis: investigations should include measurement of vitamin B12 level and radiological imaging to exclude structural lesions. Areas of ↑ T2 signal may be seen occasionally on MRI scan. CSF may be normal or show only non-specific abnormalities such as low-level pleocytosis or mildly ↑ protein levels.

Management: spasticity may require anti-spasmodic therapy such as baclofen 10–30mg 3 times a day and a dysasthesia may require amitriptyline or gabapentin. Physiotherapy and occupational therapy input may be valuable. Improvements in function may occur with HAART.

Human T lymphotropic virus type I associated (HTLV1) myelopathy

In patients from areas of significant risk for HTLV1 infection, such as Japan, the Caribbean, and parts of Central and Latin America, subacute myelopathy may result from HTLV1 infection and anti-HTLV1 antibodies should be assayed.

Acute myelopathy

Acute spinal cord disease may occasionally occur as a seroconversion event. Other important causes are spinal cord compression from lymphomatous metastases, tuberculous or bacterial abscesses, and acute infections with VZV.

Presentation: Typically rapidly developing neurological deficit, such as leg weakness and sphincter disturbance, with evidence of a sensory level.

Diagnosis: emergency investigation required with spinal MRI or CT. In the absence of compression CSF should be examined for evidence of infectious and neoplastic causes including viral PCR and cytology.

Management: supportive with specific treatment directed at the identified cause.

Peripheral nerve disease

Neuritis

- Herpes zoster (shingles)

May occur at any stage of HIV infection with a typical distribution and course. Atypical multidermatomal involvement, viraemic dissemination of lesions, and recurrences more common as CD4 counts ↓.

***Presentation*:** frequently prodromal pain of dermatomal distribution followed by an erythematous maculopapular eruption evolving into vesicles which then pustulate and crust. Bullous haemorrhagic and necrotic lesions may occur. Pain during the acute phase can be severe and disabling post-herpetic neuralgia may follow.

***Diagnosis*:** clinical picture is usually characteristic. Varicella zoster virus (VZV) can be detected in vesicular fluid by immunofluorescence.

***Management*:** pain often does not respond well to conventional analgesics and adjuvants. Amitriptyline 25–150mg/day or gabapentin up to 2.4g/day in divided doses may be required. Begin antiviral therapy with intravenous aciclovir 10mg/kg 8 hourly as early as possible and switch to oral famciclovir 500mg 3 times daily or valaciclovir 1g 3 times daily when lesions cease to progress for a total course of at least 7 days or until all lesions have dried and crusted.

- Mononeuritis multiplex

Usually occurs in patients with advanced HIV disease. Typical presentation is with subacute onset of multifocal or asymmetric sensory deficits. Nerve conduction studies show demyelination and axonal loss. May be associated with cytomegalovirus (CMV) infection in advanced immunodeficiency. Differential diagnosis includes nerve compression in severe wasting syndrome, neoplastic infiltration, and neurotropic viral infections e.g. VZV. Consider treatment with ganciclovir or foscarnet if circumstantial evidence of CMV infection (e.g. positive blood PCR).

Neuropathy

***Drug toxicity*:** the toxicity of therapeutic drugs, notably didanosine, zalcitabine, and stavudine, responsible for ↑ proportion of neuropathy.

***Distal symmetric polyneuropathy*:** occurs in ~35% of patients with advanced HIV disease. ~15% of those with asymptomatic HIV infection show abnormal nerve conduction studies. Typical symptoms are tingling, numbness, and burning pain beginning in the toes or plantar surfaces, often ascending over time. Examination shows ↓ ankle jerks, vibration sense, appreciation of temperature, and fine touch. Unexpectedly brisk reflexes should raise the question of additional spinal cord or brain disease. Differential diagnosis includes the effects of alcohol, drug toxicity and vitamin deficiency. Treatment is directed towards controlling neuropathic pain with drugs, such as amitriptyline 25–150mg daily or gabapentin starting at 300mg 8 hourly and titrating to a maximum of 2.4g daily.

***Inflammatory demyelinating neuropathy or Guillain–Barré syndrome*:** may occur during seroconversion or with changes in immune function. Manifestations as in non-HIV setting with progressive symmetric weakness in the limbs and loss of tendon jerks but CSF pleocytosis may occur.

Treatment is immunoglobulin 400mg/kg/day for 5 days or plasmapheresis, up to 6 exchanges over 2 weeks. Patients with the chronic form may need monthly cycles of treatment until stabilization.

Progressive lumbosacral polyradiculopathy: caused by CMV infection in patients with CD4 counts <50cells/μL. Bilateral leg weakness progresses over several weeks, sometimes to flaccid paraplegia. Sphincter disturbance is common and sensory loss combined with painful dysasthesia is usual. Sensory symptoms differentiate this from myopathy, and sphincter disturbance with sparing of the upper limbs distinguish it from other forms of neuropathy. Cord compression should be excluded by imaging. CSF usually has a cell count >500 x 10^6/L with 40–50% neutrophils and ↑ protein content. PCR for CMV is positive and the patient should be treated with ganciclovir or foscarnet.

Miscellaneous

Cerebrovascular disease

Strokes and transient ischaemic attacks are reported in 0.5–8% of HIV infected patients. Prevention should include attention to vascular risk factors such as smoking, hypertension, and hyperlipidaemia. Cocaine use and alcoholic binges may lead to thrombotic strokes. Embolic strokes may result from cardiac or carotid artery disease. Cardiogenic emboli may result from infective or non-infective endocarditis following myocardial infarction or from dysrhythmias. Cerebral vasculitis, particularly due to VZV or syphilis, may cause cerebral thrombosis. The hypercoagulable state that may occur with HIV may contribute. Haemorrhage may complicate VZV cerebral vasculitis, thrombocytopenia, rarely due to metastatic Kaposi's sarcoma or as a result of an incidental cerebral aneurysm.

Neurosyphilis

May affect most parts of the nervous system (see p. 96).

Neoplastic disease

Kaposi's sarcoma, although the most common systemic neoplasm in HIV infection, rarely involves the nervous system. CNS may be invaded by non-Hodgkin's lymphoma leading to malignant meningitis and compressive symptoms requiring intrathecal cytotoxic therapy and radiotherapy. 1° cerebral lymphoma occurs in patients with advanced immunodeficiency and presents with confusion, lethargy, personality change, focal neurological deficits, ataxia, and aphasia. On MRI or CT scanning lesions are ring enhancing and about 50% are associated with cerebral oedema and mass effect. The finding of a single lesion favours the diagnosis of lymphoma over cerebral toxoplasmosis. Brain biopsy should be considered and cerebral radiotherapy may improve survival.

Chapter 44

HIV: disorders of the eye

Introduction

Ocular manifestations have been reported in up to 60% of those infected with HIV, ↑ in frequency as the CD4 count ↓. Patients with CD4 count <200/μL should be closely examined for signs of ocular disease which may be asymptomatic in the early stages. Close cooperation with ophthalmology is essential to ensure timely therapeutic interventions to ↓ risk of visual impairment and blindness. Widespread use of HAART has dramatically altered the incidence and natural history of many opportunistic eye infections.

HIV-related vasculopathy

70–80% of patients with advanced HIV disease have asymptomatic transient microvascular changes that may occur simultaneously in the conjunctiva and retina. Conjunctival changes are found near the limbus and only detected by slit-lamp examination. Features include vascular narrowing, dilatation, and microaneurysms. No treatment needed.

Retinal changes are detected by fundal examination. Cotton-wool spots (infarcts of nerve fibre layer) most common feature of retinal vasculopathy. Differentiated from early CMV lesions by their small size, superficial retinal location, and transient nature with less frequent retinal haemorrhages and microaneurysms.

Iridocyclitis

Seen in association with toxoplasmic, syphilitic, bacterial, and fungal retinitis. Drugs such as rifabutin, (especially with concurrent azole and macrolide use) and cidofovir are frequent causes. Diagnosed by slit-lamp examination.

Treatment

Treat underlying infection(s) and/or ↓ or discontinue implicated drug(s). Topical steroids may be used but not if active infection.

Neurological eye manifestations

Occur in 10%. Most common features include papilloedema, cranial nerve palsies, ophthalmoplegia, and visual field defects. Caused by lymphoma and any CNS infection, most frequently cryptococcal meningitis, neurosyphilis, and toxoplasmosis. HIV encephalopathy and progressive multifocal leukoencephalopathy may have similar complications.

Investigate by magnetic resonance imaging, lumbar puncture (CSF—cell count, cytology, culture, and serology).

Immune-recovery uveitis

Mainly involves anterior uveal tract and vitreous, commonly associated with a marked disturbance of visual function due to macular oedema and epiretinal membrane formation. Believed to be a consequence of the marked reconstitution of immune function induced by HAART. Marked cellular infiltration of the vitreous (in the absence of an active retinal or chorioretinal lesion) is a hallmark of this phenomenon. Responds well to systemic steroids.

Opportunistic infections (OIs)

Cytomegalovirus infection (CMV)

CMV retinitis results from reactivation of infection acquired in childhood or early adult life. Prior to HAART it was the most common eye OI occurring in 30–40% of those with a CD4 count <50cells/μL. Bilateral in 30–50% of cases with optic nerve involvement in 5%. Serious visual complications can be avoided by the detection of its early features with regular dilated examination of the fundi for those at risk (CD4 <100cells/μL).

Clinical features

Symptoms depend on site and extent of retinal involvement. Peripheral retinal lesions are asymptomatic. Earliest and most common symptoms are multiple floaters, representing foci of inflammatory cells in the vitreous attempting to contain the infection. Other symptoms include bluring/loss of central vision, flashing lights, and scotomata. Initial focus of retinal inflammation expands peripherally inducing retinal necrosis.

Early active lesions appear as multiple granular white dots with occasional haemorrhages. With further progress areas of retinitis enlarge by following the vascular arcades, resulting in an arcuate or triangular zone of infection. Areas of active infection may also be linear, following the retinal vessels or nerve fibre layer into the periphery. Early CMV lesions may be confused with cotton-wool spots (due to HIV vasculopathy) which may coexist. Serial drawings or retinal photographs are helpful in differentiation. Continuing activity of the necrotic process results in atrophic features with thinning of the retina resulting in visualization of the underlying choroid. Other features of CMV retinitis include vascular attenuation, vessel occlusion, vitritis, and anterior uveitis (Plate 21). May be complicated by retinal detachment and cataract.

Occasionally it may be difficult to establish the cause of retinitis.

Diagnosis

Usually clinical. Confirmed by obtaining a vitreous sample for CMV using PCR testing. CMV viraemia may be a useful predictor of CMV disease. A rising CMV viral load detected by PCR is associated with ↑ eye and other organ disease.

Treatment

- HAART ↑ response to treatment, prognosis, and ↓ relapse rates.
- Oral valganciclovir 900mg twice daily for 3 weeks followed by 900mg once daily produces blood levels comparable to intravenous ganciclovir. Main side-effects are bone marrow suppression and gastrointestinal upset.
- Intravitreous ganciclovir implant is very effective but needs to be replaced after 6–9 months and does not give protection to the other eye or protect against systemic disease.
- Intravenous ganciclovir given as an induction course for 2–3 weeks (5mg/kg body weight 12 hourly) followed by maintenance therapy (5mg/kg body weight 7 days a week or 6mg/kg body weight 5 days a week). Side-effects include rigors and neutropenia that may require discontinuation of treatment or the use of granulocyte colony

stimulating factor. Oral ganciclovir (1g 3 times a day) may be given in place of intravenous formulation once retinitis has remained stable for at least 3 weeks.

- Intravenous foscarnet given as an induction course for 2–3 weeks (60mg/kg body weight 8 hourly) followed by maintenance therapy (90–120mg/kg body weight once a day). Given when ganciclovir not tolerated due to its toxicity. Side-effects include nephrotoxicity, convulsions, meatal ulceration, and electrolyte disturbance. Has ↑ infusion time and requires an infusion pump.
- Intravenous cidofovir (3–5mg/kg body weight once a week) given together with probenecid (2g orally 3 hours before the cidofovir infusion followed by 1g for 2 hours and 8 hours following its completion) and fluids. Effective in ganciclovir-resistant CMV but highly nephrotoxic and myelosuppressive.

Prognosis

Response to therapy achieved in 80–90%. Without immune reconstitution, the median time to relapse is 50–120 days using standard anti-CMV treatment. Maintenance therapy can be stopped once immune reconstitution is achieved.

Varicella zoster virus infection (VZV)

Ophthalmic herpes zoster results from involvement of the ophthalmic division of the trigeminal nerve and is recognized by characteristic vesicular eruptions. May be associated with blepharitis, conjunctivitis, keratitis, and uveitis. Complications and post-herpetic neuralgia ↑ in the immunosuppressed.

VZV is the 2nd most common cause of necrotizing retinitis which may occur at same time or follow recent herpes zoster. Early retinal lesions similar to CMV, but rapidly progressive, deep, and multifocal with ↑ risk of bilateral disease and retinal detachment which may lead to blindness in days without prompt treatment.

Diagnosis

Characteristic rash and its distribution are usually sufficient to establish the diagnosis. Serological tests and PCR rarely needed.

Treatment

Intravenous ganciclovir is the treatment of choice in addition to topical steroids. In the absence of anterior uveitis mydriatics (e.g. 1% atropine) also required.

Herpes simplex keratitis

HSV eye infection causes keratitis or rarely acute retinal necrosis. Keratitis leads to corneal ulcers, diminished corneal sensation, and ↑ intraocular pressure. Corneal ulcers are usually painful and have a dendritic appearance. Difficult to treat and relapses frequently.

Treatment

Oral aciclovir (400mg 5 times daily) or famciclovir (250–500mg 3 times daily).

Acute retinal necrosis

Commonly caused by VZV and HSV but CMV and other viruses may be implicated. Usually present with scotomata progressing rapidly to visual loss. Detailed fundal examination reveals peripheral white lesions that progress to widespread necrosis over a few days. May be complicated by proliferative retinopathy and retinal detachment.

Treatment

Responds poorly to antivirals but IV ganciclovir should be started immediately.

Toxoplasma retinochoroiditis

Rare, accounting for 1–2% of retinitis with 30–50% of patients having central nervous system involvement. Characteristically causes bilateral multifocal retinochoroidal lesions that invade the vitreous in the later stages. Majority of patients do not have pre-existing eye lesions.

Diagnosis

Fundal examination reveals characteristic extensive fluffy areas of retinal whitening with accompanying vitritis, but unlike CMV infection retinal haemorrhaging is less likely. Toxoplasma serological tests unreliable but absence of toxoplasma IgG antibodies makes its diagnosis less likely.

Treatment

Pyrimethamine in combination with sulfadiazine or clindamycin. Equally good response may be obtained with atovaquone. Long-term maintenance treatment with clindamycin and pyrimethamine usually required.

Candidal eye infection

Infection of the anterior segment of the eye results in superficial keratitis. Posterior segment infection seen in advanced HIV disease and presents as multiple often bilateral, white fluffy retinal lesions that may extend into the overlying vitreous. Majority of patients have systemic candidal infection. Culture and sensitivity of the causative yeast provides the best outcome on which to base therapy. Superficial keratitis responds well to topical antifungals. Systemic antifungals are needed for posterior segment infection e.g. voriconazole and liposomal amphotericin.

Kaposi's sarcoma (KS)

Up to 20% of patients with skin KS have eyelid and conjunctival lesions recognized by their characteristic appearance, although conjunctival lesions may resemble traumatic haemorrhages.

Treatment

Options include surgical removal, cryotherapy, and intralesional vinblastine. Systemic chemotherapy is given if there are associated skin lesions. Radiation is effective but may be complicated by loss of eyelashes and conjunctivitis.

Chapter 45

HIV: dermatological disorders

Introduction

Skin conditions are extremely common and may occur at any stage of HIV infection. Pre-existing skin conditions may worsen after its acquisition. Appearance of certain skin conditions should alert physicians to possibility of undiagnosed HIV infection. Immunodeficiency is associated with atypical presentations, severe manifestations, and a poor response to treatment. In general, improved immunity with HAART resolves or improves them.

Infections

Viral infections

Acute seroconversion (acute retroviral syndrome)

Skin rash occurs in up to 70% cases. It is often part of an infectious mononucleosis-like illness. Typically symmetrical and non-itchy extending over the trunk and upper limbs, macular or maculopapular in appearance although it can be vesicular, pustular, or urticarial. May be associated with oro-pharyngeal (highly suspicious of seroconversion illness) and genital ulceration. Resolves spontaneously within 1–2 weeks.

Herpes simplex virus (HSV)

1° and recurrent HSV present with genital and orofacial clusters of vesicles that ulcerate, crust, and heal within 2–3 weeks during the early stages of HIV infection. With advanced disease, ulcers become atypical or chronic, may coalesce to form large painful crusted lesions commonly seen perianally but may involve the perioral and rarely the periungual region. Though dissemination is rare, lesions may be auto-inoculated to distant sites. HSV infection rarely presents with necrotizing folliculitis (difficult to diagnose without biopsy).

Swabs for viral culture and immunofluorescence usually confirm the diagnosis. Polymerase chain reaction (PCR) testing of skin lesions is very sensitive and specific but not widely available. Viral culture can be performed on skin biopsy from the edge of the lesion when swab is not conclusive. Histological examination may provide a rapid diagnosis by demonstrating multinucleated giant epithelial cells.

Treatment see p. 244, p. 398.

Varicella zoster virus (VZV) infection

Those with no previous exposure to VZV develop chicken-pox that may be severe and associated with visceral involvement. Most adults have been infected by VZV so present with herpes zoster. Usually affects multiple dermatomes, commonly the thoracic and the trigeminal nerves. Vesicular eruption is normally preceded by tingling and a burning sensation. Individuals with more advanced HIV disease tend to have painful bullous, haemorrhagic, necrotic lesions that may persist for several weeks and heal with severe scarring. Recurrences and dissemination ↑. Disseminated disease is characterized by dermatomal and non-dermatomal eruptions. Rarely VZV presents with chronic widespread ulcers or hyperkeratotic lesions (if infected with aciclovir-resistant VZV).

Clinical diagnosis is usually accurate in typical dermatomal involvement but skin biopsy is required for atypical, chronic ulcerative, and hyperkeratotic lesions.

Prompt treatment with high dose aciclovir ↓ risk of dissemination and shortens its course. Clinical presentation and degree of immune deficiency determine mode and length of therapy, which is usually continued until lesions start to crust.

- Intravenous aciclovir (10mg/kg body weight 3 times a day) for disseminated infection, CD4 count <200cells/μL, and with involvement of the ophthalmic division of the trigeminal nerve. May be replaced with oral aciclovir once lesions start to crust.
- Famciclovir (500mg 3 times a day usually for 10 days) and valacilovir (1g 3 times a day usually for 7 days) have better bioavailability than aciclovir.
- Oral aciclovir (800mg 5 times a day) may be given to those with limited disease and preserved immune function.

Skin care with calamine lotion (helps pruritus) and bathing with water and mild soap is helpful. Analgesics for pain control.

Molluscum contagiosum

Caused by a pox virus and when widespread is a marker of advanced HIV disease. Lesion is typically flesh-coloured, 2–3mm domed, umblicated papule with a faint whitish core. Those with relatively preserved immune function may have mollusca on the groin which may be chronic. With advanced HIV disease, lesions may reach 1cm in size and may be widespread involving the face, trunk, eyelids, and rarely the mucous membranes (conjunctivae and lips). Mollusca are commonly seen on the beard area (related to trauma of shaving) where they are difficult to treat.

Treatment is given for cosmetic reasons as no cure is available. Usual treatment—cryotherapy. Curettage effective for recalcitrant cases.

Human papilloma virus infection (warts)

Widespread, resistant, and recurrent warts which may have atypical appearances seen more frequently in those immunosuppressed. Facial involvement, otherwise rare, well recognized in HIV infection.

Principles of therapy are as for those not infected by HIV. Ablative treatment used depending on morphology, location, and number. Plantar warts respond with variable success to topical cidofovir.

Bacterial infections

Staphylococcal skin infection

Staphylococcus aureus nasal carriage is common explaining ↑ rates of infection with this organism. *S. aureus* skin infection presents as:

- folliculitis—commonly in the hirsute areas e.g. groin, axilla, face (especially ♂), and trunk. Infection may involve deeper tissues forming abscesses.
- hidradenitis-like plaques—many adjacent follicles infected forming large discoloured lesions several centimetres deep.
- bullous impetigo—commonly seen on the groin and axillae as superficial vesicles or ulcers with yellow crusts.
- ecthyma—an eroded or ulcerated lesion with an adherent crust covering an abscess.
- scalded skin syndrome—part of systemic *S. aureus* infection.

Superficial infection responds to standard anti-staphylococcal antibiotics (e.g. flucloxacillin 500mg 4 times daily for 7–10 days).

Deep infection may require abscess drainage and prolonged courses of combined antibiotics based on bacterial sensitivities. Washing area with antiseptics helps by removing crusts and ↓ bacterial concentration.

Bacillary angiomatosis

Caused by *Bartonella henselae* and *Bartonella quintana*, small Gram-negative aerobic fastidious bacilli. In addition, *B. henselae* causes cat scratch fever and *B. quintana* trench fever. Angiogenic lesions are most often recognized in cutaneous or subcutaneous tissues and can be difficult to differentiate from Kaposi's sarcoma (KS). *B. henselae* causes lesions in lymph nodes, liver (peliosis hepatis), and spleen. *B. quintana* has a predilection for subcutaneous, deep soft tissues, and bones.

Clinical presentation

- Bacilliary angioma: friable, easy bleeding hyperpigmented papules, nodules, or plaques but in the early stages may be purplish to bright red in colour, up to several centimetres in diameter. Lesions solitary or multiple and widespread on the skin. Need to be differentiated from KS and pyogenic granuloma.
- Bacteraemia presenting as pyrexia of unknown origin.
- Organ involvement (e.g. liver, spleen, brain, and lymph nodes).

Diagnosis

- Abnormal vascular proliferation and a mixed inflammatory infiltrate on histological examination of tissues.
- Special stains (e.g. Warthin–Starry, Steiner and Steiner) required.
- Electron microscopy.
- PCR of tissue and blood samples.

Serological tests are not reliable in HIV infection.

Treatment

Prolonged course of antibiotics e.g. erythromycin 500mg 4 times a day, doxycycline 100mg twice daily, or azithromycin 0.5–1.0g daily, until lesions heal.

Mycobacterial infection

1° mycobacterial skin infection is rare. Skin may be involved in up to 10% of disseminated *Mycobacterium avium* complex infection, typically when the CD4 count is <50cells/μL. Most frequent presentations are chronic sinuses overlying an infected lymph node (scrofuloderma) and a chronic skin ulcer. Rare presentations include violaceous nodules, necrotic papules, plaques, panniculitis, and erythema nodosum.

Mycobacterial infection should be considered in any chronic non-healing skin ulcer. Diagnose by demonstration of acid fast bacilli in smears and by culture. Typical histological feature of caseating granuloma is usually absent.

Treatment see p. 416, p. 460.

Fungal infections

Cutaneous candidiasis

Skin infection with *Candida* spp. occurs in different forms including tinea unguium (leukonychia, nail ridging, flaking, onycholysis, and atrophy), acute paronychia (tender fluctuation of the nail bed), chronic paronychia, and intertrigo (an erosive painful erythematous rash on flexures associated with satellite pustules). Acute candidal paronychia must be differentiated from that caused by HSV infection using appropriate tests.

Tinea unguium requires prolonged systemic antifungals (e.g. itraconazole).

Acute paronychia and intertrigo respond well to topical antifungals (e.g. miconazole).

Dermatophytosis

Very common in HIV infection. May be atypical and extensive and may mimic inflammatory skin conditions such as seborrhoeic dermatitis or psoriasis.

- Tinea pedis—usually presents with interdigital maceration and scaling of the soles, rarely with hyperkeratosis of the soles. Usually associated with tinea unguium. Caused by *Trichophyton rubrum*. 2° bacterial infection common and may result in cellulitis.
- Onychomycosis—resulting in subungual hyperkeratosis and toenail atrophy.
- Tinea cruris—a symmetrical, erythematous scaling rash with central clearance on the groin sometimes extending to buttocks and thighs. In advanced HIV disease, it may resemble seborrhoeic dermatitis because of absence of central clearance.
- Tinea corporis—annular scaling plaques with central clearance.
- Tinea capitis—localized scaling discoid patch or generalized scaling resembling seborrhoeic dermatitis.
- Tinea faciale—differentiated from seborrhoeic dermatitis by asymmetrical distribution and well-demarcated edge.

Apart from tinea pedis, which can be treated with topical antifungals, other forms need systemic antifungals such as terbinafine (250mg daily for several weeks) or a triazole (e.g. fluconazole 50mg daily).

Cryptococcosis

Skin involvement occurs in up to 20% of systemic cryptococcal infection. Most common skin manifestation is a nodule or papule with central umbilication resembling molluscum contagiosum, usually on the face. Plaques and tender subcutaneous lesions are rare. Diagnosed by skin biopsy.

Treatment (see p. 426)

Patient should be evaluated for systemic and neurological cryptococcal infection and managed accordingly.

Penicilliosis

Endemic to S.E. Asia. Caused by *Penicillium marneffei*. Presents with fever skin lesions, anaemia, lymphadenopathy, and hepatosplenomegaly. Skin lesions resemble haemorrhagic molluscum contagiosum. Diagnosed by culture of blood, bone marrow, and skin scrapings.

Responds well to liposomal amphotericin and itraconazole but relapses are common and long-term prophylaxis with itraconazole is recommended.

Histoplasmosis

Cutaneous histoplasmosis has been reported in up to 10% of patients with systemic infection, which usually occurs in endemic areas. Diagnosis by biopsy of papules, nodules, or ulcers. Treat with liposomal amphotericin or high dose itraconazole followed by itraconazole maintenance.

Scabies

In advanced HIV disease crusted (Norwegian) scabies may occur, characterized by widespread scaly erythematous lesions on the face and scalp together with hyperkeratotic lesions on the hands and feet giving the characteristic 'breadcrumb' appearance. Highly infectious because of heavy infestation.

Treatment (see p. 288)

Patients with crusted scabies must be barrier nursed and in addition to topical treatment should be given ivermectin (200μg/kg as a single dose). Topical steroids may be needed for eczematous nodules.

Inflammatory conditions

Seborrhoeic dermatitis

Occurs in up to 85% and may be a 1st indicator of HIV infection. Severity and recurrences ↑ with ↓ CD4 count. Related to infection with *Pityrosporum* spp., ↑ sebum production, and a genetic predisposition.

Presents as an itchy erythematous rash with a yellow greasy scale but in severe cases plaques and hyperkeratotic lesions occur. Usually has a butterfly distribution but may involve eyebrows, post-auricular areas and scalp. May also affect intertriginous areas and chest. Severe cases may resemble psoriasis. Facial lesions must be differentiated from lupus erythematosus and rosacea.

Treatment

- Topical antifungals and steroids (e.g. miconazole and hydrocortisone).
- Scalp lesions—tar-containing shampoos, selenium sulfide, salicylic acid, and ketoconazole.
- Severe disease responds well but only temporarily to systemic triazoles, such as itraconazole.

Psoriasis

A chronic disease characterized by erythematous plaques or papules covered by silvery adherent scales. May appear for the 1st time or pre-existing disease may become worse with HIV infection. Psoriatic arthritis (see p. 486) ↑. Several forms of psoriasis may coexist.

- Chronic plaque psoriasis—classically involves elbows, knees, scalp, and may be associated with nail dystrophy.
- Flexural psoriasis—affecting axillae, groins, and intergluteal cleft, more common in advanced HIV disease.
- Guttate psoriasis—presents with widespread rain-drop size lesions.

Treatment

- Mild to moderate disease can be treated with a regular emollient plus moderately potent topical steroid, calcitriol, tar-containing ointments, or dithranol.
- Severe disease can be treated with methotrexate (especially in the presence of psoriatic arthritis), acitretin, cyclosporin, or hydroxyurea.

⚠ Beware of effects on the immune system of these drugs (apart from acitretin).

Eczema

Seen in up to 30%. Severity and frequency ↑ as CD4 count ↓. Xerosis (dry skin) common complaint and may be associated with an itchy, papular scaly rash on the arms and legs. Skin may be damaged as a result of excessive scratching resulting in excoriation, lichenification, eczematous changes, and discolouration.

Treatment

Treatment includes topical steroids and emollients.

Pruritic follicular and papular eruptions

Pruritus is a common occurrence. 1° follicular, popular, or nodular lesions may be altered by excoriation and lichenification.

Eosinophilic pustular folliculitis

Chronic intensely itchy follicular rash affecting face, upper trunk, and extensor surfaces of the arms, usually seen when CD4 count <200cells/μL. Sterile papular, papulo-pustular, or urticarial papules centred around hair follicles found. May be ↑ IgE with eosinophilia.

Treatment

Responds best to phototherapy. Emollients for eczematous lesions. Antihistamines usually not helpful. HAART may produce some improvement.

HIV-associated pruritus

Diagnosis of exclusion of other causes of pruritus. No 1° lesions. Clinical features 2° to scratching—excoriation, linear lesions, lichenified eczematous changes, and post-inflammatory pigmentation.

Treatment

Regular emollients, topical steroids for eczematous changes and antihistamines.

Malassezia furfur folliculitis

Yeast overgrowth producing folliculitis through production of fatty acids and scale formation blocking follicular ostea. Presents with chronic or relapsing pruritic follicular-centred papules on the scalp, flexures, upper trunk, and face.

Treatment

Oral itraconazole (preferred option) 200mg daily for 7 days. If patient has AIDS, maintenance (200mg once or twice daily) or intermittent 'pulse' therapy should be considered. Other options are oral fluconazole and 2% ketaconazole cream. Scalp relapses are best treated with intermittent ketoconazole shampoo.

Neoplasia

Kaposi's sarcoma (KS)—see p. 498

Incidence ↓ since the introduction of HAART. Human herpes virus-8 (HHV-8) identified in 1994 as the causative agent. Although the skin is usual site, KS may develop in visceral organs.

Typically, KS lesions appear on the nose and hard palate but may arise anywhere on the skin. Disease usually has an insidious course with new lesions appearing as existing ones enlarge. Rapidly aggressive disease may occur but is rare. Initially starts as a painless, non-pruritic pink or red macule or a papule which gradually darkens to resemble a bruise. Surrounded by a yellow halo due to extravasated red cells (Plate 22). May be dark and difficult to recognize in black people. KS lesions vary in size from a few millimetres to several centimetres. Extensive plaques with scaling can develop on the legs and may break down producing local pain and oedema. Lesions on the soles may be particularly troublesome interfering with walking. Facial and genital KS is cosmetically unsightly. With treatment, lesion becomes flat, colour fades but some pigmentation persists even in absence of residual tumour.

Non-pitting oedema is commonly associated with KS, especially affecting the lower limbs. May be due to skin lymphatic involvement or 2° to vasoactive substances produced by KS. Degree of oedema occasionally disproportionate to size of KS lesions (i.e. feature of the disease itself rather than 2° to lymph node enlargement/lymphatic obstruction).

Diagnosis

Typical skin KS lesions are diagnosed clinically, but biopsy provides an absolute diagnosis in atypical lesions. Patients with symptoms or signs suggestive of other organ involvement should be evaluated by imaging techniques. Patients with severe oedema may require computerized tomography (CT) to exclude localized obstruction or accompanying pathology.

Treatment (see p. 502)

Treatment for skin KS is for cosmetic reasons and to alleviate symptoms.

Lymphomas (see p. 504)

Extranodal cutaneous involvement occurs in up to 8% of those with B-cell non-Hodgkin's lymphoma. Presents with an enlarging violaceous nodule or plaque, which may ulcerate.

Cutaneous T-cell lymphoma presents as a scaly patch or plaque with erythema, hypopigmentation or hyperpigmentation, and atrophy. It may be misdiagnosed as chronic eczema.

The skin may be involved when lymphoma (usually B-cell) involves an underlying lymph node.

Treatment (see p. 504)

The principles of management of non-Hodgkin's lymphoma are same as lymphoma elsewhere and chemotherapy is usually given.

Drug reactions

Cutaneous drug reactions ↑, as does the development of hypersensitivity reactions to previously tolerated drugs. Mild drug eruptions do not always necessitate the cessation of the causative drug especially if it is the most effective agent and is given for a short time e.g. co-trimoxazole for *Pneumocystis jiroveci* (*carinii*) pneumonia. Desensitization may be possible for essential drugs. Cross-sensitivities may occur e.g. between dapsone and co-trimoxazole.

Hypersensitivity reactions are common with certain antiretroviral drugs such as nevirapine and abacavir which may cause a fatal reaction. Special attention with counselling to patients on these treatments is important to ensure early recognition and prompt action.

- Morbilliform (erythematous maculopapular) drug eruption—is common and may be associated with systemic symptoms. Most frequent causative drugs are amoxicillin and sulfonamides. Progresses in a caudocephalic direction, resolving within 3–5 days occasionally persisting for weeks after its withdrawal. Many viral infections cause a similar rash.
- Erythroderma—occurs when a morbilliform rash becomes confluent and involves the whole body. May result in hypothermia and shock.
- Erythema multiforme, Stevens–Johnson syndrome, and toxic epidermal necrolysis—↑ in HIV infection. Offending drug must be stopped, patients best managed in high-dependency units where attention to electrolyte and fluid balance and skin care are of paramount importance.
- Nail and oral pigmentation—2° to zidovudine.
- Penile ulceration—due to foscarnet.

HIV: pyrexia of unknown origin

Introduction

Pyrexia of unknown origin (PUO) was defined by Petersdorf and Beeson (1961) as a temperature of >38.3°C on multiple occasions over a period of >3 weeks with failure to reach a diagnosis after 1 week of investigation.

HIV-related diseases are an important cause of prolonged fever and must be considered in patients with PUO. In patients with known HIV infection PUO may arise during follow-up. Durack and Street (1991) produced a definition of HIV associated PUO, including temperatures >38.3°C on multiple occasions over a period of >4 weeks for out-patients or 3 days for inpatients, with negative microbiological results after at least 2 days incubation.

PUO occurs predominantly in the late stages of infection with CD4 counts <100cells/μL and is less common in patients on effective HAART. In the general population, infections account for only 33% of PUO. However, in HIV positive patients, infectious diseases are the predominant aetiology accounting for 80–90% with neoplasia and drug reactions accounting for most of the others.

A cause can be found in 80%. In those with undetermined diagnoses fever may settle spontaneously. In the general population a single pathology is almost universal but two or more simultaneous pathologies may be found in about 20% of HIV-related cases. Even if patients are taking standard prophylaxis against agents, such as *Pneumocystis jiroveci* (*carinii*) or *Mycobacterium avium* complex (MAC), these cannot be excluded without appropriate investigation.

There are important geographical differences e.g. tuberculosis and leishmaniasis are much more common in Europe compared with USA. It is also important to consider non-HIV-related causes and other infections, e.g. gonorrhoea, whose presentation may be modified by immunodeficiency. Strenuous diagnostic efforts are important in PUO as it may enable the diagnosis and treatment of infections before the onset of specific organ dysfunction, e.g. a *Pneumocystis jiroveci* infection. A careful history including sexual, travel, and drugs (prescribed and non-prescribed) is mandatory.

HIV-related aetiology (data from Europe and USA)

- Mycobacterial infection
  - *Mycobacterium tuberculosis*: 7% (USA)–37% (Europe). CD4 count may be normal
  - *Mycobacterium avium* complex: 12–31% (CD4 count <100cells/μL)
  - Others (e.g. *M. kansasii*, *M. genavense*): 1–5%.
- *Pneumocystis jiroveci*: 5–13% (CD4 count <200cells/μL)
- Viral
  - Cytomegalovirus: 5–9% (CD4 count <50cells/μL)
  - HIV itself, herpes simplex virus, varicella zoster virus, parvovirus B19, adenovirus, hepatitis virus B and C: 2–7%.

- Bacterial: 5–7%.
- Fungal (cryptococcosis, candidaemia, disseminated histoplasmosis, aspergillosis, *Penicillium marneffei*: 2–8% (CD4 count <200cells/µL)
- Parasitic
  - Leishmaniasis: ~0% (USA)—12% (Europe)
  - Toxoplasmosis: 1–3%
  - Others (isosporiasis, cryptosporidiosis): <1%.
- Neoplasia
  - Lymphoma: 5–10% (CD4 count may be normal)
  - Kaposi sarcoma: isolated reports.
- Drugs: <1%.
- Other unusual causes include Reiter's syndrome, non-specific hepatitis, Castleman's disease, angiofollicular hyperplasia.

Diagnosis

Careful history taking followed by examination especially for lymphadenopathy, hepatosplenomegaly, and retinal abnormalities (through dilated pupils). All patients should have 1st level (non-invasive) investigation proceeding to 2nd level (invasive) if diagnosis is not established.

1st level includes

- Full blood count/differential white count, liver function tests, C-reactive protein, urinalysis
- Pulse oximetry
- Chest X-ray
- Repeated cultures of blood, sputum, urine, and faeces as indicated for bacteria, mycobacteria, and fungi
- Blood film examination
- Serum cryptococcal antigen
- Other specific serologies indicated by travel or exposure history

2nd level includes

- Abdominal and thoracic computerized tomography (CT)
- Exercise oximetry
- Gallium scan
- Bronchoscopy with broncho-alveolar lavage
- Biopsy (histology and microbiology)—bone marrow, liver, lymph node (including mediastinoscopic), skin, intestinal/oesophageal mucosa
- Lumbar puncture
- PCR for CMV

Causes of PUO unrelated to HIV must not be forgotten and may require other investigations e.g. auto-antibody screen.

Management

This depends on the underlying cause. Cases where no underlying additional pathology is found may respond to HAART. As in any fever, general measures such as good hydration, antipyretics, and reassurance are important. In patients with late stage HIV disease and limited treatment options, palliation with steroids may be necessary. MAC infections and, less commonly, leishmaniasis often present with unexplained pyrexia without focal organ involvement. Other causes of HIV-related PUO that may present with clinical features specific to their 1° infection site are described elsewhere in this book.

Non-HIV-related causes of PUO

Infection

Bacterial

- Site specific
  - abscesses, urinary tract infection, endocarditis, hepatobiliary infection, osteomyelitis.
- General
  - syphilis, relapsing fever, Lyme disease, gonorrhoea, lymphogranuloma venereum, psittacosis, salmonellosis, Q fever.

Viral

- CMV, Epstein–Barr virus, hepatitis viruses.

Fungi (usually only if immunosuppressed)

- Candidiasis.

Parasites

- malaria, toxoplasmosis.

Connective tissue/autoimmune diseases

- Rheumatoid arthritis, Still's disease, systemic lupus erythematosis.

Vasculitis

- Giant cell arteritis, polymyalgia rheumatica, polyarteritis nodosa.

Granulomatous diseases

- Sarcoidosis, regional enteritis, granulomatous hepatitis.

Neoplasia

- Lymphomas, Hodgkin's disease, leukaemias, solid tumours especially renal cell carcinoma, malignant histiocytosis.

Inherited diseases

- Familial Mediterranean fever.

Drugs

- Antibiotic reactions.

Endocrine

- Hyperthyroidism.

Factitious

Mycobacterium avium complex

Ubiquitous and frequently isolated from soil, food, and water. Infection usually affects those with CD4 counts <100cells/μL (median 1° 10cells/μL). Any organ can be affected, most commonly lymph nodes, spleen, gastrointestinal tract, lungs, and bone marrow but most patients develop disseminated infection without prior localization. Symptoms may be severe.

Clinical features

Most common is pyrexia (in ~90%) with night sweats, diarrhoea/abdominal pain/nausea and vomiting/weight loss, lymphadenopathy, and hepatosplenomegaly.

Investigations and diagnosis

- FBC—anaemia (common and often severe).
- LFTs—↑ alkaline phosphatase (common).
- Blood cultures.
- Culture of material from bone marrow, lymph nodes, and liver.
- Staining of material from bone marrow, lymph nodes (Plate 23), liver for mycobacteria (marrow provides rapid diagnosis in ~30%).
- PCR testing of potentially infected material (if available).
- X-rays may show internal lymphadenopathy with a typical abscess pattern on CT.

Management

3–4 drug regimens are recommended as multiresistance is usual.
A macrolide (clarithromycin 500mg daily twice or azithromycin 500mg daily) plus ethambutol 15mg/kg daily plus a rifamycin (rifabutin 450–600mg/day or rifampicin 450–600mg/day) and/or a quinolone (e.g. ciprofloxacin 500mg daily twice). Data is lacking to advise on the duration of treatment. HAART should also be commenced taking into account potential drug interactions. Steroids may be required to ameliorate severe fever.

1° prophylaxis is now rarely required because of the effectiveness of HAART, but may be considered for those with a CD4 count <50cells/μL. Effective drugs include azithromycin (1.2g weekly), clarithromycin 500mg daily twice and rifabutin (less effective).

Visceral leishmaniasis

Caused by *Leishmania* spp., protozoa transmitted by sandflies from rodents, small carnivores, dogs, foxes, and humans. Typically presents with fever, malaise, weight loss, hepatosplenomegaly, and lymphadenopathy.

Diagnosed by identifying organism in tissue by microscopy (Leishman–Donovan bodies in macrophages), culture, or PCR. Fine-needle aspiration of spleen is most sensitive (about 98%) but bone marrow aspiration safer with 54–86% sensitivity. Serology (immunofluorescent antibody test and direct agglutination test) insensitive (up to 76%) unless high protozoal load.

Treated with sodium stibogluconate 20mg/kg/day IV/IM for 28 days or liposomal amphotericin B.

Chapter 47

HIV: endocrine and metabolic disorders

Introduction

Metabolic disturbances and alterations in endocrine functions occur at all stages of HIV disease. HIV may directly infect endocrine glands but more commonly endocrine abnormalities are due to functional disturbances or 2° to drugs and intercurrent severe illnesses.

Endocrine disturbances

Pituitary function

Panhypopituitarism is rare but selective failure can occur e.g. gonadotrophins. Pituitary infarction is found in up to 10% of autopsies of AIDS patients. The pituitary may also be involved by opportunistic infection (OI) such as toxoplasmosis, cytomegalovirus (CMV), and *Mycobacterium avium* complex (MAC).

Thyroid disease

Autopsy studies have shown infiltration by lymphoma, Kaposi's sarcoma, and OIs such as MAC and CMV. These pathologies are not usually associated with abnormal thyroid function tests. Thyroid binding globulins are high and should be taken into consideration when interpreting total thyroid hormone levels.

Thyroid dysfunction may occur in those with advanced HIV disease during intercurrent illnesses. Overt hypothyroidism is rare.

Gonadal function

Dysfunction occurs in both sexes especially in the late stages of HIV disease and in those with weight loss. Sex hormone binding globulin levels are ↑ in 30–50%. Free testosterone levels are more reliable in the assessment of hypogonadism. Panhypopituitarism from hypothalamic and/or pituitary destruction causing gonadal failure is rare. The aetiology of gonadal dysfunction is often multifactorial. Severe systemic illness, OIs, malnutrition, weight loss, recreational drug use, chronic alcoholism, and abnormal levels of cytokines may be contributory. HIV-related gonadal failure results in loss of muscle mass, fatigue, sexual dysfunction, and ↓ quality of life. Unlike HIV negative men there is no ↑ in fat mass.

Testicular function

Total testosterone levels may be elevated in the early stages of HIV infection but tend to decline with disease progression. Erectile dysfunction is common in AIDS. Low testosterone levels may be due to a functional disorder of the hypothalamus, 1° testicular failure, or a combination of both. Testicular function is affected by drugs such as:

- opiates—associated with hypogonadotropic hypogonadism.
- ketoconazole—causing oligospermia and gynaecomastia.
- megestrol acetate—inhibiting gonadotropin secretion.

Testosterone replacement ↑ lean body mass, body weight, well-being.

Ovarian function

Irregular periods, oligomenorrhoea, and amenorrhoea occur with ↑ frequency as HIV disease progresses. ↓ muscle mass is associated with androgen deficiency. Up to 67% of ♀ with AIDS wasting syndrome have ↓ levels of free testosterone. The mechanism of this is not known.

Adrenal function

The adrenal gland is the most commonly affected endocrine gland leading to glucocorticoid, and less commonly, aldosterone deficiency. Hypothalamic–pituitary–adrenal axis abnormalities in HIV are usually due to medications, destruction of the adrenals, or the anterior pituitary by OIs and malignancies, autoimmune adrenalitis, and abnormal cytokine levels.

Adrenals may be directly infected by HIV. CMV adrenal gland involvement (found in 40–85% of autopsies) may lead to acute adrenal insufficiency.

Features of adrenocortical disturbances found in HIV infection:

- ↓ levels of dehydroepiandrosterone with ↑ cortisol.
- low basal adrenal androgen levels.
- ↓ adrenal responses to adrenocorticotrophic hormone (ACTH).

Drugs may also compromise adrenal function:

- megestrol acetate (used as an appetite stimulant) ↓ plasma cortisol level and may lead to acute adrenal crisis if stopped abruptly after prolonged use.
- ketoconazole results in ↓ cortisol and testosterone levels.
- rifampicin enhances hepatic cortisol metabolism and causes adrenal insufficiency in patients with Addison's disease who are on replacement therapy or in those with limited adrenal function.

Patients with fatigue, loss of weight, postural hypotension, hyponatraemia, and hyperkalaemia should be assessed with a short synacthen test. 1° adrenal insufficiency can be identified by measuring ACTH simultaneously with serum cortisol. Any severe illness may disturb the hypothalamic–pituitary–adrenal axis resulting in minor abnormalities of adrenal function tests.

Aldosterone deficiency may occur (often with glucocorticoid deficiency) leading to persistent hyponatraemia, hyperkalaemia, and metabolic acidosis requiring replacement therapy.

Management

Patients with glucocorticoid insufficiency should receive replacement therapy with hydrocortisone 30mg/day in divided doses.

Patients with aldosterone deficiency should receive fludrocortisone 50–300μg/day.

Pancreatic function

Both exocrine and endocrine functions are affected during HIV disease.

Pancreatic endocrine function

Insulin resistance occurs more frequently in HIV infection especially in those treated with protease inhibiters (PIs) and those with wasting syndrome. Diabetes is more likely to occur in those with other predisposing factors e.g. family history.

Pentamidine, used in the treatment of *Pneumocystis jiroveci* (*carinii*) pneumonia (PCP), is toxic to pancreatic β cells inducing hypoglycaemia in 15–28% (2–3 times more common than in HIV –ve patients). The reason for this is unknown. Substantial destruction of β cells may later lead to diabetes mellitus. Management of diabetes should follow the same principles as for HIV –ve individuals.

Pancreatic exocrine function ***(see p. 400)***

Reduced exocrine pancreatic function is common in HIV infection and may be asymptomatic. Severe chronic pancreatic insufficiency results in malabsorption.

Metabolic disorders

Lipodystrophy syndrome

Lipodystrophy, dyslipidaemia, and hyperglycaemia (from insulin resistance) are often combined although each component may occur in isolation. May arise spontaneously but much more commonly associated with the use of HAART, especially if containing PIs.

Lipodystrophy

Found in ~4% of those with untreated HIV infection. Rate for those taking HAART is difficult to determine because of inconsistent diagnostic criteria but ranges from 20% up to 75% (median development time—18 months). Magnitude varies with individual PIs. Prevalence also related to long-term nucleoside reverse transcriptase inhibitor (NRTI) use, especially stavudine (D4T). More common in whites and almost twice as common in ♀.

Lipohypertrophy (especially associated with PIs)
- Dorsocervical fat pad—buffalo hump
- Increased neck circumference (by 5–10cm)
- Breast hypertrophy (♀ and ♂)
- Central truncal adiposity—pot belly due to ↑ intraperitoneal fat.

Lipoatrophy (especially associated with NRTIs, particularly stavudine)
- Loss of subcutaneous fat from cheeks—emaciated appearance
- Peripheral subcutaneous fat loss from arms, shoulders, thighs, buttocks.

Dyslipidaemia

HIV infection (especially when advanced) may cause abnormalities in lipid metabolism which include:
- ↑ serum triglyceride
- ↓ total cholesterol—both high-density lipoprotein (HDL) and low-density lipoprotein (LDL)
- ↓ triglyceride clearance
- predominance of small, dense LDL particles.

It is reported in up to 80% of those taking HAART and especially prevalent in those taking a PI-based regimen. Typical abnormalities:
- hypercholesterolaemia—mostly very-LDL but also intermediate density lipoproteins. HDL unchanged or ↑
- hypertriglyceridaemia.

More frequent and severe with ritonavir and lopinavir–ritonavir, followed by amprenavir and nelfinavir with indinavir and saquinavir having the fewest effects. Atazanavir appears to have little, or no, effect although further data is required.

NRTIs are much less liable to be implicated although stavudine is more likely to be associated with ↑ in cholesterol and triglycerides. The nucleotide reverse transcriptase inhibitor, tenofovir, may ↑ cholesterol and triglyceride levels but less than with stavudine.

Non-NRTIs can cause alterations in the lipid profiles but to a much lesser extent than PIs. Nevirapine produces marginally smaller changes than efavirenz and improvements in lipid levels when switching from PIs.

Hyperglycaemia

New-onset diabetes mellitus, diabetic ketoacidosis, and exacerbations of pre-existing diabetes mellitus have all been reported with ↑ rates of other risk factors e.g. family history, pregnancy. Diabetes is directly associated with HIV infection, reported in 3.3% although this is increased to 5.9% with concomitant hepatitis C virus infection. Strongly linked to the use of PIs occurring in up to 17% with a median onset of symptoms about 60 days after starting treatment. Although, discontinuation of PIs may reverse hyperglycaemia there is insufficient data to estimate this likelihood. Its incidence does not vary substantially by PI used.

Assessment

Patients on antiretroviral therapy should have body weight, lipids, and blood sugar measured at regular intervals. Clinical examination and self-reporting of body shape changes help detect early signs. Photographs may aid in the early recognition of facial lipoatrophy. Additional cardiovascular risks, such as life style, smoking, hypertension, family history, and age, should also be assessed.

Management

- General advice
    - Nutrition: assessment, dietetic advice (low fat), possible benefit from dietary supplements (fibre, omega-3 fatty acids).
    - Exercise: ↑ physical activity and exercise to build muscles, improve abdominal shape and combat peripheral wasting.
- Start HAART before CD4 <200cells/μL or AIDS is diagnosed.
- Care with choice of initial regimen if possible:
    - avoid PIs and NRTI combinations with highest risk
    - use zidovudine or tenofovir instead of stavudine.
- Switch to drugs with low or no association. Benefit of switching is inconsistent, morphological changes being more resistant.
- Fibrates and statins—used according to lipid profile.
    - Hypercholesterolaemia managed with low-fat diet and statins.
    - Hypertriglyceridaemia responds best to low-fat diet, fibrates, and statins.
    - Pravastatin is the preferred statin as it is least likely to interact with PIs. Lovastatin may also be suitable. Atorvastatin must be used with caution and simvastatin avoided because of substantial risks of PI interaction.
    - Fibrates (gemfibrozil, bezafibrate, fenofibrate) are usually used in combination with statins as more effective than fibrate monotherapy. Seek advice from lipidologist before starting. ↑ risk of rhabdomyolysis and hepatoxicity.
- Other drugs
    - Metformin for insulin resistance, dyslipidaemia, and fat accumulation.
    - Growth hormone for fat accumulation.
    - Glitazones for insulin resistance with weight loss.
- Invasive methods for lipodystrophy.
    - Plastic surgery e.g. liposuction and breast reduction.
    - Polylactic acid (New-Fill®) and Bio-Alcamid™ injections for lipoatrophy.

Electrolytes and water imbalance

Sodium and water

Hyponatraemia is a common finding in patients with advanced HIV disease. Up to 60% of hospitalized patients have low plasma sodium levels, mostly due to gastrointestinal loss associated with hypovolaemia. Respiratory and central nervous system infections or certain drugs, e.g. antidepressants, may cause the syndrome of inappropriate secretion of antidiuretic hormone. This is characterized by hyponatraemia, inappropriately ↑ urinary osmolality for the degree of serum hypo-osmolality and normal blood volume in the context of normal adrenal and thyroid functions. Severe hyponatraemia causes confusion, seizures, and coma.

Decreased water clearance from HIV-related nephropathy may exacerbate hyponatraemia. Hyporeninaemic hypoaldosteronism should be considered when hyponatraemia is associated with hyperkalaemia, providing normally functioning kidneys and adrenals.

Hyponatraemia may be caused by miconazole and pentamidine and hypernatraemia (and nephrogenic diabetes insipidus) by foscarnet.

Potassium

High dose co-trimoxazole may result in hyperkalaemia especially with pre-existing renal impairment. Other causes include pentamidine-associated tubular nephropathy, HIV-nephropathy, and 1° adrenal insufficiency.

Calcium and phosphate

Up to 20% of patients will have hypocalcaemia at some stage. Causes include:

- HIV enteropathy (most common).
- Vitamin D deficiency.
- Severe intercurrent illness.
- Drugs
  - foscarnet binds calcium resulting in decreased ionized calcium.
  - ketoconazole inhibits 1,25-dihydroxy cholecalciferol (vitamin D) synthesis.
  - pentamidine causes renal loss of magnesium with 2° hypocalcaemia.

Hypophosphataemia may occur with intercurrent illness. Tenofovir can lead to hypophosphataemia as a result of effect on tubular function.

HIV-associated wasting syndrome

Defined by CDC as involuntary loss of >10% of body weight, plus >30 days of either diarrhoea or weakness and fever in the absence of concurrent illness other than HIV infection. An AIDS defining illness, less common since the introduction of HAART, when it accounted for up to 37% of AIDS diagnoses. Still a common problem independently associated with an increased risk of OIs, disease progression and death. Weight loss is mainly due to muscle wasting and to a lesser extent, loss of fat.

Additional factors that exacerbate wasting include:
- depression
- nutritional balance e.g. anorexia, dysphagia, poor nutrient absorption
- OIs
- metabolism e.g. increased resting metabolic rate, increased protein turnover, increased production of cytokines, and low testosterone.

Assessment

- Weight and body mass index at regular intervals help with early recognition and monitoring.
- Specialist nutritional review.
- Testosterone measurement.
- Measurement of body composition (bioimpedence analysis and anthropometry are useful in monitoring changes over time).
- Techniques such as dual energy x-ray absorptiometry (DEXA) scan, magnetic resonance imaging (MRI), and total body electrical conductivity provide more accurate measurement of body composition.

Management

- Treatment of contributing factors.
- Improving food intake by appropriate strategies including dietary supplements, enteral and parentral feeding.
- Pharmacologic agents:
  - Testosterone may be considered to reverse muscle loss but there is concern about the adverse effects of long-term administration.
  - Megestrol an appetite stimulant (side-effects include hypogonadism, adrenal insufficiency, deep venous thrombosis, and avascular necrosis).
  - Growth hormone administration results in increase in lean body mass but is expensive and benefit may be lost after discontinuation.
  - Thalidomide results in significant weight gain but has strict prescribing guidelines and has potential serious side-effects.
  - Anabolic hormones e.g. oxymetholone is beneficial, side-effects include liver toxicity.

Chapter 48

HIV: renal disorders

Introduction

Relatively common in those with HIV infection and may just amount to proteinuria (in up to 30%). Necropsy studies in the USA have shown renal pathological abnormalities in 3–7%. Initial presentation may be as acute renal failure, especially in advanced HIV disease, 2° to:

- Dehydration and electrolyte disturbances (e.g. following vomiting and diarrhoea).
- Acute tubular necrosis due to:
  - sepsis
  - hypotension
  - drug nephro-toxicity (e.g. tenofovir, adefovir, aminoglycosides, pentamidine, aciclovir, cidofovir, foscarnet, amphotericin B).
- Obstruction (2° to nephrolithiasis and crystalluria)
  - indinavir—~4% develop nephrolithiasis, prevented by ample fluid intake (>2L a day)
  - sulfadiazine and aciclovir—can cause crystalluria especially in high dosage and with dehydration.

HIV-related 2° infection (e.g. tuberculosis) can involve the kidney but HIV infection itself may cause 1° renal disease.

The general management of renal failure should follow the same principles as HIV –ve patients, i.e. fluid/dietary restriction, renal replacement therapy, erythropoietin, vitamin D analogues, etc.

HIV-associated nephropathy (HIVAN)

First described in 1984. Studies from USA and some European centres suggest that it is the most common HIV-related renal disease. Renal glomerular and tubular epithelial cells have been shown to be infected by HIV, though mechanisms of viral-induced injury are unclear.

Predominantly found in black ♂ of African origin and currently the 3rd most common cause of end stage renal disease (ESRD) in African-Americans, aged 20–64 years.

Clinical features

Presents with nephrotic syndrome—proteinuria >3.5g/day, hypoalbuminaemia, oedema, and hyperlipidaemia. Leads to progressive renal insufficiency. Typically no hypertension.

Diagnosis

- CD4 count is usually <200cells/μL.
- Urinalysis shows leucocytes, hyaline casts, oval fat bodies but no cellular casts.
- Renal ultrasound typically shows normal or enlarged renal size with ↑ echogenicity.
- Definitive diagnosis by renal biopsy showing focal segmental glomerulosclerosis with 'collapsing' features and tubular atrophy.

Management

Initial reports of dismal prognosis (inexorable progression to ESRD within 6–12 months) have improved with treatment that at least delays disease progression.

- HAART.
- Prednisolone (improves renal function by ↓ HIV initiated inflammatory process).
- Angiotensin converting enzyme inhibitors—treatment of choice for hypertension, but may also be beneficial in the normotensive.

Immune-mediated renal disease

Less common than HIVAN but reported as the main cause of HIV-related renal disease in non-African Americans based on studies from France, Italy, and Thailand. Found in 25–50% of those having a biopsy for renal disease. The types of glomerular involvement found include:

- IgA nephropathy—HIV directly implicated, reported almost exclusively in Caucasians and Hispanics;
- membranous nephropathy;
- membranoproliferative, mesangial proliferative, diffuse proliferative, or crescentic glomerulonephritis.

Hepatitis B virus (HBV) and hepatitis C virus (HCV) both more common in injecting intravenous drug users, are important co-infections and may individually cause renal disease.

HCV-associated cryoglobulinaemic glomerulonephritis is found in both HIV and non-HIV infected patients but is much more aggressive in the former. Typical presentation includes purpura, arthralgias, and peripheral neuropathy in addition to renal insufficiency. Circulating cryoglobulins and ↓ complement levels may be found.

HBV, syphilis, and malignancy may all cause membranous nephropathy and are all found more frequently in those with HIV infection.

Clinical features

Slowly progressive and mild compared with HIVAN. Typical early features are asymptomatic proteinuria and haematuria (on urinalysis), with mild renal insufficiency.

Diagnosis

- Detection of other infection(s) e.g. syphilis, HBV, and HCV.
- Renal biopsy.

Management

- Treat any co-infection or malignancy.
- HAART.

Interstitial nephritis

Not uncommon and may be associated with other renal pathology such as HIVAN. Equal prevalence in blacks and whites. May present with proteinuria, renal failure, or nephrotic syndrome.

Acute interstitial nephritis 2° to allergic drug reactions presents with acute renal failure, skin rash, and eosinophilia. Non-steroidal anti-inflammatory drugs are a common cause.

Acute renal failure and HIV seroconversion

Acute renal failure and nephrotic syndrome may be presenting features of acute HIV seroconversion. Renal biopsy typically shows acute tubular necrosis and mesangioproliferative glomerulonephritis, with tubuloreticular inclusions.

Drugs and renal disease

- Indinavir: nephrolithiasis, interstitial nephritis
- Ritonavir: interstitial nephritis
- Tenofovir: renal tubular dysfunction with hypophosphataemia, normoglycemic glycosuria, and proteinuria. Fanconi's syndrome and acute renal failure also reported.

Other diseases (less commonly reported)

Minimal change disease, amyloidosis, haemolytic uraemic syndrome, and renal malignancy.

End stage renal disease

Dialysis should be considered (haemodialysis currently the preferred method). May only be required on a temporary basis until HAART is introduced. Cadaver renal transplantation has been performed in small numbers of selected patients with no evidence of ↑ rate of opportunistic infection.

Chapter 49

HIV: cardiovascular disorders

Introduction

Reports of the prevalence of cardiac involvement in patients with AIDS vary from 28–73%, with the first case, myocardial Kaposi's sarcoma (KS) found at autopsy in 1983. With HAART, cardiac manifestations directly related to HIV have fallen although ↑ cardiovascular problems related to drug side-effects are anticipated.

Pericardial effusion

Found in about 20% with AIDS. Often small with no haemodynamic consequences, although if large may cause tamponade. Associated with low CD4 count and reported causes include bacteria, especially *Mycobacterium* spp., *Cryptococcus neoformans*, cytomegalovirus, tumours (lymphoma, KS) and multiple unusual organisms. Clinically similar to non-HIV infected patients and although usually seen in advanced HIV infection rarely causes death.

Myocarditis

Prior to HAART autopsy evidence was found in ~33% of those with AIDS with a specific cause found in <20% (the most common being *Toxoplasma gondii*, *Mycobacterium tuberculosis*, and *C. neoformans*). HIV alone can probably cause myocarditis as HIV or its proteins have been found in the myocardium of patients with or without cardiac disease.

Dilated cardiomyopathy

Prevalence in patients with AIDS is 10–30% by echocardiographic and autopsy studies. Associated with advanced disease, low CD4 counts and myocarditis, which may act as a trigger. Several studies have supported a direct role for HIV-1 causing cardiac injury, but the mechanism remains unclear. It may be related to co-infection with cytomegalovirus, coxsackievirus group B, or Epstein–Barr virus. The overall prognosis is poor.

Endocarditis

Non-bacterial thrombotic endocarditis

Friable, fibrinous clumps of platelets and red blood cells adherent to cardiac valves (usually tricuspid in HIV infection) without an inflammatory reaction. Occurs in 3–5% of those with AIDS, usually aged >50 years. Associated with malignancy, hyper-coagulable states, and chronic wasting disease. Emboli may occur in up to 42%, involving the brain, lung, spleen, kidneys, and coronary arteries. They are usually asymptomatic though rarely may be fatal.

Infective endocarditis

Occurs most commonly in injecting drug users (IDUs), usually affecting the tricuspid valve. The main causative organisms are *Staphylococcus aureus* (75%) and *Streptococcus viridans* (20%). Usually presents with fever, sweats, weight loss, and coexisting pneumonia and/or meningitis with increased mortality in advanced HIV disease in comparison to asymptomatic infection.

Pulmonary hypertension

Pulmonary hypertension

HIV is an independent risk factor for the development of pulmonary hypertension. The stage of HIV infection is unrelated to the development and progression of pulmonary hypertension and it may predate the diagnosis of HIV disease. Found most commonly in young ♂. Progressive dyspnoea followed by ankle oedema are the usual presenting features. Diagnosed after excluding other causes e.g. thrombo-embolism, talc granuloma (particularly in IDUs). The response to pulmonary vasodilator agents, antiretroviral drugs, and anticoagulation therapy is variable.

Venous thrombosis

↑ risk of venous thrombo-embolic disease leading to deep venous thrombosis and consequently pulmonary embolism. Related to changes in coagulation (see p. 495).

Cardiac neoplasia

Kaposi's sarcoma

In autopsy studies (mostly homosexual ♂) incidence of cardiac KS prior to HAART was 12–28% (usually part of disseminated involvement). Typical cardiac sites are the visceral layer of serous pericardium or subepicardial fat (especially beside a major coronary artery). Clinical features are often negligible. May cause pericardial effusion which can produce cardiac tamponade requiring emergency paracentesis. If suspected, diagnosis can be confirmed by biopsy through a pericardial window which also provides decompression.

Non-Hodgkin's lymphoma

Usually part of disseminated neoplasia rather than primary cardiac lymphoma (very rare). Typically high grade with spread often early in those with AIDS. Usually no specific symptoms but may present with progressive congestive heart failure, pericardial effusion, cardiac arrhythmia, or cardiac tamponade. Nodular or polypoid lymphomas may appear predominantly involving the pericardium with variable myocardial infiltration. Their removal may alleviate mechanical obstruction. Prognosis is poor, although clinical remission has been observed with combination chemotherapy.

Vascular disease

May be directly caused by HIV with infected monocytes and macrophages producing atheroma by adhesion or angiitis. HAART, especially containing protease inhibitors (PIs), all except atazanavir, may cause hyperlipidaemia leading to atherosclerosis and thrombosis. Hyperlipidaemia is found to a lesser extent with the nucleoside/nucleotide reverse transcriptase inhibitors (especially stavudine) and the non-nucleoside reverse transcriptase inhibitors. Insulin resistance (associated with PIs) is an independent risk factor for myocardial infarction and death. The risk of myocardial infarction is ~3 times that of ♂ in the general population if PIs are used for ≥30 months. Other cardiovascular risk factors are important to consider, especially cigarette smoking as higher rates have been reported in homosexual and bisexual men with HIV infection. Therefore, advice on low-fat diets, regular exercise, blood pressure control, lipid lowering drugs, and smoking cessation are important in patient care.

Drug associated

Cardiomyopathy may be caused by zidovudine (also myocarditis), doxorubicin, amphotericin B, and foscarnet; dysrhythmias by ganciclovir and α-interferon; conduction defects by co-trimoxazole, pentamidine, and pyrimethamine.

Chapter 50

HIV: musculo-skeletal disorders

Introduction

Prevalence of joint manifestations is uncertain. However, studies show that they are likely to be influenced by HIV risk factors:

- injecting drug users (IDUs) and haemophiliacs are more susceptible to septic arthritis and osteomyelitis
- homosexual ♂ are more likely to develop sexually acquired reactive arthritis (SARA).

Joint symptoms may also be a feature of other conditions found more commonly in those with HIV infection, e.g. haemophilia (with haemarthrosis), syphilis, gonorrhoea, hepatitis B and C virus, and chlamydial infections. They may also be due to the side-effects of drugs used to treat HIV and related conditions.

Autoantibodies are commonly produced, except when CD4 counts are very low and may re-appear with immune reconstitution by HAART. When CD4 counts are >500cells/μL (early after seroconversion or immune restoration with treatment) autoimmune diseases may occur. Diseases reported include systemic lupus erythematosus, vasculitis, polymyositis, Raynaud's phenomenon, Behçet's disease, primary biliary cirrhosis, and Graves' disease. Immune complex vasculitis is associated with counts 200–499cells/μL and spondyloarthropathy with counts <200cells/μL.

Inflammatory arthropathies

Arthralgia

Most common joint manifestation occurring in up to 45%. Pathology is unclear but may involve cytokines or transient bone ischaemia. Can occur at any stage of HIV disease and may be the first manifestation, being reported in 50–70% of those presenting with 1° HIV infection. Usually mild to moderate in intensity.

In up to 10% of those with advanced HIV infection a painful transient articular syndrome, characterized by an acute onset of severe pain in up to four joints, has been described. Knee most commonly affected, with shoulder and elbow also involved. Symptoms may mimic acute septic arthritis but no effusion, synovitis, or ↑ in joint fluid white cells. Radiology normal or may show periarticular osteopenia. Treated with standard analgesics/non-steroidal anti-inflammatory drugs (NSAIDs) though narcotics may be required.

Diffuse idiopathic lymphocytic syndrome

Similar to Sjögren's syndrome and found at any stage of HIV infection. Presents with salivary gland enlargement (parotid swelling may be massive), xerostomia, xerophthalmia, and arthralgia. Treat with artificial saliva and tears. Zidovudine in HAART ↓ parotid enlargement.

Acute symmetrical polyarthritis

Resembles rheumatoid arthritis (RA). Characterized by involvement of small joints of the hand leading to ulnar deviation of the digits and swan-neck deformities. May be differentiated from RA by acute onset and negative rheumatoid factor. Radiological appearances similar to RA with periarticular osteopenia, joint-space narrowing, and marginal erosions. Gold treatment may be required.

HIV-associated arthritis

Asymmetrical, oligoarticular arthritis. Possibly caused by effects of local infection (HIV detected in joint fluid). More common in ♂. Typically presents with sudden onset of severe pain, mainly affecting knees and ankles. Self-limiting, usually lasting from a few weeks to 6 months. Synovial fluid commonly contains up to 2500 white blood cells/μL. Radiology may show osteopenia but no erosions. A chronic mononuclear cell infiltrate is found on synovial biopsy. Treat with NSAIDs or intra-articular corticosteroid injections for symptomatic relief.

Hypertrophic osteoarthropathy

May appear as a complication of *Pneumocystis jiroveci* (*carinii*) pneumonia (PCP). Affects bones, joints, and soft tissues. Presents with severe pain in the lower limbs, arthralgia, non-pitting oedema, and finger clubbing. Skin over affected areas (ankle, knees, and elbows) is shiny, warm, and oedematous. Extensive periosteal reaction and subperiosteal proliferative changes in the long bones of the legs are found on radiology with bone scans showing ↑ uptake along the cortical surfaces. Usually responds to treatment of underlying PCP.

Reactive arthritis

Probably no more frequent in those with HIV infection but tends to be more severe. Lower limb peripheral arthritis predominates. Synovial fluid is inflammatory (a few thousand polymorphonuclear leucocytes/mL), sterile with a glucose level at least 66% of the serum level. Treat initially with NSAIDs (as in HIV –ve). Other drugs may be required e.g. phenylbutazone, gold, methotrexate (with caution as immunosuppressive) and other disease modifying agents. HAART is likely to be beneficial.

Psoriatic arthritis

More common and severe than in HIV-negative individuals usually polyarticular and asymmetrical. Extra-articular manifestations occur in ~50%. Usually insidious with the appearance of bone erosions within weeks or months. Radiologic findings of the distal interphalangeal joints are pathognomonic. Joint and tendon involvement in HIV-associated psoriatic arthritis tends to be less responsive to NSAIDs (still 1st line therapy). Methotrexate and azathioprine are effective but require careful monitoring because of myelosuppression. Sulfasalazine may be helpful but skin rash occurs in 30%. Low-dose systemic corticosteroids ineffective and high doses may produce many side-effects. Gold, retinoids, phototherapy, cyclosporine, and zidovudine reported to improve the skin and joints in some.

Osteonecrosis (avascular necrosis)

Result of direct damage to the vascular supply, leading to death of subchondral bone. Additional risks are prior use of corticosteroid, testosterone, or anabolic steroids, hyperlipidaemia, hypercoagulability, sickle cell disease, alcohol abuse, and smoking. Most common site is femoral head followed by humeral head, with bilateral involvement in 40%. May be asymptomatic or cause severe disabling deep pain. As plain x-rays may be normal magnetic resonance imaging (MRI) recommended. In early stages rest may be adequate, but in advanced disease joint replacement or other surgery may be required.

Infections

Septic arthritis

Usually mono-articular, with the hip being most frequently affected, although in IDUs there may be sternoclavicular joint involvement. *Staphylococcus aureus* followed by *Streptococcus pneumoniae* are the most common causative organisms. If CD4 count <100cells/μL multiple joint involvement and associated skin infection may occur with opportunistic infections (e.g. *Mycobacterium avium* complex, cryptococcosis, sporotrichosis). Diagnosed by Gram-stain and culture of synovial fluid. Blood cultures may be positive before synovial cultures. Treat with appropriate antibiotics, usually IV and monitor inflammatory markers.

Osteomyelitis

- Septic: may follow direct extension or haematogenous spread from an infected joint. Suspect if septic arthritis fails to respond despite adequate treatment.
- Tuberculous: develops from the haematogenous spread of an acute or reactivated infection. The spine, especially the thoracic and lumbar, is most commonly affected, starting in the vertebral body and spreading to the adjacent disk spaces. Vertebral wedging leads to gibbus formation. In addition to antibiotics surgical intervention with irrigation and debridement may be required.
- Bacillary angiomatosis due to *Bartonella henselae* may cause osteomyelitis. Occurs in the immunosuppressed and characterized by vascular proliferation involving the nervous system (aseptic meningitis, intracerebral mass lesions), liver (peliosis hepatitis), lymph nodes (adenitis) and bone.

Osteopenia/osteoporosis

HIV infection is associated ↓ bone mineral density (BMD) determined by measurement of x-ray absorption e.g. dual energy x-ray absorptiometry (DEXA) scan. A DEXA scan T-score (number of standard deviations from the mean value in young, healthy individuals) is diagnostic. Scores between –1 and –2.5 indicate osteopenia (pre-symptomatic) and –2.5 or less osteoporosis. Osteopenia found in up to 65% and osteoporosis up to 25% of those with HIV infection. Duration of infection significantly associated. Other factors are HIV wasting, low body mass index, malnutrition, immobilization, hypogonadism, menopause, steroids, alcohol excess, and smoking. HAART, especially with protease inhibitors, suggested as a contributor but conflicting evidence.

Occur mainly in the vertebrae, lower arms, and hips. Osteoporosis often asymptomatic but may cause pain (low back, neck, hip), loss of height, kyphosis, and fractures. Bone metabolism should be assessed (serum calcium, phosphate, and alkaline phosphatase). Management should include advice on diet, exercise, and avoidance of alcohol/nicotine. Osteopenia can be managed with vitamin D (400–800IU daily) and calcium supplements (calcium-rich diet or calcium tablets 1.2g/day). Osteoporosis should be treated with bisphosphonates (with additional vitamin D and calcium supplementation).

Neoplasia

Non-Hodgkin lymphoma

1° or 2° bone involvement occurs in 20–30%. May present as a pathological fracture, especially of the lower limbs. Radiology shows an area of osteolysis with cortical destruction. A periosteal reaction and soft tissue mass may also be present. Findings similar to bacterial osteomyelitis, therefore biopsy recommended. Treated with chemotherapy, radiation, and possibly surgical debridement.

Kaposi's sarcoma

Rarely reported and usually associated with widespread dissemination. Frequently asymptomatic, otherwise bone pain, with radiology either normal or demonstrating lesions usually lytic, occasionally sclerotic. Diagnosis by biopsy. Radiotherapy may alleviate bone pain.

Muscle disease

1° myopathy is uncommon and a polymyositis syndrome occurs very rarely. The most important cause of 2° myopathy is prolonged zidovudine therapy, associated with ↑ creatinine kinase level in 16% and symptomatic weakness in 6%. Probably caused by mitochondrial dysfunction because of the inhibition of mitochondrial DNA γ-polymerase by zidovudine. Muscle weakness and wasting is proximal with preserved reflexes and sensory function. Electromyographical evidence of myopathy found in >90%. Ragged, red fibres (due to the accumulation of abnormal mitochondria) may be seen on muscle biopsy. Treatment involves discontinuation of the drug but for some patients prednisolone (starting with 60–80mg daily, reducing over several months) may be required to restore muscle strength.

Chapter 51

HIV: reticulo-endothelial disorders

Haematological disorders

Common haematological abnormalities may lead to consideration of HIV as the cause.

Direct effect of HIV itself or 2° to concurrent infection, malignancy, and therapeutic agents. ↓ haemopoiesis, altered coagulation, and immune-mediated cytopenias with ↓ bone marrow cellularity and dysplasia common findings.

Anaemia

Most common form of cytopenia and an independent prognostic factor. Usually due to ↓ erythropoiesis but other mechanisms e.g. infection, drug toxicity, malignancy, dietary deficiencies, and blood loss may contribute. Chronic anaemia causes fatigue, exertional dyspnoea and a hyperdynamic state which, if severe, may lead to angina, congestive cardiac failure, and confusion.

Diagnosis and evaluation

Examine and test for iron, vitamin B12 and folate deficiencies, haemolysis and blood loss according to red cell indices. Eliminate possible causes by excluding infection and malignancy and reviewing drug therapy. Bone marrow examination may be required.

- HIV-related. Normocytic, normochromic anaemia ↑ frequency and severity as HIV progresses. May be a direct effect of HIV on bone marrow progenitor cells, ↓ erythropoietin production and ↑ cytokines (inhibit haemopoiesis). Improves or normalizes with HAART providing drug effects do not supervene.
- Drug toxicity
  - Macrocytosis and normal haemoglobin—typical with zidovudine (AZT).
  - Macrocytic anaemia—caused by AZT and stavudine. AZT exerts broader myelosuppressive effects, more frequent in patients receiving higher doses (in ~1% receiving 500mgs a day) and those with advanced disease. Anaemia may require blood transfusion following discontinuation of AZT. In patients with a low level of endogenous erythropoietin (<500IU/L), recombinant human erythropoietin may resolve anaemia thereby ↓ need for transfusion.
  - Normocytic, normochromic anaemia—associated with normal or ↓ reticulocyte count, 2° to bone marrow suppression. Causes include anaemia of chronic infection and drugs (e.g. ganciclovir, cotrimoxazole, amphotericin, and interferons).
  - Haemolytic anaemia—features are macrocytosis, ↓ haptoglobin, and ↑ lactic dehydrogenase, indirect bilirubin, and reticulocyte count. Common causes include drugs e.g. dapsone (with methaemoglobinaemia), ribavirin, and primaquin. Glucose-6-phosphate dehydrogenase (G6PD) deficiency predisposes to dapsone and primaquin haemolysis. Autoimmune haemolytic anaemia (AIHA) with positive Coomb's test also occurs.

- Bone marrow infiltration (usually causes pancytopenia)
  - Opportunistic infection (OI)—most commonly *Mycobaterium avium* complex, (also tuberculosis and cytomegalovirus).
  - Tumours—lymphoma and rarely Kaposi's sarcoma.
- B19 parvovirus infects erythroid precursors. In immune deficiency persistent infection may result in severe chronic normocytic normochromic anaemia. Diagnosed by detecting B19 parvovirus antibodies and DNA (by polymerase chain reaction) in serum and/or bone marrow. Responds well to high dose intravenous immunoglobulins (0.4g/kg/day) which contain parvovirus antibodies but may require repeated blood transfusions.

Thrombocytopenia

Occurs in up to 30%. May be result of drug toxicity, immune and non-immune destruction, or defective platelet production. Commonly an isolated haematological abnormality with ↑ levels of anti-platelet immunoglobulin. HIV-related immune thrombocytopenia frequent early finding tending to deteriorate as HIV progresses. Results from clearance of immunoglobulin coated platelets by reticulo-endothelial system.

Diagnosis and evaluation

Exclude underlying causes e.g. drug toxicity, liver disease, and lymphoma. In their absence the presence of normal or ↑ megakaryocytes on bone marrow examination is sufficient to diagnose HIV-induced thrombocytopenia.

Treatment

- Mild and asymptomatic—HAART, switch/discontinue implicated drugs.
- Symptomatic or before surgical procedures—intravenous immunoglobulins, steroids, and HAART.
- Substantial bleeding—packed red cells and platelet transfusion.

Thrombotic thrombocytopenic purpura

Rare, of unknown aetiology, usually seen in early stages of HIV infection. Characterized by hyaline microvascular deposits. Clinical features include fever, renal impairment, neurological deficit, and microangiopathic haemolytic anaemia. Good response to plasmapheresis, steroids, and anti-platelets.

Neutropenia

HIV directly implicated, especially in advanced stages. More commonly due to drug toxicity, associated infection, and bone marrow infiltration. Risk of bacterial infection ↑ significantly when absolute neutrophil count <500cells/μL. Drugs causing neutropenia include AZT, ganciclovir, co-trimoxazole, pentamidine, α-interferon, and chemotherapeutic agents.

Diagnosis and evaluation

Careful review of medication. Withdraw offending drug/s if absolute neutrophil count is <500cells/μL. If cause uncertain consider bone marrow examination.

Treatment

- HAART—variable response
- Granulocyte colony stimulating factor:
  - HIV-induced
  - drug-induced (if implicated drug cannot be reduced or stopped).

Coagulation disorders

↑ risk of thrombotic disease associated with low CD4 counts, OIs, neoplasms, and HIV-associated autoimmune disorders such as AIHA.

- Lupus anticoagulant may be detected with thrombo-embolic disease.
- ↓ levels of active protein S frequently found, although not associated with immune suppression.
- Contributing prothrombotic factors include; ↓ plasminogen activator inhibitor level, abnormal platelet aggregation and ↑ von Willebrand factor.

Persistent generalized lymphadenopathy

Generalized lymphadenopathy involving ≥2 extra inguinal sites persisting for more than 3 months. Of no prognostic significance but other causes of generalized lymphadenopathy should be excluded. Occurs in up to 70% of patients within 1 year of seroconversion but may co-exist with other manifestations of HIV infection. Lymph nodes usually symmetrical, >1cm in size, rubbery, and non-tender. May be accompanied by hepatosplenomegaly. Mediastinal lymphadenopathy usually has other causes.

Important diagnoses to consider in HIV associated lymphadenopathy

- Persistent generalized lymphadenopathy
- Bacterial infections (including mycobacteria)
- 2° syphilis
- Lymphoma
- Histoplasmosis
- Multicentric Castleman's disease

Chapter 52

HIV: malignancies

Introduction

Incidence of malignancy is ↑ with impaired cell mediated immunity, observed before HIV epidemic. Applies most commonly to a narrow spectrum of more unusual tumours, especially those induced by viral co-infections, rather than those most commonly seen in the general population. Some occur much more frequently in HIV infection, especially when immunosuppressed, with the following designated as AIDS defining illnesses:

- Kaposi's sarcoma
- non-Hodgkin's lymphoma
- invasive cervical carcinoma.

Other associated malignant conditions include squamous cell carcinoma (anogenital, conjunctival, labial, and glossal), testicular tumours, melanomas, Hodgkin's disease, multiple myeloma, leiomyosarcoma in children, and lung cancer.

The following viral infections contribute to the induction of malignant disease in the immunosuppressed:

- human herpes virus 8 (HHV-8)—KS and body cavity lymphomas. Found in ~100% in multicentric Castleman's disease
- human papilloma virus (HPV)—anogenital and possibly oral carcinomas
- Epstein–Barr virus (EBV)—certain forms of lymphoma
- hepatitis B and C viruses—hepatocellular carcinoma

Other factors such as specific sexual practices and cigarette smoking (which should therefore be discouraged) may play a part.

Overall risk of malignancy is doubled in an HIV-infected population. Natural history of malignancy may be altered in HIV infection with advanced, rapidly progressive disease more likely. Treatment may be made difficult because of ↑ sensitivity to side-effects of chemotherapy if immunosuppressed and ↓ bone marrow reserve. HAART has had a dramatic effect on the incidence of some tumours, particularly 1° cerebral lymphoma.

Kaposi's sarcoma (KS)

Initially described in 1872 by Moritz Kaposi and rare before HIV epidemic. Four different types:

- classic—usually elderly ♂ from eastern Mediterranean/Europe causing multiple skin lesions of lower limbs.
- endemic—children and young ♂ in equatorial Africa. More virulent than classic.
- acquired—people on immunosuppressant therapy. Resolves when drugs stopped.
- epidemic—associated with HIV infection. Variable but generally more aggressive than other types.

Caused by HHV-8 (found in >90% of KS lesions) spread sexually, by mother-to-child contact and organ transplant. High viral levels in saliva suggest oral contact as a route of transmission. In homosexual ♂ new HHV-8 infection is associated with an HIV-positive partner. No evidence to support transmission by semen (HHV-8 rarely detected) and conflicting data on the role of rimming.

Epidemic KS

Most common malignancy associated with HIV infection. Before HAART, was the AIDS defining disease in 15–20% of homosexual ♂ (found in up to 50% with AIDS early in the epidemic). Incidence decreasing prior to HAART but substantially ↓ since HAART. Predominantly found in homosexual ♂ and rare among IV drug users and haemophiliacs. Also rare in ♀ (possible hormonal factor) but if found often more aggressive and usually associated with HIV acquisition from a bisexual ♂. Mean time from HHV-8 seroconversion to KS development—33 months. KS found more commonly in those with advanced disease. Rarely sole cause of death unless there is pulmonary involvement when respiratory failure may supervene. Prevalence of KS in different HIV populations reflects the background seroprevalence for HHV-8.

Clinical features

Skin lesions

May occur on any part of the body but facial (margin of nostrils, tip of the nose, and eyelids) involvement common. Typical pigmented macules, papules, plaques, nodules ranging in size from several millimetres to many centimetres. Colour varies from pink to deep purple with a yellow or green halo (extravasated erythrocyte pigments) characteristically surrounding them. Colourless subcutaneous nodules may also be found. In dark-skinned people the lesions are dark brown or black. Ulceration of nodules may lead to bleeding or infection. Large painful plaques may appear, especially on thighs and soles of feet.

Oral lesions

Found in ~33% of those with epidemic KS usually affecting hard palate (also gingiva, tongue, uvula, tonsils, pharynx, trachea). Often asymptomatic, although may cause local symptoms related to their site and extent. Usually appear as focal or diffuse red/purple plaques which may become nodular and ulcerate.

Others

- Gastrointestinal (GI) tract: prior to HAART found in 40% of at initial KS diagnosis. Unless symptomatic their presence does not influence prognosis. May occur without skin lesions and may cause GI bleeding or obstruction.
- Respiratory: may involve lung parenchyma, bronchial tree, and pleura leading to large blood-stained pleural effusions. Usually symptomatic (dyspnoea, haemoptysis, cough, wheezing, and radiology often shows ill-defined nodules or areas of infiltration.
- Lymph nodes: modest lymphadenopathy common. Rarely massive lymphadenopathy (possibly without KS elsewhere) necessitating diagnostic biopsy.
- Lymphoedema: non-pitting, most commonly affecting feet and legs and may be complicated by ulceration and infection. May result from direct KS dermal lymphatic involvement.
- Hepatic, splenic, cardiac, pericardial, bone marrow involvement all rarely reported, usually at autopsy.

Social/emotional implications

Lesions often obvious and disfiguring acting as a constant reminder leading to isolation, anxiety, and depression.

Diagnosis and assessment

- Clinical appearance and biopsy
- Other specific investigations depending on site (e.g. radiology, scan, endoscopy).
- HHV-8 antibody and viral load (VL) tests developed but not widely available. VL ↓ when KS treated with chemotherapy and HAART.

Staging based on distribution of KS, CD4 count, and other HIV associated symptoms/opportunistic infections (OIs) to determine level of risk for disease progression. Poor prognosis if both advanced tumours and systemic disease.

Management

HAART often significantly improves KS (in up to 80%) without further intervention. Treatment options depend on site, KS extent/activity, CD4 count, presence of systemic symptoms, and other OIs, past or present.

No interventional treatment

Consider if few skin lesions and no problems. Disfiguring lesions can be cosmetically camouflaged.

Local therapy

- Cryotherapy—small flat lesions on thin skin (e.g. face, genitals). Repeat treatment usually required. May leave hypopigmented scar.
- Radiotherapy—for lesions that are painful, causing lymphatic obstruction, oropharyngeal, or ophthalmic. Side-effects include local erythema, hair loss, mucositis, and pigmented scarring. Although lesions regress with irradiation, regrowth within 6 months common.
- Intralesional vinblastine, vincristine, or alpha interferon—limited mucocutaneous disease. Painful injections causing inflammatory response before lesions shrink or disappear leaving a scar. Repeat injections required and relapse within 6 months common.

Liposomal chemotherapy

Liposomal doxorubicin and liposomal daunorubicin now standard of care for KS. Preferentially absorbed by vascular KS lesions producing targeted chemotherapy with ↓ side-effects. Liposomal doxorubicin (20mg/m^2 every 2–3 weeks) appears to be more effective (response rate 90%) and is licensed for extensive skin or visceral KS and CD4 counts <200cells/μL. Bone marrow suppression occurs in 50% but the associated neutropenia can be treated with granulocyte-colony-stimulating factor (G-CSF).

Cytotoxic chemotherapy

Now largely superseded by liposomal chemotherapy. Usually a combination of 3 or more of—bleomycin, doxorubicin, etoposide, tenoposide, vinblastin, vincristine. Paclitaxel has a 50% response rate.

▶ Prophylaxis against *Pneumocystis jiroveci* (*carinii*) pneumonia (PCP) should be provided during chemotherapy because of 2° immunosuppression.

Alpha interferon

Best results in early KS if limited to the skin, CD4 count >200cells/μL, no systemic symptoms or history of OIs. Improvement in ~40%. Flu-like symptoms are usual, depression can occur, and neutropenia may develop (ameliorated by G-CSF though this ↑ constitutional symptoms).

Retinoic acid (oral and topical)

Variable data with ~33% showing some response.

Non-Hodgkin's lymphoma (NHL)

First cases of NHL in homosexual ♂ reported in 1982. Prior to HAART accounted for 2–3% of AIDS defining illnesses with haemophiliacs/those with other clotting disorders having the highest incidence. Occurs in up to 10% of those with AIDS although not necessarily as the presenting disease. Conflicting data on incidence since HAART introduced but survival improved.

NHL immunoblastic lymphoma in 60% (↑ with age), Burkitt's lymphoma 21% (most common 10–19 years), and 1° lymphoma of the brain in 19% (any age). Each type found twice as commonly in whites as in blacks and in ♂ as in ♀. ~95% are of B-cell origin with aggressive histological appearances. EBV episome is found in 40–50% overall, ranging from ~100% of 1° brain lymphoma to 20% of immunoblastic tumours.

Systemic lymphoma

Wide range of CD4 count at presentation including normal levels but median is 100cells/μL. Typically presents with lymphadenopathy, fever, weight loss (>10%), and night sweats. Extranodal disease (any site) usual with GI tract, CNS, bone marrow, and liver being frequently affected. GI presentation most common and NHL should be considered if suspicious symptoms (e.g. dysphagia, GI bleeding/pain).

Diagnosis and staging

- Biopsy of 1° lesion
- Staging by CT/MRI scanning and bone marrow biopsy

Management

- Chemotherapy (improved tolerance if CD4 count >200cells/μL) usually cyclical. PCP prophylaxis should be taken as treatment causes immunosuppression. Regimen examples include:
  - CHOP (cyclophosphamide, hydroxydaunomycin [doxorubicin], oncovin [vincristine], prednisolone). Addition of G-CSF reduces neutropenia. Reported response rate—67%
  - m-BACOD (methotrexate, bleomycin, doxorubicin, cyclophosphamide, vincristine, dexamethasone). Reported response rate—46%.
- Rituximab (monoclonal antibody causing B-cell lysis)—if resistance to chemotherapy. Has also been used in combination with CHOP.

Survival better than with 1° brain lymphoma and has ↑ since the introduction of HAART, although its optimal use during chemotherapy has not been established. Alternatives and their consequences are to:

- discontinue HAART—↑ HIV replication and exaggerated CD4 ↓
- continue HAART (with close monitoring)—risk of ↓ drug levels (with indinavir, didanosine, efavirenz, nevirapine) and ↑ side-effects
- modify HAART to ↓ interaction/side-effects.

Primary CNS lymphoma

An EBV induced tumour 1000× more frequent in those with HIV infection. Associated with very low CD4 count (<50cells/μL in 75%) and a history of OIs. Usually presents with confusion, amnesia, and lethargy. In addition focal symptoms may appear (e.g. seizures, hemiparesis, cranial nerve palsies, aphasia).

Diagnosis

Difficult to distinguish from cerebral toxoplasmosis.

- Computerized tomography (CT)/magnetic resonance imaging (MRI) Single (~50%) or multiple lesions. (Former suggests NHL as ~20% of those with toxoplasmosis have a single lesion).
- Fundal and slit lamp examination (20% have ocular involvement).
- Lumbar puncture for:
  - lymphoma cells
  - EBV DNA using PCR.
- Toxoplasma serology (toxoplasma unlikely if negative serology).
- Brain biopsy—usually delayed until failure of response to anti-toxoplasma therapy is demonstrated.

Management

- HAART ↑ survival.
- Whole brain radiotherapy (usually with short-term dexamethasone to reduce oedema)—response reported in up to 75% but median survival only up to 4.8 months.
- Combined radiotherapy and chemotherapy (no evidence of ↑ benefit).

Prognosis poor and partly dependant on control of other OIs. Has improved with HAART.

Primary effusion lymphoma (body cavity lymphoma)

Account for 5% of HIV associated lymphoma. Usually seen in homosexual ♂ and associated with HHV 8. Presents with effusions (pleural, pericardial, ascites).

Treat with chemotherapy (similar to systemic lymphoma) but poor prognosis (2–5 months).

Multicentric Castleman's disease

Induced by HHV-8 in HIV infection. Characterized by recurrent lymphadenopathy, fevers, hepatosplenomegaly, and sometimes KS. May be fatal even without frank malignant transformation.

Treat with combination chemotherapy, e.g. CHOP, steroids, anti-CD20 monoclonal antibodies. Prognosis is poor with a median survival of less than 30 months.

Hodgkin's disease

Although not an AIDS defining diagnosis found 8 times more commonly in those with AIDS. Tends to be more aggressive with the mixed cellularity subtype predominating. Associated with EBV infection, usually developing with CD4 counts 200–300cells/μL.

Presents with lymphadenopathy (glands often very large), Pel-Ebstein fever, anaemia, and weakness. Bone marrow and systemic involvement common. Diagnosed by lymph node or bone marrow histology (Reed–Sternberg cells).

Stages I/II most frequently treated with radiotherapy and stages III/IV with combination treatment, e.g. MOPP (mechlorethamine, oncovin [vincristine], procarbazine, prednisolone).

Invasive cervical carcinoma (ICC)

Added to the AIDS case definition in 1993 following reports showing ↑ prevalence of cervical dysplasia with HPV infection and immunosuppression (usually severe). However, no substantial clinical evidence demonstrating a ↑ incidence of ICC in ♀ with HIV not explained by other risk factors. May be due to the possibility of longer latency, improved screening and treatment to those at risk, and improved immunity with HAART.

Annual cervical cytology is advised. ICC should be managed as for ♀ without HIV infection. Abnormal cytology should be investigated by colposcopy with biopsy of suspicious areas. Mild dyskaryosis (CIN1) should be followed every 3–6 months as spontaneous regression is common. Standard treatment for moderate/severe dyskaryosis (CIN II and III) consists of lesional ablation or excision. Recurrence rate is higher in HIV infected ♀.

Anal carcinoma

Relation with HIV infection difficult to assess as both are associated with unprotected anal intercourse and multiple partners. Strongly linked with high grade HPV infection. Prior to the HIV epidemic the relative risk of anal carcinoma in homosexual ♂ was estimated to be 80-fold higher than heterosexual controls. Recent data suggests that HIV infected individuals with anal HPV infection are significantly more likely to develop high grade dyskaryosis or anal carcinoma if they acquire other local infections (e.g. gonorrhoea, syphilis, HSV). HAART does not appear to be protective. Although not routine clinical practice, anal cytology may be used to detect dyskaryosis. High/moderate grade lesions can be further investigated by anoscopy using a colposcope having pre-treated the anal canal with 3% acetic acid to allow identification of tissue for biopsy. Anal carcinoma is treated as for those without HIV infection. Limited data available on management of anal dyskaryosis but current practice suggests that treatment (by excision or laser ablation) should only be considered if severe dyskaryosis (AIN3).

Leiomyosarcoma

↑ rate in children with HIV when, unlike in HIV uninfected children, tumours are EBV induced.

Lung cancer

Eight-fold increase in HIV infection compared with age and gender matched controls and is not explained by smoking alone. Current rising incidence results from improved survival with HAART (its development is not immunodeficiency dependent). Compared to those HIV negative lung cancer usually occurs at a younger age and with advanced disease. Presentation similar with cough, chest pain, haemoptysis, and dyspnoea common symptoms and typical changes on x-ray. Both small cell and non-small cell tumours occur. Progression and response to treatment worse than with HIV negative patients and not improved by HAART. Chemotherapy poorly tolerated. Radiotherapy has a high rate of radiation oesophagitis. Prognosis can only be significantly improved with early diagnosis followed by curative surgical resection.

Chapter 53

HIV: management

Introduction

Highly active antiretroviral therapy (HAART) has produced dramatic improvements in the prognosis of HIV infection with ↓ rates of mortality and opportunist infections (OIs).

Important principles to consider in those under regular review are:

- treat before symptomatic disease or critical immunological damage;
- avoid treating earlier than necessary to ↓ long term drug side-effects;
- regimen choice must consider patient lifestyle, potential drug interactions, and side-effects while ensuring adequate antiviral potency.

Patient's commitment to starting treatment is essential. Pre-treatment adherence education is vital as adherence must be >95% to obtain both maximum magnitude and duration of antiviral effect. HAART rarely needs starting as an emergency.

Drug resistance should be assayed pre-treatment, ideally at diagnosis, because of possible resistant viral transmission.

When to start

Primary infection

Prime indication for treatment is severe symptoms (which may indicate risk of more rapid progression to symptomatic disease). These may resolve with HAART. Treatment duration is undefined and its influence on subsequent clinical course is uncertain.

Chronic infection

In the asymptomatic patient, the likelihood of developing clinical AIDS over a 3 year period can be predicted from a combination of viral load (VL) and CD4 count (see Fig. 53.1). CD4 counts give the best indication of OI risk but high VLs are associated with more rapid rates of CD4 ↓.

HAART should be offered:

- if HIV-related symptoms (independent of VL and CD4 count) are observed
- before CD4 counts have fallen <200cells/μL (if asymptomatic). The point of maximal 'cost-effectiveness' has not been defined by trial data but the consensus is that treatment should be commenced with CD4 counts 200–350cells/μL depending on:
  - rapidity of CD4 ↓
  - VL level
  - patient preference.

Other factors e.g. older age (↑ speed of development immunodeficiency) should also be considered. In pregnancy, treatment may be given to ↓ risk of mother to child transmission when such therapy may not be indicated in the non-pregnant state.

Starting HAART at very low CD4 counts ↑ drug side-effects although with nevirapine hepatotoxicity is ↑ by CD4 counts >250cells/μL. In patients with active OIs commencement of HAART should be deferred if possible until after completion/simplification of treatment for the OI, particularly tuberculosis (TB) as major drug interactions may occur.

Once started, treatment (except when given for fetal protection) should be continued indefinitely.

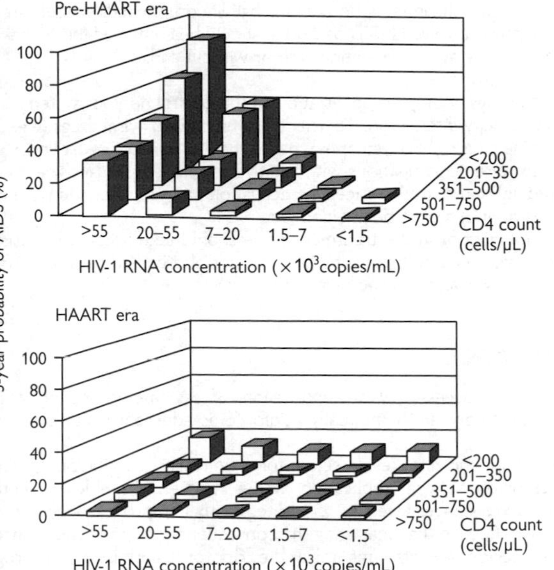

Fig. 53.1 Prognosis according to CD4 cell count and viral load in the pre-HAART and HAART eras. *Source*: Reprinted with permission from Elsevier (Egger M et al., *Lancet* 2002, 360, 119–29).

How to start

Initial treatment influences the pattern of resistance mutations. If it fails, the range of drugs available for 2nd line therapy is restricted. Therefore the following are important aims of the first treatment.

- Maximize adherence—especially important for regimens containing drugs where resistance may be produced by single mutations (e.g. lamivudine and NNRTIs).Treatment based on a ↓ CD4 count should be continued long term. Intermittent therapy should only be considered in those achieving full viral suppression. For fully informed patients insisting on this option the interruption of long half-life drugs needs special care. If efavirenz is involved NRTI backbone should be continued for 2 weeks at least after efavirenz cessation with or without a PI.
- Minimize drug reactions.
- Include drugs with good penetration to the central nervous system.
- Avoid toxicity/interaction. Toxicity of some antiretroviral drugs (e.g. stavudine causing lipodystrophy) makes them unsuitable as 1st line therapy. Drug combinations with additive toxicity (e.g. didanosine + stavudine) and shared intracellular activation pathways (e.g. zidovudine and stavudine) should be avoided (see p. 517).

Drug combinations in the treatment naïve should take account of resistance testing, co-pathologies, risk factors for diabetes and cardiovascular disease, lifestyle, and informed patient choice.

Adherence

Essential for successful viral suppression. Stress importance prior to starting treatment and continually reinforce as adherence may diminish with time.

Sub-therapeutic drug levels select for HIV resistant mutations arising from error-prone viral replication. Some regimens have low genetic barrier to resistance. Investing in strategies that improve adherence is more cost effective than managing the consequences of poor compliance. Such strategies will also minimize the risk of transmission of drug-resistant virus which may adversely affect HAART response in the newly infected.

Factors influencing adherence

- Patient
  - Commitment
  - Religious/cultural/health beliefs
  - Poor diet (may be related to socio-economic difficulties)
  - Need to take medication (seen by family/workmates)
  - Drug and alcohol use
  - Psychological (depression associated with low adherence)
  - Presence of symptoms/side-effects (may encourage/discourage adherence, respectively)
  - Relationship with healthcare team.

- Provider
  - Provision of adherence support services
  - Patient education.
- Regimen
  - Lifestyle assessment and compliance with regimen
  - Dosing frequency, pill burden, and food/fluid requirements.

How to improve adherence

Multi-factorial approach should be adopted, taking account of the patient's perceptions of the benefits as well as the practicalities of treatment. The individual's commitment to taking drugs should be assessed before starting therapy and at regular intervals. Concerns about drug side-effects should be explored. Motivational techniques can help patients strengthen their intentions and adherence behaviour. Psychosocial aspects including relationships, alcohol and drug use, housing, employment, and immigration status should be considered, with appropriate professional involvement. Measures that may improve adherence:

- programmable wristwatches, text messaging, telephone reminders, pill diaries and charts, medication containers, and help of family and friends;
- input from nurses, health advisers, psychologists, and pharmacists;
- written information.

There is no ideal and accurate method to monitor adherence. Self-reporting, pill counting, self-completed questionnaires, and drug levels have all been used with varying success.

What to start with

Current classes of antiretroviral drugs inhibit the virus at different stages of its cellular lifecycle (see Fig. 53.2):

- interaction with CD4/chemokine receptors—fusion inhibitors
- inhibition of reverse transcription (conversion of viral RNA to pro-viral DNA)
  - nucleoside/nucleotide reverse transcriptase inhibitors (NRTIs)
  - non-nucleoside reverse transcriptase inhibitors (NNRTIs)
  - inhibition of protease processing of viral sub-units leading to assembly of infective virions—protease inhibitors (PIs).

Other therapeutic targets in the viral lifecycle are under investigation.

Combination treatment

Triple combinations are the standard of care. The drug, classes have differing side-effects, drug interactions, and impact on co-pathologies. Individual drugs, within classes, may have significantly better convenience, tolerability, or side-effect profiles than others e.g. atazanavir (PI)—↓ effect on lipids and once a day therapy.

Standard regimens for both asymptomatic and late diseases

- 2 NRTIs (beware inadvisable combinations—see p. 517) plus a NNRTI;
- 2 NRTIs plus a PI (usually boosted with low dose ritonavir);
- Triple nucleoside analogue combinations (e.g. Trizivir®). Lack potency at high (>100,000copies/mL) VLs but have the advantages of simplicity and ↓ risks of drug interactions (useful in patients requiring simultaneous treatment for TB). Initial therapy should be restricted to patients with special adherence or drug interaction problems.

	NNRTI	PI
Advantages	1. Low pill burden 2. ↓lipid abnormalities/ central fat accumulation 3. Once daily doage possible	1. ↓skin rash/hepatotoxicity 2. ↓broad class resistance 3. High barrier to genetic resistance e.g. Kaletra®
Disadvantages	1. Class resistance with single mutations 2. Ineffective against HIV-2 (inherent resistance)	1. Heavy pill burden (most) 2. Hyperlipidaemia, insulin resistance, lipodystrophy, central fat distribution if predisposed 3. ↑ drug interactions 4. ↑ food/fluid requirements/ restrictions especially when unboosted

Currently most treatment naïve patients are started on NNRTI regimens. Efavirenz and nevirapine have different side-effect profiles but are of equivalent potency. Nevirapine is associated with skin rash and hepatic reactions and efavirenz, neuropsychological side-effects and potential teratogenicity.

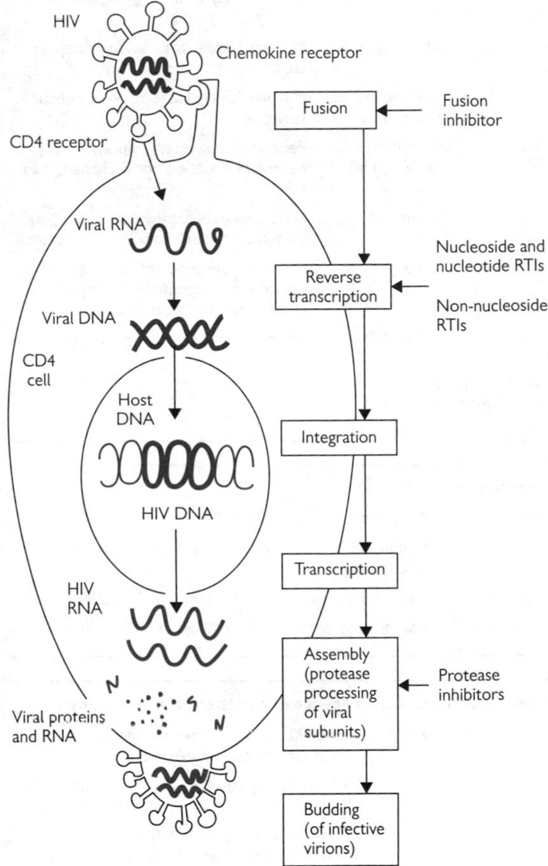

Fig. 53.2 HIV lifecycle and points of drug action

NRTIs (nucleotide—tenofovir). All oral

Abacavir* (ABC)	300mg bd	Hypersensitivity (may be fatal) in 4%: fever, malaise, rash, GI. **Do not rechallenge.**
Didanosine (DDI)	400mg if >60kg (or 300mg) daily	Take on empty stomach. Peripheral neuropathy, pancreatitis, nausea, diarrhoea. Rarely lactic acidosis, hepatic steatosis.
Emtricitabine (FTC)	200mg daily	Minimal. Rarely lactic acidosis, hepatic steatosis.
Lamivudine* (3TC)	150mg bd or 300mg daily†	Minimal. Rarely lactic acidosis, hepatic steatosis.
Stavudine* (D4T)	40mg if >60kg (or 30mg) bd	Peripheral neuropathy, lipodystrophy, pancreatitis, lactic acidosis, hepatic steatosis.
Zalcitabine (DDC)	0.75mg tid	Peripheral neuropathy, stomatitis, pancreatitis, lactic acidosis, hepatic steatosis.
Zidovudine* (AZT)	250–300mg bd	Bone marrow suppression (anaemia, neutropenia), myopathy. Rarely lactic acidosis, hepatic steatosis.
Tenofovir (TDF)	300mg daily	Asthenia, headache, GI, rarely renal insufficiency.

* Consistent CSF penetration.
† Reduce to 250mg when combined with TDF.

NRTI combined preparations

Combivir®	1 tablet bd, contains AZT 300mg + 3TC 150mg.
Trizivir®	1 tablet bd, contains AZT 300mg + 3TC 150mg + ABC 300mg.
Truvada®	1 tablet daily, contains TDF 300mg and FTC 200mg.
Kivexa®/Epzicom®	1 tablet daily contains ABC 600mg and 3TC 300mg.

NNRTIs. All oral and show evidence of consistent CSF penetration

Efavirenz (EFZ)	600mg daily	CNS effects (advise take at night), hepatitis, contra-indicated in pregnancy.
Nevirapine (NVP)	200mg bd or 400mg/day	Initially 200mg/day ↑ to 400mg/day after 2/52 Rash, Stevens–Johnson syndrome, hepatitis.
Delavirdine (DLV)	400mg tid	Diarrhoea, itching, and rash Not routinely available in the UK.

Boosted PI dosages with ritonavir (RTV), 100mg bd (except Kaletra® which already includes RTV) or 100mg daily with ATZ. All oral. When boosted, food restrictions are not critical. Only indinavir shows evidence of consistent CSF penetration		
Amprenavir (APV)	600mg (if >50kg) bd	GI, rash, oral pararthesia, lipodystrophy.
Atazanavir (ATZ)	300mg daily	Indirect hyperbilirubinaemia, cardiac conduction defect (prolonged PR interval).
Fosamprenavir (FPV)	700mg bd	GI, rash, lipodystrophy (less than other PIs).
Indinavir (IDV)	800mg bd	Nephrolithiasis, GI, indirect hyperbilirubinaemia lipodystrophy. ↑ fluids by 2L.
Kaletra® Lopinavir (LPV) 133.3mg + RTV 33.3mg	3 capsules bd	GI, ↑ transaminases, asthenia, lipodystrophy.
Saquinavir tabs	1.0g bd	GI, headache, ↑ transaminase, lipodystrophy.

PIs used without additional PI boosting. Both oral		
Nelfinavir (NFV)	1.25g bd	Take with food Diarrhoea, ↑ transaminase, lipodystrophy.
Ritonavir (RTV)	600mg bd	Take with food GI, parasthesia, hepatitis, raised transaminase, pancreatitis, lipodystrophy.

Fusion inhibitor (FI). Licensed for treatment failure. Subcutaneous administration		
Enfuvirtide (ENF)	90mg bd	Injection site reaction, ↑ pneumonia, hypersensitivity reaction (may recur on re-challenge)

Antiretroviral drug combinations to avoid

- D4T+AZT—thymidine analogues compete for the same intracellular enzyme plus antagonistic effect;
- FTC+3TC—cytosine analogues—no additive activity;
- ABC+3TC+TDF—↑ virological failure.
- DDI + TDF + EFZ—↑ virological failure in treatment naive patients.

Caution with

- DDI and D4T—↑ peripheral neuropathy, lactic acidosis, and acute pancreatitis, especially in pregnancy;
- DDC+DDI—↑ peripheral neuropathy;
- DDC+D4T—↑ peripheral neuropathy.

Monitoring therapy

Side-effects are very common with HAART although most spontaneously resolve after a few weeks. Patients should be asked to report side-effects and be given written information about serious complications e.g. abacavir hypersensitivity reactions. Consideration should be given to providing anti-emetics and anti-diarrhoeal agents for the common early gastrointestinal symptoms. Sedatives may be needed for severe EFZ associated insomnia/vivid dreams.

Routine tests

- Full blood count, liver function (LFTs)/renal function tests—should be checked 2 weeks into treatment and then at subsequent clinic visits. Patients who develop abnormal LFTs or a significant anion gap should have plasma lactate level checked.
- VL—the rate of fall on therapy is a useful prognostic indicator. Whatever the pre-treatment VL, suppression to a level of 1,000copies/mL or less is achievable in most patients by 4 weeks. When not attained associated with longer term failure. The success of a treatment combination can be judged by achieving a VL of <50copies/mL within 3–6 months, then maintained for 48 weeks.
- CD4 count—usually ↑ with viral suppression initially as a result of re-circulated existing reserves. Further ↑ and maintenance of continuous production of CD4 cells dependant on ability of thymus to produce new T cells. Complete restoration does not occur in most chronically infected patients but immune reconstitution occurs to varying degrees even in those who achieve limited viral suppression. Prophylaxis against PCP can be discontinued in those responding to therapy (CD4 count >200cells/μL for at least 3–6 months).

Both CD4 and VL should be checked and repeated at 4 weeks and 12 weeks into therapy and then at 3 monthly intervals if virological control is achieved.

- Lipid profiles—should be checked 3 monthly and major abnormalities addressed. Monitor for the development of lipodystrophy and consider early treatment switches if apparent. Elevated random lipids should be re-measured while fasting.
- Blood sugar levels—should be monitored, particularly with PI therapy. Fasting blood sugar should be measured if random level elevated.

Adherence reinforcement should be undertaken at each visit. Risk of acquisition of co-infections and STIs should be assessed and tested for when appropriate.

Therapeutic drug monitoring (TDM)

Up to 35% of patients taking PIs have sub-optimal drug concentrations with ~50% developing virological failure. A fixed drug dose may not be appropriate for all patients. Measuring drug levels to determine therapeutic dose may help promote durable viral suppression and ↓ resistance. Dose–response and concentration–response relationships have been identified for PIs and NNRTIs (some data for NRTIs).

Potential use of TDM

Only of value if highly adherent (>95%) and at steady-state conditions (after at least 14 days of therapy). Blood samples should be obtained at the end of the dosing interval, as close to minimum concentration (Cmin) as possible, to enable comparison with product monograph concentrations. TDM can be of benefit in:

- pregnant ♀ and children—may have altered/highly variable pharmacokinetics;
- highly adherent individuals who have poor initial or transient viral responses not explained by viral resistance. In these situations Cmin values may assist in assessing genetically determined high hepatic metabolic rates, poor absorption, or drug interactions that prevent adequate drug levels. Adjusting antiretroviral doses to achieve Cmin values within 30% of the mean/median value of the product monograph may ↑ likelihood of adequate therapeutic levels and viral response;
- those on new drug therapy with unknown/potential drug interactions;
- those on once daily PI—ensures adequate 24 hour drug concentration.

Major drug side-effects and interactions

Mitochondrial toxicity

A mechanism by which NRTIs may cause myopathy, peripheral neuropathy, hepatic steatosis, lactic acidosis, and, in infants, neurological disease. However, the link is strongest with lactic acidosis. This has been reported in infants born to mothers receiving AZT or 3TC+AZT. D4T+DDI has been associated with lactic acidosis in pregnancy and should be avoided/switched. Caused by inhibition of mitochondrial γ DNA polymerase, the enzyme responsible for DNA synthesis, but effects on other mitochondrial enzymes may contribute. D4T, DDC, and DDI inhibit γ DNA polymerase whereas AZT inhibits other mitochondrial enzymes. Hence toxicity induced by D4T improves on switching to AZT or ABC.

Hyperlactataemia

Clinical significance of isolated hyperlactataemia (venous lactate between 2.5 and 5.0mmol/L) unknown. Routine measurement of venous lactate and anion gap in asymptomatic patients not recommended.

Lactic acidosis

Characterized by arterial pH <7.35 and venous lactate >5mmol/L (sample taken without tourniquet into tube containing fluoride-oxalate, transported immediately on ice to laboratory). Occurs most frequently with D4T and in ♀. Usually develops after several months of treatment. Main features are nausea, vomiting, weight loss, fatigue, abdominal pain, tender hepatomegaly, and respiratory failure. Laboratory findings:

- venous lactate >5.0mmol/L, metabolic acidosis, high anion gap (usually >18mmol/L);
- ultrasound and CT abdomen—hepatomegaly with fatty infiltration (microvascular steatosis found on liver biopsy);
- may find—↑ hepatic transaminases, creatine kinase, lactate dehydrogenase, and amylase.

Management

Diagnosis must be considered in any patient presenting with nausea, vomiting, abdominal pain, and abnormal LFTs. Essential to discontinue antiretroviral medication and to exclude other causes. Supportive therapy required with fluid replacement, oxygen therapy and, if necessary, assisted ventilation and haemodialysis. Benefit from carnitine, thiamine, co-enzyme Q, and riboflavin is limited.

Peripheral neuropathy

Risk of drug induced peripheral neuropathy ↑ with HIV disease progression. Reported with NRTIs, more frequent with DDC, D4T, and DDI. Presents with distal symmetric polyneuropathy (DSP), which may be difficult to differentiate from HIV-related DSP but tends to be painful, more sudden and progressive. Discontinuation of the offending NRTI may result in improvement but symptoms may deteriorate for several weeks. Pain relief may be obtained with acetyl-L-carnitine, tricyclic antidepressants, anticonvulsants (gabapentin and lamotrigine), and recombinant human nerve growth factor.

Important antiretroviral interactions with other drugs

Drug	ART	Effect	Action
Terfenadine	All PIs and NNRTIs	Dangerous arrhythmias	Use loratidine or cetirizine
Midazolam and triazolam	All PIs and EFZ	Increased sedating effect	Use alternative sedative
Rifampicin	All PIs and NNRTIs	Complex effect on cytochrome P450	Use rifabutin instead
Rifabutin	SQV	↓ SQV by 40%	Do not use SQV unless RTV boosted
Rifabutin	RTV	↑ rifabutin 4-fold,	↓ rifabutin dose to 150mg/day, continue same dose of RTV
Rifabutin	Other PIs	↑ rifabutin level and ↓ PI level	↓ rifabutin to 150mg/day and ↑ PI dose as appropriate
Phosphodiesterase-5 inhibitors (used for erectile dysfunction)	All PIs	↑ blood levels and side-effects	Use smallest possible dose
Methadone	NNRTIs	↑ metabolism of methadone leading to withdrawal symptoms	↑ methadone dose
Simvastatin	All PIs and DLV	Large ↑ in simvastatin levels—↑ myositis	Use pravastatin

* All PIs are substrate and inhibitors of cytochrome P450 (CYP450)—RTV the strongest, SQV the weakest.

* NNRTIs, NVP and EFZ induce CYP450.

* St John's wort (*Hypericum perforatum*) is a strong inducer of CYP450 and should not be used with PIs or NNRTIs.

Abnormal liver function test and hepatotoxicity

Reported with all classes of antiretrovirals. ↑ in ♂ and in those with other predisposing risk factors e.g. excessive alcohol consumption, hepatitis B (HBV) and hepatitis C virus (HCV) infections. Abnormal LFTs graded from 1 (ALT 2–3 x upper limit of normal) to 4 (ALT >10 x upper limit of normal). Minor abnormalities do not require intervention apart from monitoring.

Abnormal LFTs found in those on antiretroviral treatment:

- NRTIs—commonly reported with DDI, D4T, and AZT. Hepatotoxicity—part of ABC hypersensitivity (usually associated with skin rash, fever, and eosinophilia)
- NNRTIs—8% with EFZ and 15% NVP (hepatotoxicity in 4%). ♀ and those with higher CD4 count at ↑ risk.
- PIs—up to 30%, most frequent with RTV containing regimens. Co-infection with HCV infection reported in most.

Avoidance and management

Careful history including alcohol intake. Screen for HBV and HCV. Important to measure LFTs before starting HAART. Asymptomatic ↑ of ALT (especially grade 1–3) does not normally require any action apart from close monitoring, exclusion, and treatment of underlying aggravating factors. Isolated hyperbilirubinaemia 2° to IDV and ATZ not clinically significant.

Specific action required with:

- grade 4 ALT ↑—stop offending drugs;
- symptomatic hepatotoxicity—stop all drugs until symptoms resolve. NVP should not be re-started if it was the cause;
- symptomatic ↑ of ALT with hyperlacataemia—stop offending drugs;
- ABC hypersensitivity reaction—stop immediately and do not rechallenge (fatal reaction).

Acute pancreatitis

Most commonly implicated NRTIs are DDI (up to 7%) and D4T. They should not be combined. Possibly caused by mitochondrial toxicity or direct toxic effect of the pancreas. Risk ↑ in ♀ especially with CD4 <200cell/μL, excessive alcohol use and nutritional deficiencies.

Presents with acute abdomen ± nausea and vomiting. Differentiate from other causes of acute abdomen e.g. cholecystitis and intestinal obstruction. Serum amylase usually ↑, may be normal (can also be ↑ in other causes of acute abdomen). DDI can ↑ salivary amylase, usually associated with sicca syndrome. Diagnostic accuracy higher if serum lipase also ↑. Ultrasound and CT scan of the abdomen may help establish diagnosis, extent of disease, and complications e.g. pancreatic abscess, pseudocyst.

Management

Monitor circulatory, renal, and liver functions (in a high dependency unit if necessary). Support with analgesia, fluid, and nutrition. Stop antiretrovirals or substitute the implicated drug with TDF or a non-NRTI regimen.

Drug-related skin rash

Skin reactions are common. Most frequently found with NNRTIs (NVP 16%, EFZ 4%) and ABC 8%. NVP induced rash typically occurs in first two weeks of therapy. An induction dose of half the maintenance dose for two weeks minimizes this risk. Typically maculopapular, affecting the trunk. Systemic symptoms occur with more severe reactions seen especially with ABC. Toxic epidermal necrolysis and Stevens–Johnson syndrome reported in 0.5%.

Management

Mild skin rash does not require intervention and will often settle spontaneously (with continuation of antiretrovirals). Antihistamines may be needed for symptomatic relief. More severe reactions need drug switching e.g. EFZ may replace NVP.

ABC hypersensitivity reaction

Occurs in ~4%, usually in the first 6 weeks of therapy (94%), median 11 days. Normally presents with ≥2 of following features: GI tract (nausea, vomiting, diarrhoea, pain), headache, fever, malaise, maculopapular or urticarial rash, abnormal LFTs, myalgia, dyspnoea, cough, respiratory distress, and eosinophilia. Once suspected, ABC should be stopped promptly and supportive treatment instituted. Symptoms, except rash resolve in 24–48 hours.

⚠ ABC should not be used again as mortality from rechallenge is 4%.

Lipodystrophy

See p. 466.

Immune reconstitution

CD4 count ↑ on HAART mainly due to CD4 memory cells in first 4 months then followed by ↑ naïve cells associated with ↓ CD4 activation markers, due to ↓ viral replication. Initial phase of CD8 ↑ followed by a second phase of ↓. Most studies demonstrate ↓ HIV-specific immune responses and ↓ CD8 responses towards HIV. This contrasts with ↑ immune responses against other pathogens. ↓ incidence of OIs in patients who have higher CD4 counts from HAART. HIV damages thymus and lymphoid tissue at an early stage and may ↓ immune recovery. ↓ immune response may in part be due to failure of the thymus, as demonstrated by ↓ thymus emigrants measured in peripheral blood. The lower the CD4 nadir the slower and less complete immune reconstitution is likely to be.

Immune recovery inflammatory response (IRIS)

Inflammatory response induced by HAART occurring at sites of clinical and subclinical disease, usually seen in patients with CD4 count <100cells/μL at the initiation of therapy. The enhanced immunity is the likely mechanism converting a subclinical infection to an apparent symptomatic one due to the expansion of CD4 memory cells. Examples of IRIS include:

- cytomegalovirus retinitis—4–8 weeks after HAART. Immune recovery uveitis may occur in patients with previous CMV retinitis. Patients with active and subclinical infection and those with CD4 <50/μL are at special risk.
- HCV—restoration of HCV-specific responses occurs during HAART in patients with pre-existing HCV infection. Patients with negative HCV antibody but detectable HCV–RNA seroconvert with immune restoration. HCV–RNA levels ↑ with HAART especially if treatment is started when CD4 count >350cells/μL. Accompanied by transient ALT ↑.
- *Mycobacterium avium* complex (MAC)—presents with localized disease e.g. painful lymphadenopathy or inflammatory masses associated with suppuration, unlike classical MAC where it is a disseminated infection. Due to the restoration of delayed hypersensitivity.
- Herpes zoster—↑ by 5 times the expected rate, occurring in the first 4 months of HAART. Seen more frequently in those who develop a significant CD8 ↑.
- TB—paradoxical tuberculous reaction e.g. ↑ in lymph node size, fever, and appearance of TB at other sites. Usually occurs in first 2 months (often 2–4 weeks) of starting TB therapy. Medication should not be routinely stopped. Steroids may be beneficial in controlling inflammatory process.
- Herpes simplex virus—more frequent and severe disease occurs in patients responding to HAART.
- Progressive multifocal leukoencephalopathy—may present for the first time or become worse in patients responding to HAART. Inflammatory brain changes (perivascular lymphocyte, macrophage, and plasma cell infiltrate) are more severe. CD8 seems to mediate the immunopathological process to JC virus.

Frequently asked questions

When do I start treatment?

Treatment is usually started when the CD4 level ↓, ideally before itreaches 200cells/μL. The aim of treatment is to suppress viral replication, measured by the viral load (VL), and this should later be followed by ↑ in CD4 count. A combination of 3 antiretroviral drugs is usually used termed HAART (highly active antiretroviral therapy).

What is drug resistance?

The HIV virus can develop resistance by mutating so that it can replicatein spite of the antiretroviral treatment. This most commonly arises when medication is not taken reliably. If a person is infected with a drug resistant strain of HIV virus their treatment options will be ↓ (some times severely).

Do I need to use condoms even if my partner is also known to be HIV positive?

Yes, it is important to practice safe sex to avoid superinfection (becoming infected with another strain of HIV) which may adversely affect the immune system and carry drug resistance.

Does it matter if I forget to take my medication for a few days?

Yes. It is very important that you take your anti-HIV drugs regularly. If doses are missed the virus may not be suppressed and there is ↑ risk of viral mutations and drug resistance.

If my VL is undetectable, does it mean I am no longer infectious?

No. An undetectable VL does not mean that there is no virus in the blood. It just means that there are too few particles to be detected on the test. There is still a risk of transmission with a low VL and so you must continue to practise safe sex.

When will I get AIDS?

Current therapy has had a dramatic effect in improving the well-being and life expectancy of people with HIV. Effective therapy makes HIV a chronic rather than a life-threatening infection. Therefore it is likely that you may not develop AIDS. Some people never need treatment but if it is started it must be taken consistently and probably for life.

HIV drug resistance

May be intrinsic, e.g. HIV-2 resistance to NNRTIs, or acquired as a result of mutations in viral proteins targeted by antiretroviral agents. Two factors drive mutations: high rate of viral replication (10^{8-10} virions produced daily) and error-prone reverse transcription (1 base pair substitution, deletion, insertion, recombination for every genome transcription).

1° mutation predates antiretroviral treatment which selects for it. 2° mutation develops during HAART and may be additive to 1°. HAART ↓ development of resistance by suppressing viral replication and thus generation of new variants. It can also suppress existing mutants if they are not resistant to all drugs in the regimen. However, resistance emerges if drug levels are insufficient to block viral replication but high enough to exert a positive selective pressure on these mutants. Even with undetectable VL low-level replication may allow resistance to develop. Drug resistance has been demonstrated in up to 25% of patients on HAART. Compensatory (2°) mutation reverses ↓ viral fitness resulting from other mutations. Some mutations induce resistance to certain agents while simultaneously producing hypersusceptibility to others (e.g. M184V ↑ sensitivity to AZT).

Mutations

Many mutations ↓ viral fitness. However, resistance mutations confer a selective advantage by ↓ susceptibility to antiviral agents, thereby enabling the mutant quasispecies to proliferate under treatment with those agents. Resistance mutations are described using a number referring to the affected codon (group of 3 nucleotides coding for an amino acid). A letter may be added after the number to denote amino acid in the mutant e.g. 74V ('V'aline). This may be coupled with another preceding the number to show the wild type amino acid, e.g. L74V ('L'eucine → 'V'aline). Resistance develops rapidly (within weeks of commencing treatment) if only a single mutation is required e.g. M184V (3TC, FTC) and K103N (NVP). It evolves more gradually if multiple mutations are required e.g. AZT, ABC, or PIs. Additional requirements may include a compensatory mutation e.g. 30N (NFV).

K65R mutation (selected by TDF, ABC, DDI, and DDC) confers resistance to TDF, ABC, and 3TC and ↑ susceptibility to AZT and D4T. This mutation develops rapidly when regimens combining TDF with 2 of ABC, DDI or 3TC are given to the treatment naïve. Co-existence of K65R and M184V ↑ resistance to ABC and DDI but retains susceptibility to TDF, AZT, and D4T. Regimen with TDF must include AZT or a PI/NNRTI.

Multiple mutations may interact. Prediction of resulting resistance patterns may be made by matching with resistance profile databases. This is provided by commercial resistance tests (e.g. *Virtual* Phenotype™).

Databases of resistance profiles available at:

http://hivdb.stanford.edu (Stanford-Database)

www.hiv.lanl.gov/content/index (Los Alamos-Database)

www.hivfrenchresistance.org (HIV-1 genotypic drug resistance interpretation's algorithms).

Examples of resistance mutations (affected codons)

Nucleoside and nucleotide		
3TC/FTC	184, 44, 118	
ABC	65, 74, 115, 184	
AZT/D4T	41, 44, 67, 70, 118, 210, 215, 219	
	(Thymidine analogue mutations—TAMs, now known as multi-NRTI associated—NAMs)	
DDI	65, 74	
TDF	65, ≥3 NAMs including 41 or 210	
Multi-nucleoside		
'151 complex'	62, 75, 77, 116, 151	
69 insertion complex	41, 62, 67, 69 (insertion), 70, 210, 215, 219	
NNRTI		
Multi-NNRTI single	103, 106, 188	
requiring 2	100, 181, 190, 230	
EFV or NVP	Any of above alone, 108, 188	
Protease inhibitors		
	major	**minor**
APV	50V	10, 32, 46, 47, 54, 73, 90
ATV	50L	32, 46, 54, 71, 82, 84, 88, 90
IDV	46, 82, 84	10, 20, 24, 32, 36, 54, 71, 73, 77, 90
NFV	30, 90	10, 36, 46, 71, 77, 82, 84, 88
SQV	48, 90	10, 54, 71, 73, 77, 82, 84
RTV	82, 84	10, 20, 32, 33, 36, 46, 54, 71, 77, 90
LPV/RTV (4–6 required)	10, 20, 24, 32, 33, 46, 47, 50V, 53, 54, 63, 71, 73, 82, 84, 90	
Multiple (if >4)	10, 46, 54, 82, 84, 90	10, 54

Persistence of mutation/resistance

When treatment that selected for resistant quasispecies is discontinued wild-type virus usually becomes predominant within 2 months. Drug-resistant mutants occasionally remain dominant, e.g. 41L (zidovudine) but usually cease to be detectable by standard assay. However, they may still persist as minority quasispecies e.g. 90M (PI) or latent integrated proviral DNA (archived resistance). Standard assays therefore may not exclude drug resistance if carried out >1 month after stopping failing regimen. Interpretation of resistance mutations must take into account previous treatment history including evidence of viral persistence.

Resistance testing

Standard resistance assays require VL of ≥1000copies/mL and cannot detect minority species. Expert advice needed in interpreting results.

Genotyping

Viral genes sequenced to identify key mutations known to confer (alone or with others) resistance. Current methodology only detects viral mutants comprising at least 20–30% of the total population. Analysis is based on known correlation between genotype and phenotype from previous studies. Results normally available in ~4 weeks.

Phenotyping

Viral cell cultures are set up with increasing concentrations of antiretroviral drugs to determine IC50, the concentration of drug required to inhibit viral replication by 50%. Cut-off value indicates by which factor the IC50 of an HIV isolate can be ↑ while still being classified as susceptible (when compared with a wild-type control). IC50 above this value indicates resistance. Usually takes longer than genotyping.

Efflux pumps

P-glycoprotein (P-gp) and multi-drug resistance associated protein 1 (MRP1) are human cell membrane constituents, known as efflux pumps. Found in the lining of intestine, renal tubules, biliary canaliculi, capillaries in brain, testes, placenta; stem cells, lymphocytes, and macrophages. Their function is to protect tissues by actively transporting foreign substance out of cells. Cell membrane expression of P-gp/MRP1 and resulting activity of efflux pump vary depending on genetic polymorphism and induction or inhibition by various factors including HIV infection (↑ P-gp in advanced stage). PIs may be subject to efflux action resulting in ↓ absorption (intestinal P-gp) or ↓ levels in CD4 cells leading to ↓ response to treatment with ↑ likelihood of resistance mutations.

Clinical application of resistance testing

Now recommended soon after diagnosis of HIV infection. It is particularly required in the following situations:

- 1° infection (to identify transmitted resistance);
- pregnancy (to ↑ likelihood of viral suppression in the short time scale);
- virological failure of HAART (to guide choice of next regimen).

Studies suggest that HAART achieves better viral suppression when guided by resistance testing (with expert interpretation).

When to switch and options

Treatment switches may be required for intolerance, side-effects, metabolic disorders, or virological failure (defined as viral rebound or failure to achieve initial viral suppression).

In patients where new 3-drug options (that are likely to fully suppress viral replication) are available, switches should be considered when there have been 2 or more consecutive viral loads >400copies/mL having excluded other explanations (e.g. intercurrent infection). Also important to exclude poor adherence or factors leading to ↓ drug levels before switching. Viral resistance testing should be done. Results may allow partial regimen change. If, due to previous treatment, decisions are difficult it may be wise to wait until VL has reached an amplifiable level before switching. Single drug switches can be made for drug related problems (e.g. side-effects) if satisfactory viral suppression.

In the absence of resistance data first treatment switches are influenced by initial therapy. Options to consider for:

- 2 NRTIs + PI regimens:
  - switch to 2 new NRTIs + a NNRTI;
  - if there is likely to be NRTI cross-resistance—a new boosted PI + a NNRTI and a new NRTI.

Amprenavir may retain activity after other PI failures and boosted lopinavir requires multiple resistance mutations to lose efficacy.

- 2 NRTI + NNRTI regimens—switch to a boosted PI and 2 new NRTIs.
- triple NRTI—switch to a PI + a NNRTI + a new NRTI.

Failing regimens may be continued if no viable treatment change possible. If viral load moderate and immune function stable residual antiviral activity is likely to be beneficial.

Enfuvirtide—a complex 36 amino acid peptide that inhibits HIV (syncytium and non-syncytium inducing) fusion to CD4 cells. Its sequence is derived from HIV gp41. Has low potential for metabolic complications or drug interactions because of extracellular site of action. Resistance can develop by amino acid sequence changes in binding region of gp41 but unlikely to have cross resistance with other drug classes. Administered by sub-cutaneous injection (injection site reactions may occur). May be used as add-on therapy when no other options available for treatment change but in this situation resistance may develop quickly. The best use is in combination with conventional drugs optimized on the basis of resistance profiling.

Other options include structured treatment interruptions to allow re-emergence of wild type virus and then to re-treat. However, there is likely to be a significant ↓ in CD4 count which may not recover on re-treatment (response may be limited due to the re-emergence of the resistant strains). Use of multiple drug combinations may have some medium term effect but suffer from major problems of tolerability.

In addition to therapies aimed directly at the virus, treatments improving CD4 numbers or stimulating immune responses are options.

Adjuvant therapy

Immune therapy

Pathogenesis of HIV is complex involving interactions between virus and immune system. Precise immune control of HIV infection not fully understood. HIV infection characterized by ↑ production of certain cytokines (e.g. interleukin (IL)1, IL6, tumour necrosis factor) and ↓ production of others (e.g. IL2, IL12, and interferon gamma).

HAART partially reverses some immune abnormalities but most patients, even with full viral suppression, lack effective HIV-specific responses. Especially common if treatment commenced in advanced disease. Immune therapy may improve these responses.

Cytokine therapy

HIV infection results in gradual ↓ production and response to endogenous IL2. Synthesized by CD4 cells it induces proliferation and differentiation of CD4 and CD8 cells. IL2 given subcutaneously as an intermittent course produces ↑ CD4 count if given alone but more enhanced when combined with HAART. Viral load does not ↑ but long term effects unknown. Side-effects such as fever, tachycardia, hypotension, and respiratory failure are typically dose-dependent and can limit its use.

Immune stimulation

Endogenous (structured treatment interruptions) or exogenous antigens (therapeutic vaccination) are other ways of stimulating immune responses. Remune (Th1 stimulant) and ALVAC vcp 1452 are examples of therapeutic vaccines which have shown immunological benefit.

Structured treatment interruptions

Failure of HAART to restore HIV-specific immune responses may be related to loss of antigen presentation. Viral rebound following treatment interruption presents fresh HIV antigens to the immune system facilitating rapid response by resting memory cells. Structured treatment interruption allows for emergence of wild-type virus, more responsive to antiretrovirals. It may be considered as a salvage therapeutic intervention for multi-drug resistance. Main drawbacks are a rapid rebound of virus, re-emergence of archived drug resistant virus, ↓ CD4 count and development of an acute retroviral syndrome.

Hydroxyurea

Acts by reducing cellular adenine (a nucleotide necessary for DNA synthesis) by inhibiting the enzymes needed for its production. It enhances antiretroviral activity (and toxicity) of adenosine analogues, such as DDI and induces cellular kinases that phosphorylate NRTIs, ↑ their antiretroviral activity (and toxicity). Main side-effects are bone marrow suppression (dose dependant), pancreatitis, and liver toxicity. Optimum dose unknown (usually given as 500mg twice daily) and so far no major trial evidence of benefit.

Post-exposure prophylaxis (PEP)

Following occupational or non-sexual contact

Case-control study conducted by the US Centers for Disease Control (CDC) has shown that zidovudine PEP given to those occupationally exposed to HIV was associated with an 80% ↓ in infection. Combination treatment, demonstrably more potent and less likely to be affected by viral resistance, now recommended.

Therefore consider if contact with HIV likely through:

- percutaneous injury (e.g. from needles, instruments, bone fragments, bites which break the skin);
- exposure of broken skin (e.g. abrasions, cuts, eczema);
- exposure of mucous membranes (including the eye).

Average risk for HIV transmission after percutaneous exposure to HIV-infected blood in health care settings is ~3/1000 injuries. ↑ with large volumes of blood, deep injury, and high VL. After mucocutaneous exposure average risk is ~1/1000. No risk of HIV transmission if intact skin exposed to HIV-infected body fluids.

If HIV status of source is unknown a designated doctor (not exposed worker) should obtain consent for HIV and other blood-borne virus testing.

Management

Wash skin or exposed wound with soap and water, without scrubbing and antiseptics. Bleeding of puncture wounds should be encouraged. Exposed mucous membranes, including conjunctivae, should be liberally irrigated with water, before and after removing any contact lenses.

Following a discussion of risks and benefits, PEP should be recommended to HCPs if they have had a significant occupational exposure to blood or other high risk body fluid from someone either known to be HIV infected, or considered to be at high risk of HIV infection. PEP should be commenced as soon as possible after the event and should be continued for 4 weeks. UK DoH guidance states that PEP may still be worth considering even if 2 weeks have elapsed following exposure however studies suggest that delays >72 hours may render PEP ineffective.

Following sexual contact

Limited data but reports from Brazil and S. Africa suggest that PEP may provide some protection. Use of PEP following sexual exposure to HIV is only recommended within 72 hours of exposure (as early as possible).

Risk benefit assessment should be made considering risk of transmission according to coital act (see box) and likelihood of source being HIV +ve (see p. 347). Other factors to consider include possibility of pre-existing HIV infection, and ability to adhere to/tolerate proposed antiretroviral regimen.

Situations when PEP following sexual exposure is recommended (from BASHH guidelines)

- Unprotected contact with known HIV +ve individual
  - receptive and insertive anal sex
  - receptive and insertive vaginal sex.
- Unprotected contact with unknown HIV status where prevalence is >10%.
  - receptive anal sex.

PEP regimens

- Combivir® (AZT 300mg + 3TC 150mg) twice daily + NFV 1.25g twice daily.
- Alternatives for AZT are D4T or TDF and for NFV is LPV/RTV (Kaletra®).

PEP continued for 1 month. A negative antibody test 6 months after completing PEP confirms that infection has been avoided.

HIV: pregnancy

Preconception

Advise HIV discordant couples wishing to conceive on maximizing the chance of conception while minimizing the risk of sexual transmission.

♀ HIV +ve/♂ HIV –ve

Advise on how to perform artificial insemination at the time of ovulation, using quills, syringes, and Gallipots.

♂ HIV +ve/♀ HIV –ve

- Transmission risk ~1:500 per unprotected sexual act, therefore after discussion of risk advise unprotected sexual intercourse around the time of ovulation.
- Sperm washing, spermatozoa separated from surrounding HIV-infected seminal plasma by a sperm swim-up technique, is available in a number of centres in the UK. To date, there have been no cases of seroconversion in ♀ inseminated with washed sperm.
- If ♂ has low sperm count, intracytoplasmic sperm injection following sperm washing may be offered.

In vitro fertilization

Now considered ethically acceptable for subfertility because of vertical transmission rates of <2% and ↑ life expectancy for parents taking HAART.

The effectiveness of pre-conceptual folic acid for those requiring such prophylaxis is unknown although a higher, 5mg dose is recommended.

Contraception

See p. 332.

Mother to child (vertical) HIV transmission without intervention

Vertical transmission rates vary from 15 to 20% in non-breastfeeding European ♀ to 25–40% in African ♀ who breastfeed. Although transmission is associated with advanced HIV disease and low antenatal CD4 count a high maternal VL is the strongest individual predictor.

In ♀ who do not breastfeed >80% of vertical transmission occurs late in the 3rd trimester (from 36 weeks), during labour and at delivery, with <2% during the 1st and 2nd trimesters. The main obstetric risk factors are vaginal delivery, duration of membrane rupture, chorioamnionitis, and preterm delivery. It is estimated that breastfeeding ↑ the mother to child transmission rate by 14% for ♀ infected with HIV before birth and by 30% in those infected postnatally.

In ♀ without advanced disease N. American and European studies suggest no ↑ risk of accelerated immunosuppression during pregnancy. CD4 counts may fall but return to pre-pregnancy levels after delivery.

Frequently asked questions

Can I get pregnant?

It is possible for an HIV +ve ♀ to have a baby. The risk of vertical transmission is 15–40% but this is ↓ to <2% with retroviral treatment, caesarean section (if viral suppression inadequate) and avoidance of breastfeeding. Also the parents' life expectancy is ↑ with treatment if it is required. Artificial insemination techniques avoid the risk of transmission to an HIV –ve ♂ partner and sperm washing ↓ the risk of a positive ♂ infecting a ♀.

Can I have a vaginal delivery?

It is generally advisable to have an elective caesarean section as it ↓ the risk of vertical transmission by 50%. However, if there is good viral suppression vaginal delivery may be acceptable.

Can I breast feed?

No. There is a high risk of mother to child transmission with breastfeeding.

Vertical HIV transmission with intervention

Transmission rate has been reduced to <2% by:
- anti-retroviral therapy, given antenatally and intrapartum to the mother and to the neonate for the first 4–6 weeks of life
- delivery by elective caesarean section
- avoidance of breastfeeding.

Management

▶ Guidance on the management of HIV infection changes rapidly with new evidence. It is therefore important to consult contemporary guidelines (see useful resources).

Identification

Routine antenatal HIV antibody testing should be advised and offered to all pregnant ♀ in early pregnancy (usually at booking). Midwives must be able to provide information on the benefits of early diagnosis ensuring that an expert sees newly diagnosed cases promptly. Management during pregnancy should be multidisciplinary involving an obstetrician, HIV physician, midwife, paediatrician, and appropriate others (e.g. social worker, psychologist). Partner notification should be managed with the ♀'s co-operation and support. However, in the absence of this, the ♀'s HIV status may be disclosed to an at-risk sexual contact (for his protection) although the ♀ must be informed and the clinician able to justify this action. Otherwise assurances should be given regarding confidentiality especially relating to friends and relatives accompanying the ♀ who may be unaware of her HIV diagnosis.

Advice should be given about avoiding unprotected sexual intercourse both for the benefit of partner(s) and the safety of the ♀.

Assessment and screening

Repeat HIV antibody test, to confirm and assess as for any newly diagnosed case (see p. 370) with close monitoring of CD4 counts and plasma viral loads (VLs).

HIV infection is associated with presence of other STIs that may ↑ genital HIV VL potentially increasing the risk of vertical transmission. Screening should include:
- serological testing for syphilis, hepatitis B and C viruses (if not already done at booking)
- specimens for *Chlamydia trachomatis*, *Neisseria gonorrhoeae*, *Trichomonas vaginalis*, and bacterial vaginosis.

Anti-retroviral treatment

▶ Advised for all ♀ during pregnancy and at delivery.

The AIDS Clinical Trials Group protocol 076 (1994) demonstrated that zidovudine monotherapy, initiated between 14 and 34 weeks of pregnancy, intravenously during delivery and to infants for 6 weeks, ↓ risk of HIV-1 infection if not breastfeeding from 25.0% to 7.6%. In the UK zidovudine is currently the only antiretroviral drug specifically indicated for use during pregnancy (excluding 1st trimester) but monotherapy does not fully suppress plasma viraemia, leading to ↑ risk of viral resistance. Therefore HAART, involving 3 or more drug combinations should be used if the mother requires it for her own health. It should be considered if the CD4 count falls below 350cells/μL but may be deferred, especially with a low VL (<10,000copies/mL). Its introduction before the CD4 count falls <200cells/μL is important as opportunistic infections develop more commonly. Prophylaxis against *Pneumocystis jiroveci* (*carinii*) should be considered for those presenting with a CD4 count <200cells/μL. 1st line prophylaxis is co-trimoxazole, a folate antagonist, therefore potential benefits have to be balanced with the risks of fetal neural tube defects. If used in early pregnancy folic acid supplements should be provided and ultrasound scanning arranged after the 1st trimester.

To prevent vertical transmission only (♀ does not requiring HIV treatment for own health)

UK (RCOG) guidelines recommend starting treatment between 28 and 32 weeks of gestation (may be earlier if multiple pregnancy or history of preterm labour), US (CDC) guidelines from 14 to 34 weeks. Options are:

- short-term anti-retroviral therapy (START), especially with a high VL (>10,000copies/mL).
  - During pregnancy: HAART regimen, if possible containing zidovudine, which may be stopped shortly after pregnancy providing that the maternal VL is <50copies/mL.
  - Pre-delivery: intravenous zidovudine infusion, 2mg/kg for 1st hour reducing to 1mg/kg/hour until delivery. If stavudine is part of the HAART regimen it should be stopped as it competes with zidovudine for the same phosphorylation pathway
  - Delivery: requirement for caesarean section uncertain if VL<50copies/mL.
  - Neonate: oral zidovudine syrup, 2mg/kg four times a day for 6 weeks.
- zidovudine monotherapy
  - During pregnancy: 300mg twice daily or 200mg three times a day by mouth, stopping immediately after delivery
  - Pre-delivery: start intravenous zidovudine infusion, 2mg/kg for 1st hour reducing to 1mg/kg/hour until delivery
  - Delivery: caesarean section
  - Neonate: oral zidovudine syrup, 2mg/kg four times a day for 6 weeks.

Consensus appears to be moving away from monotherapy as combination treatment is more likely to suppress VLs to undetectable levels with a ↓ risk of viral resistance. However, its use must be balanced against the risks to mother and fetus of exposure to multiple potentially toxic drugs. Evidence suggests that pre-eclampsia is more common among pregnant treated ♀ with HAART, but there is no apparent ↑ rate of premature delivery, ↓ birth weight, ↓ Apgar scores, or stillbirths with such regimens with or without protease inhibitors.

Treatment in advanced HIV infection

Ideally resistance testing should be performed before commencing HAART, if possible deferring its introduction until the end of the 1st trimester or beginning of the 2nd. It should be continued after delivery. A zidovudine containing regimen is recommended unless there is resistance or other contraindication (extensive safety data in pregnancy). Zidovudine should be given intrapartum, even if not used as part of the maternal regimen, by infusion, until the cord is clamped. Treatment as described above should be given to the neonate for 6 weeks.

Women conceiving while taking HAART

Continue regimen if effective viral suppression. If failing, consider changing therapy after 1st trimester following resistance testing.

Women presenting in late pregnancy or during labour

If immunological and virological assessment is not possible, HAART, including zidovudine (intravenously intrapartum), should be started. Continue HAART intrapartum and postpartum until the results of the CD4 count and VL are known.

Delivery should be by caesarean section with consideration given to its timing to allow peak fetal concentrations.

If this is not available a single 200mg oral dose of nevirapine can be given during labour and the neonate treated with nevirapine, 2mg/kg 48 hours post-delivery. Nevirapine monotherapy may lead to non-nucleoside reverse transcriptase inhibitor resistant mutations which could compromise future treatment options for the ♀ as well as ↑ risk of further transmission of resistant virus. ⚠

Options in countries with limited resources

- Zidovudine/lamivudine combination: from 36 weeks of gestation, intrapartum and for 1 week postpartum—50% ↓ in vertical transmission for African breastfeeding ♀.
- Nevirapine (long half-life): single 200mg dose at onset of labour and 2mg/kg single dose to the neonate 48 hours post-delivery. Relative efficacy at 14–16 weeks—47%.

All ♀ who receive antiretroviral therapy in pregnancy should be registered prospectively with the Anti-retroviral Pregnancy Registry, which in Europe is managed by GlaxoSmithKline (www.uk.gsk.com).

Obstetric arrangements

Elective caesarean section before labour or rupture of membranes

Overall provides 50% ↓ in vertical transmission persisting when anti-retroviral treatment used. Effective even with low VL (1000copies/mL) but additional benefit uncertain in those taking HAART if VL <50copies/mL. US (ACOG) guidelines recommend elective caesarean section if maternal VL near delivery is >1000copies/mL. It should be timed to take place after 38 weeks of gestation. 'Bloodless' technique (using a staple gun) may further reduce transmission rates. Prophylactic antibiotics are recommended.

A zidovudine infusion should be started 4 hours before beginning the caesarean section and continued until the umbilical cord has been clamped. Maternal VL should be checked at delivery. The cord should be clamped as soon as possible after delivery and the baby bathed immediately after birth.

Vaginal delivery

If a woman chooses a vaginal delivery:

- membranes should be left intact for as long as possible
- fetal scalp electrodes and fetal blood sampling should be avoided
- emergency caesarean section may be required for other obstetric reasons including prolonged rupture of membranes (in pre-HAART era transmission rate doubled after 4 hours).

The neonate

All infants born to ♀ who are HIV +ve should be treated with anti-retroviral therapy from birth. Unless the mother started anti-retroviral therapy late in pregnancy (within 4 weeks of delivery) treatment of the infant may be discontinued after 4–6 weeks.

Zidovudine monotherapy should be used if the infant's mother received zidovudine antenatally or intrapartum, either as monotherapy or in HAART regimen. Consider HAART for neonates of mothers starting antiretroviral therapy late in pregnancy, with a high VL at delivery or a complicated delivery. Preterm or sick infants may not tolerate oral therapy and zidovudine is the only anti-retroviral drug available as an intravenous preparation.

Maternal antibodies crossing the placenta are detectable in most neonates of mother who are HIV-positive. Therefore nucleic acid amplification, by an ultrasensitive polymerase chain reaction technique, is used for the early diagnosis of infant infection. Typically tests are carried out at birth, then at 3 weeks, 6 weeks, and six months. At 6 months this test will detect >99% of infected babies if not breastfed. Final confirmation is a negative HIV antibody test at 18 months of age, following decay of maternal antibodies.

Infant feeding

All HIV positive mothers should be advised to avoid breastfeeding. Mixing breast with artificial feeding appears to ↑ risk of viral transmission compared with breastfeeding alone (African data).

There is no ↑ incidence of adverse reactions to inactivated va although their protective efficacy may be ↓. Live vaccines may ↑ risks of adverse reactions and in general should be avoided (except measles). Yellow fever vaccine is a live attenuated vaccine with uncerta safety and efficacy in HIV infection. The World Health Organization recommends immunization for asymptomatic HIV infected people travelling to endemic areas but there is insufficient evidence to advise those with symptomatic infection. Those who became asymptomatic with CD4 >200cells/μL following HAART may be offered immunization (evidence supports safety and efficacy). A certificate of exemption is needed for those who cannot be immunized if travel is necessary and advice should be given on the risk and methods to avoid bites of mosquitoes (vector of yellow fever).

Cholera vaccine has little protective value.

Food and water

Those with CD4 >250 cells/μL are at ↑ risk from gastrointestinal pathogens (cryptosporidiosis, salmonella, etc.). Particular care should be taken with raw fruit/vegetables, undercooked or raw seafood/meat, tap water/ice, unpasteurized milk/dairy products, and food/ beverages purchased from street vendors. Safe products include thoroughly cooked food, fruit peeled by the traveller, bottled/canned drinks (especially carbonated), hot coffee/tea, or water brought to the boil and simmered for 1 minute. If local tap water must be used and cannot be boiled the use of a water filtration unit, with added chlorine or iodine, ↑ its safety. Waterborne infections (e.g. cryptosporidiosis, giardiasis) may also result from ingesting water during recreational water activities therefore swimming in contaminated water (sewage, animal waste) should be avoided.

Travellers' diarrhoea

Prophylactic antimicrobials against travellers' diarrhoea are not routinely recommended (side-effects/promotion of drug resistant organisms) but if risk/benefit analysis favour their use, options include fluoroquinolones, e.g. ciprofloxacin 500mg daily and co-trimoxazole (trimethoprim/sulfamethoxazole) 960mg daily (resistance common in tropical areas). Antibiotics may be carried for empirical therapy if significant diarrhoea develops (e.g. ciprofloxacin 500mg twice daily for 3–7 days). Antiperistaltic agents, e.g. loperamide, are useful (except if diarrhoea is bloody or associated with pyrexia) but should be discontinued if symptoms persist >48 hours. Seek medical advice if failure to respond, blood in the stool, pyrexia/ rigors, or dehydration.

Other precautions

Advice should be given about other preventive measures for anticipated exposure e.g. malaria prophylaxis and protection against arthropod vectors. Avoid direct soil and sand contact with skin by wearing shoes, protective clothing, and using towels on beaches to avoid hook worm, strongyloidosis, and cutaneous larva migrans. Avoid swimming in fresh water in areas of risk for schistosomiasis.

Recreational travel is commonly associated with sexual encounters. Newly acquired STIs, including HIV superinfection, can compromise the underlying HIV infection. A supply of condoms should be carried, as availability at the destination may be limited and of dubious quality.

Bon voyage.

Useful resources

Books

Cohen PT, Merle AS, and Volberding PA 1999 *The AIDS Knowledge Base*. Philadelphia: Lippincott, Williams & Wilkins.

Holmes KK, Mårdh P-A, Sparling PF, Lemon SM, Stamm WE, Piot P, and Wasserheit JN 1999 *Sexually Transmitted Diseases*. New York: McGraw-Hill.

McMillan A, Young H, Ogilvie MM, and Scott GR (2002) *Clinical Practice in Sexually Transmissible Infections*. London: Saunders.

Websites

International/national bodies

- Department of Health: www.dh.gov.uk
- Medical Foundation for AIDS and Sexual Health: www.medfash.org.uk
- National Institutes of Health: www.nih.gov
- World Health Organization: www.who.int
- Health Protection Agency (England and Wales): www.hpa.org.uk
- Scottish Health Statistics: www.isdscotland.org
- Centers for Disease Control: www.cdc.gov
- Joint United Nations Programme on HIV/AIDS: www.unaids.org
- National AIDS Trust, UK www.nat.org.uk

Colleges and faculty

- Royal College of Physicians (London): www.rcplondon.ac.uk
- Royal College of Physicians (Edinburgh): www.rcpe.ac.uk
- Royal College of Physicians and Surgeons (Glasgow): www.rcpsglasg.ac.uk
- Royal College of Obstericians and Gynaecologists: www.rcog.org.uk
- Faculty of Family Planning and Reproductive Healthcare: www.ffprhc.org.uk

Professional organizations

- General Medical Council: www.gmc-uk.org
- British Medical Association: www.bma.org.uk
- British Association for Sexual Health and HIV: www.bashh.org
- International Union against Sexually Transmitted Infections: www.iusti.org
- British HIV association: www.bhiva.org
- International AIDS Society—USA: www.iasusa.org
- Society of Sexual Health Advisers: www.ssha.info
- Genito-urinary Nurses Association: www.guna.org.uk

Management guidelines

- UK STI management guidelines: www.bashh.org/guidelines/ceguidelines.htm
- US STI management guidelines: www.cdc.gov/std/treatment/rr5106.pdf
- UK HIV treatment guidelines: www.bhiva.org/guidelines/2003/hiv/index.html

- Other HIV guidelines—pregnancy, hepatitis B/C co-infection, TB, adherence at BHIVA website)
- RCOG management of HIV in pregnancy guidelines: www.rcog.org.uk/resources/Public/RCOG_Guideline_39_low.pdf
- US HIV treatment guidelines: www.aidsinfo.nih.gov/guidelines
- WHO STI management guidelines: www.who.int/reproductive-health/publications/rhr_01_10/01_10.pdf
- European STD guidelines: www.iusti.org/guidelines.pdf
- National Institute for Clinical Excellence: www.nice.org.uk

HIV/AIDS information

- Medscape: www.medscape.com
- AIDSinfo—US Department of Health and Human Services (also HIV management guidelines): www.aidsinfo.nih.gov
- John Hopkins AIDS Service: www.hopkins-aids.edu
- AIDSmap: www.aidsmap.com
- AIDS Education Global Information System: www.aegis.com
- HIV i-Base: www.i-base.info
- HIV drug resistance
  - Stanford HIV drug resistance database: www.hivdb.stanford.edu
  - HIV-1 genotypic drug resistance interpretation's algorithms: www.hivfrenchresistance.org
  - Los Alamos-Database: www.hiv.lanl.gov/content/index.
  - Also at AIDSinfo—see above.
- HIV drug interactions: www.hiv-druginteractions.org

Miscellaneous

- e-medicine: www.emedicine.com
- Chlamydia professional: www.chlamydiae.com
- International Herpes Management Forum: www.ihmf.org
- National electronic Library for Health: www.nelh.nhs.uk
- British National Formulary: www.bnf.org
- NHS sexual health information: www.playingsafely.co.uk

Self-help

- UK Self Help: www.ukselfhelp.info
- Herpes viruses association: www.herpes.org.uk
- International herpes alliance: www.herpesalliance.org
- Vulval pain society: www.vul-pain.dircon.co.uk
- Sexual dysfunction association: www.sda.uk.net
- Terence Higgins Trust: www.tht.org.uk
- +ve: www.plusve.org

Index

D

E

F

G

H

R